Teen Health Series

Adolescent
Health
SOURCEBOOK

Second Edition

Health Reference Series

Second Edition

Adolescent Health
SOURCEBOOK

Basic Consumer Health Information about the Physical, Mental, and Emotional Growth and Development of Adolescents, Including Medical Care, Nutritional and Physical Activity Requirements, Puberty, Sexual Activity, Acne, Tanning, Body Piercing, Common Physical Illnesses and Disorders, Eating Disorders, Attention Deficit Hyperactivity Disorder, Depression, Bullying, Hazing, and Adolescent Injuries Related to Sports, Driving, and Work

Along with Substance Abuse Information about Nicotine, Alcohol, and Drug Use, a Glossary, and Directory of Additional Resources

Edited by
Joyce Brennfleck Shannon

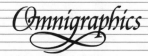

Omnigraphics

615 Griswold Street • Detroit, MI 48226

Bibliographic Note

Because this page cannot legibly accommodate all the copyright notices, the Bibliographic Note portion of the Preface constitutes an extension of the copyright notice.

Edited by Joyce Brennfleck Shannon

Health Reference Series

Karen Bellenir, *Managing Editor*
David A. Cooke, M.D., *Medical Consultant*
Elizabeth Collins, *Research and Permissions Coordinator*
Cherry Stockdale, *Permissions Assistant*
Laura Pleva Nielsen, *Index Editor*
EdIndex, Services for Publishers, *Indexers*

* * *

Omnigraphics, Inc.

Matthew P. Barbour, *Senior Vice President*
Kay Gill, *Vice President—Directories*
Kevin Hayes, *Operations Manager*
David P. Bianco, *Marketing Director*

* * *

Peter E. Ruffner, *Publisher*
Frederick G. Ruffner, Jr., *Chairman*
Copyright © 2007 Omnigraphics, Inc.
ISBN 0-7808-0943-2

Library of Congress Cataloging-in-Publication Data

Adolescent health sourcebook : basic consumer health information about the physical, mental, and emotional growth and development of adolescents, including medical care, nutritional and physical activity requirements, puberty, sexual activity, acne, tanning, body piercing, common physical illnesses and disorders, eating disorders, attention deficit hyperactivity disorder, depression, bullying, hazing, and adolescent injuries related to sports, driving, and work; along with substance abuse information about nicotine, alcohol, and drug use, a glossary, and directory of additional resources / edited by Joyce Brennfleck Shannon. -- 2nd ed.
     p. cm. -- (Health reference series)
  Summary: "Provides basic consumer health information about physical, mental, and emotional health issues specific to adolescents. Includes index, glossary of related terms, and other resources""--Provided by publisher.
  Includes bibliographical references and index.
  ISBN 0-7808-0943-2 (hardcover : alk. paper) 1. Teenagers--Health and hygiene. 2. Adolescent psychology. 3. Consumer education. 4. Adolescence.
  RJ140.A335 2006
  613'.0433--dc22
                                                                              2006022877

The information in this publication was compiled from the sources cited and from other sources considered reliable. While every possible effort has been made to ensure reliability, the publisher will not assume liability for damages caused by inaccuracies in the data, and makes no warranty, express or implied, on the accuracy of the information contained herein.

This book is printed on acid-free paper meeting the ANSI Z39.48 Standard. The infinity symbol that appears above indicates that the paper in this book meets that standard.

Printed in the United States

Table of Contents

Visit www.healthreferenceseries.com to view *A Contents Guide to the Health Reference Series*, a listing of more than 12,000 topics and the volumes in which they are covered.

Part IV: Reproductive and Sexual Health during Adolescence

Part V: Adolescent Injury

Part VI: Physical Disorders and Illnesses That May Affect Adolescents

Preface

About This Book

Adolescence is a time of significant physical, mental, and emotional development, and the choices teens make can impact their health and well-being in adulthood. Unfortunately, many teens choose to experiment with behaviors that have serious, long-term consequences. For example, nearly half of 8th graders and more than three-fourths of 12th graders have tried alcohol even though underage drinking is illegal and has been linked to increased learning problems, injuries, risky sexual activity, violence, and death.

Other choices teens make include whether or not to use tobacco, try illicit drugs, participate in sexual activities, alter their appearance, or take safety precautions at work, at play, or behind the wheel. Even food and activity choices carry consequences. A survey of U.S. youth found that more than nine million are overweight, making them vulnerable to chronic conditions such as diabetes and hypertension.

Adolescent Health Sourcebook, Second Edition offers parents and their teens basic information about the growth and development of adolescents and the issues that impact them as they move from childhood, through puberty, to adulthood. It offers guidelines regarding nutrition, physical activity, and weight management, and it discusses concerns related to appearance, reproduction, and injury. Physical and mental disorders that commonly affect teens are described. Social concerns—such as bullying, hazing, online abuse, dating violence, and substance abuse—are discussed. The book's end section provides a glossary and directory of resources for further help and information.

How to Use This Book

This book is divided into parts and chapters. Parts focus on broad areas of interest. Chapters are devoted to single topics within a part.

Part I: Adolescent Health and Development Overview describes the normal physical and mental development of teens. It offers parental guidelines and includes information about puberty, adolescent medical care, sleep needs, educational disabilities, and mortality.

Part II: Adolescent Nutrition and Weight Management describes calorie needs and nutrient requirements for optimal health and growth. It discusses the impact of marketing on food choices and provides tips for helping young people make wise decisions about food and physical activity.

Part III: Appearance, the Skin, and Related Issues during Adolescence answers health-related questions about appearance, including acne causes and treatments, cosmetic use, tanning, body piercing, and tattoos. It also discusses other concerns that impact teen health and self-perception, including antiperspirants, warts, athlete's foot, jock itch, and plastic surgery.

Part IV: Reproductive and Sexual Health during Adolescence describes reproductive systems, normal sexual development, and possible problems. Information about sexually transmitted diseases, contraception, and teen pregnancy is also provided.

Part V: Adolescent Injury discusses accidents and injuries that teens experience during recreation or sports activities or in motor vehicles or the workplace. Statistical information and injury prevention tips are also included.

Part VI: Physical Disorders and Illnesses That May Affect Adolescents provides facts about common medical issues that may arise during the teen years, including asthma, cancer, diabetes, growth problems, infectious mononucleosis, juvenile rheumatoid arthritis, meningitis, and scoliosis.

Part VII: Abuse and Violence Affects Adolescent Health offers practical information to help parents and teens recognize and respond to bullying, online solicitations, cyberbullying, abuse in dating relationships, hazing, and sexual assault. Guidelines for safety and abuse prevention are described.

Part VIII: Adolescent Mental Health discusses stress management and the warning signs of mental illness. Individual chapters describe symptoms and treatments for mental illnesses that may begin or intensify during the teen years, including anxiety, mood, personality, behavioral, and psychotic disorders.

Part IX: Teens and Substance Abuse provides information about drugs and other chemical substances. It describes health consequences related to the abuse of alcohol, anabolic steroids, tobacco, inhalants, illicit drugs, and prescription and over-the-counter medications. The part concludes with a chapter of tips to help parents talk to teens about alcohol and other drugs.

Part X: Additional Help and Information includes a glossary of terms related to adolescent health and a directory of organizations able to provide more information.

Bibliographic Note

This volume contains documents and excerpts from publications issued by the following U.S. government agencies: Centers for Disease Control and Prevention (CDC); Federal Bureau of Investigation (FBI); Health Resources and Services Administration (HRSA); National Adoption Information Clearinghouse; National Cancer Institute (NCI); National Clearinghouse on Child Abuse and Neglect Information; National Diabetes Education Program (NDEP); National Dissemination Center for Children with Disabilities; National Heart, Lung, and Blood Institute (NHLBI); National Institute of Arthritis and Musculoskeletal and Skin Diseases (NIAMS); National Institute of Child Health and Human Development (NICHD); National Institute of Diabetes and Digestive and Kidney Diseases (NIDDK); National Institute of Mental Health (NIMH); National Institute on Alcohol Abuse and Alcoholism (NIAAA); National Institute on Drug Abuse (NIDA); National Institutes of Health (NIH); National Library of Medicine (NLM); National Women's Health Information Center (NWHIC); National Youth Violence Prevention Resource Center; Occupational

Safety and Health Administration (OSHA); Substance Abuse and Mental Health Services Administration (SAMHSA); U.S. Department of Agriculture (USDA); U.S. Department of Health and Human Services (HHS); U.S. Department of Justice (DOJ); U.S. Department of Transportation (DOT); and the U.S. Food and Drug Administration (FDA).

In addition, this volume contains copyrighted documents from the following organizations: A.D.A.M., Inc.; American Academy of Facial Plastic and Reconstructive Surgery; American Academy of Family Physicians (AAFP); American Heart Association (AHA); American Obesity Association (AOA); American Osteopathic College of Dermatology; American Urological Association; Asthma and Allergy Foundation of America (AAFA); Child and Adolescent Bipolar Foundation (CABF); Columbia University Health Education Program; National Academies Press; National Adolescent Health Information Center (NAHIC); National Campaign to Prevent Teen Pregnancy; Nemours Foundation; Partnership for a Drug-Free America; and the Think First National Injury Prevention Foundation.

Full citation information is provided on the first page of each chapter. Every effort has been made to secure all necessary rights to reprint the copyrighted material. If any omissions have been made, please contact Omnigraphics to make corrections for future editions.

Acknowledgements

In addition to the listed organizations, agencies, and individuals who have contributed to this *Sourcebook*, special thanks go to managing editor Karen Bellenir, research and permissions coordinator Liz Collins, and document engineer Bruce Bellenir for their help and support.

About the Health Reference Series

The *Health Reference Series* is designed to provide basic medical information for patients, families, caregivers, and the general public. Each volume takes a particular topic and provides comprehensive coverage. This is especially important for people who may be dealing with a newly diagnosed disease or a chronic disorder in themselves or in a family member. People looking for preventive guidance, information about disease warning signs, medical statistics, and risk factors for health problems will also find answers to their questions in the *Health Reference Series*. The *Series*, however, is not intended to serve as a tool for diagnosing illness, in prescribing treatments, or as a substitute for the physician/patient relationship. All people concerned about medical symptoms or the possibility of disease are encouraged to seek professional care from an appropriate health care provider.

Locating Information within the Health Reference Series

The *Health Reference Series* contains a wealth of information about a wide variety of medical topics. Ensuring easy access to all the fact sheets, research reports, in-depth discussions, and other material contained within the individual books of the *Series* remains one of our highest priorities. As the *Series* continues to grow in size and scope, however, locating the precise information needed by a reader may become more challenging.

A Contents Guide to the Health Reference Series was developed to direct readers to the specific volumes that address their concerns. It presents an extensive list of diseases, treatments, and other topics of general interest compiled from the Tables of Contents and major index headings. To access *A Contents Guide to the Health Reference Series*, visit www.healthreferenceseries.com.

Medical Consultant

Medical consultation services are provided to the *Health Reference Series* editors by David A. Cooke, M.D. Dr. Cooke is a graduate of Brandeis University, and he received his M.D. degree from the University of Michigan. He completed residency training at the University of Wisconsin Hospital and Clinics. He is board-certified in Internal Medicine. Dr. Cooke currently works as part of the University of Michigan Health System and practices in Brighton, MI. In his free time, he enjoys writing, science fiction, and spending time with his family.

Our Advisory Board

We would like to thank the following board members for providing guidance to the development of this *Series*:

- Dr. Lynda Baker, Associate Professor of Library and Information Science, Wayne State University, Detroit, MI

- Nancy Bulgarelli, William Beaumont Hospital Library, Royal Oak, MI

- Karen Imarisio, Bloomfield Township Public Library, Bloomfield Township, MI

- Karen Morgan, Mardigian Library, University of Michigan-Dearborn, Dearborn, MI

- Rosemary Orlando, St. Clair Shores Public Library, St. Clair Shores, MI

Health Reference Series *Update Policy*

The inaugural book in the *Health Reference Series* was the first edition of *Cancer Sourcebook* published in 1989. Since then, the *Series* has been enthusiastically received by librarians and in the medical community. In order to maintain the standard of providing high-quality health information for the layperson the editorial staff at Omnigraphics felt it was necessary to implement a policy of updating volumes when warranted.

Medical researchers have been making tremendous strides, and it is the purpose of the *Health Reference Series* to stay current with the most recent advances. Each decision to update a volume is made on an individual basis. Some of the considerations include how much new information is available and the feedback we receive from people who use the books. If there is a topic you would like to see added to the update list, or an area of medical concern you feel has not been adequately addressed, please write to:

Editor
Health Reference Series
Omnigraphics, Inc.
615 Griswold Street
Detroit, MI 48226
E-mail: editorial@omnigraphics.com

Part One

Adolescent Health and Development Overview

Chapter 1

A Parent's Guide to Surviving the Teen Years

You've lived through 2:00 A.M. feedings, toddler temper tantrums, and the "but I don't want to go to school today" blues. So why is the word teenager causing you so much anxiety?

When you consider that the teen years are a period of intense growth, not only physically but morally and intellectually, it's understandable that it's a time of confusion and upheaval for many families. Despite some adults' negative perceptions about teens, they are often energetic, thoughtful, and idealistic, with a deep interest in what's fair and right. So, although it can be a period of conflict between parent and child, the teen years are also a time to help children grow into the distinct individuals they will become.

Understanding the Teen Years

So when, exactly, does adolescence start? The message to send your kid is: Everybody's different. There are early bloomers, late arrivals, speedy developers, and slow-but-steady growers. In other words, there's a wide range of what's considered normal.

But it's important to make a (somewhat artificial) distinction between puberty and adolescence. Most of us think of puberty as the

This information was provided by KidsHealth, one of the largest resources online for medically reviewed health information written for parents, kids, and teens. For more articles like this one, visit www.KidsHealth.org, or www.Teens Health.org. © 2004 The Nemours Center for Children's Health Media, a division of The Nemours Foundation.

development of adult sexual characteristics: breasts, menstrual periods, pubic hair, and facial hair. These are certainly the most visible signs of impending adulthood, but children between the ages of 10 and 14 (or even younger) can also be going through a bunch of changes that aren't readily seen from the outside. These are the changes of adolescence.

Many kids announce the onset of adolescence with a dramatic change in behavior around their parents. They're starting to separate from mom and dad and become more independent. At the same time, kids this age are increasingly aware of how others, especially their peers, see them and they're desperately trying to fit in. Kids often start "trying on" different looks and identities, and they become acutely aware of how they differ from their peers, which can result in episodes of distress and conflict with parents.

Butting Heads

One of the common stereotypes of adolescence is the rebellious, wild teen continually at odds with mom and dad. Although that extreme may be the case for some kids and this is a time of emotional ups and downs, that stereotype certainly is not representative of most teens.

But the primary goal of the teen years is to achieve independence. For this to occur, teens will start pulling away from their parents— especially the parent to whom they're the closest. This can come across as teens always seeming to have different opinions than their parents or not wanting to be around their parents in the same way they used to.

As teens mature, they start to think more abstractly and rationally. They're forming their moral code. And parents of teens may find that kids who previously had been willing to conform to please them will suddenly begin asserting themselves—and their opinions—strongly and rebelling against parental control.

You may need to look closely at how much room you give your teen to be an individual and ask yourself questions such as: Am I a controlling parent? Do I listen to my child? Do I allow my child's opinions and tastes to differ from my own?

Tips for Parenting during the Teen Years

Looking for a roadmap to find your way through these years? Here are some tips.

Educate Yourself

Read books about teenagers. Think back on your own teen years. Remember your struggles with acne or your embarrassment at developing early—or late. Expect some mood changes in your typically sunny child, and be prepared for more conflict as he or she finds his or her way as an individual. Parents who know what's coming can cope with it better. And the more you know, the better you can prepare your child.

Talk to Your Child Early Enough

Talking about menstruation or wet dreams after they've already started means you're too late. Answer the early questions your child has about bodies, such as the differences between boys and girls and where babies come from. But don't overload your child with information—just answer their questions.

You know your child. You can hear when your child is starting to tell jokes about sex or when attention to personal appearance is increasing. This is a good time to jump in with your own questions such as:

- Are you noticing any changes in your body?

- Are you having any strange feelings?

- Are you sad sometimes and don't know why?

A yearly physical exam is a great time to bring up these things. A doctor can tell your preadolescent child—and you—what to expect in the next few years. The exam can serve as a jumping-off point for a good parent/child discussion. The later you wait to have this discussion, the more likely your child will be to form misconceptions or become embarrassed about or afraid of physical and emotional changes.

Furthermore, the earlier you open the lines of communication on these subjects, the better chance you have of keeping them open throughout the teen years. Give your child books on puberty written for kids going through it. Share memories of your own adolescence with your child. There's nothing like knowing that mom or dad went through it too, to put your child more at ease.

Put Yourself in Your Child's Place

Practice empathy with your growing child. Help your child understand that it's normal to be a bit concerned or self-conscious. Tell your child it is okay to feel grown-up one minute and like a little child the next.

5

Pick Your Battles

If teenagers want to dye their hair, paint their fingernails black, or wear funky clothes, it may be worth thinking twice before you object. Teens want to shock their parents and it's a lot better to let them do something temporary and harmless; leave the objections to things that really matter, like tobacco, drugs, and alcohol.

Maintain Your Expectations

Teens will likely act unhappy with expectations their parents place on them. However, they usually understand and need to know that their parents care enough about them to expect things from them. Appropriate grades, behavior, and adherence to the rules of the house are important standards to maintain. If parents have appropriate expectations, teens will likely try to meet them.

Inform Your Teen—and Stay Informed Yourself

The teen years often are a time of experimentation, and sometimes that experimentation includes risky behaviors. Don't avoid the subjects of sex, or drug, alcohol, and tobacco use; discussing these things openly with your child before he or she is exposed to them increases the chance that your teen will act responsibly when the time comes.

Know your child's friends—and know your child's friends' parents. Regular communication between the parents of adolescents can go a long way toward creating a safe environment for all the children in a peer group. Parents can help each other keep track of the kids' activities without making the kids feel that they're being watched.

Know the Warning Signs

A certain amount of change may be normal during the teen years, but too drastic or long-lasting a switch in a child's personality or behavior may signal real trouble—the kind that needs professional help. Watch out for one or more of these warning signs:

- extreme weight gain or loss
- sleep problems
- rapid, drastic changes in personality
- sudden change in friends
- skipping school continually

- falling grades
- talk or even jokes about suicide
- signs of tobacco, alcohol, or drug use
- run-ins with the law

Any other inappropriate behavior that lasts for more than six weeks can be a sign of underlying trouble too. You may expect a glitch or two in your child's behavior or grades during this time, but your A/B student shouldn't suddenly be failing, and your normally outgoing kid shouldn't suddenly become constantly withdrawn. Your child's doctor or a local counselor, psychologist, or psychiatrist can help you find proper counseling.

Respect Your Child's Privacy

Some parents, understandably, have a very hard time with this one. They may feel that anything their child does is their business. But to help your teen become a young adult, you'll need to grant some privacy. If you notice warning signs of trouble, then you might want to invade your child's privacy until you get to the heart of the problem. But otherwise, it's a good idea to back off.

In other words, your teenager's room and phone calls should be private. You also shouldn't expect your teen to share all thoughts or activities with you at all times. Of course, for safety reasons, you should always know where your child is going, what they're doing, and with whom, but you don't need to know every detail, and you definitely shouldn't expect to be invited along.

Monitor What Your Child Sees and Reads

Television shows, magazines and books, the Internet—kids have access to tons of information. Be aware of what your child is watching and reading. Don't be afraid to set limits on the amount of time spent in front of the computer or the television. Know what your child is learning from the media and who he or she may be communicating with over the Internet.

Make Appropriate Rules

Bedtime for a teenager should be age appropriate, just as it was when your child was a baby. Reward your teen for being trustworthy. Does your child keep to a 10:00 P.M. curfew? Move it to 10:30 P.M.

And does a teen always have to go along on family outings? You decide what your expectations are, and don't be insulted when your growing child doesn't always want to be with you anymore. Think back. You probably felt the same way about your mom and dad.

Will This Ever Be Over?

As your child continues to progress through the teen years, you'll notice a slowing of the highs and lows of adolescence. Eventually you'll have an independent, responsible, communicative child. So remember the motto of many parents with teens: We're going through this together, and we'll come out of it—together!

Chapter 2

Normal Growth and Development during Adolescence

Growth Charts: United States

Growth charts are widely used as a clinical and research tool to assess nutritional status and the general health and well-being of children and adolescents. Multipurpose growth charts developed in the 1970s by the National Center for Health Statistics have been used to evaluate and monitor the growth of children in the United States. These growth charts were also adapted by the World Health Organization (WHO) for worldwide use. The growth charts have been revised to include children and adolescents to 20 years of age.

Biomarkers for Assessing Pubertal Reproductive Development and Health:

Anatomical Markers for Staging Pubertal Development

Puberty is a developmental period associated with tremendous change. The timing of the onset of puberty varies among adolescents as does, most likely, the interval between onset of pubertal markers.

This chapter includes: Excerpts from "CDC Growth Charts: United States," Centers for Disease Control and Prevention (CDC), May 30, 2000; and excerpts from "Biomarkers for Assessing Reproductive Development and Health: Part 1–Pubertal Development," *Environmental Health Perspectives* Volume 112, Number 1, January 2004, National Institute of Environment Health Sciences (NIEHS).

CDC Growth Charts: United States

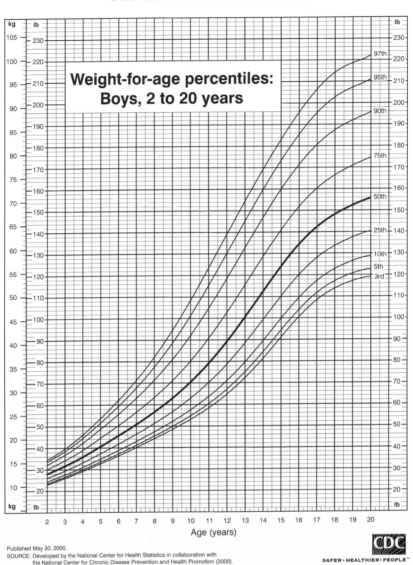

Weight-for-age percentiles: Boys, 2 to 20 years

Age (years)

Published May 30, 2000.
SOURCE: Developed by the National Center for Health Statistics in collaboration with
the National Center for Chronic Disease Prevention and Health Promotion (2000).

SAFER · HEALTHIER · PEOPLE™

Figure 2.1. *Weight-for-Age Percentiles: Boys, 2 to 20 Years*

CDC Growth Charts: United States

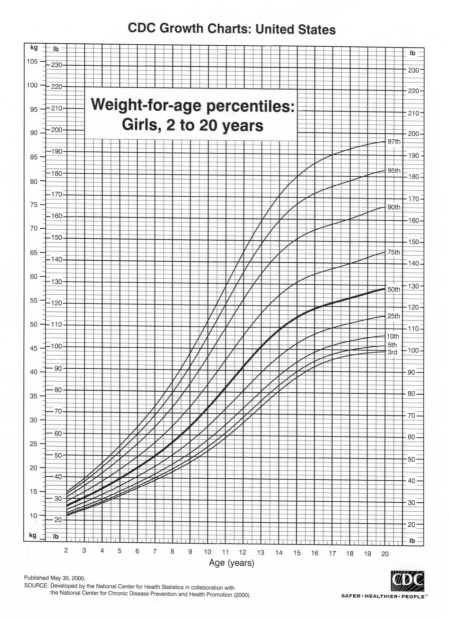

Figure 2.2. Weight-for-Age Percentiles: Girls, 2 to 20 Years

CDC Growth Charts: United States

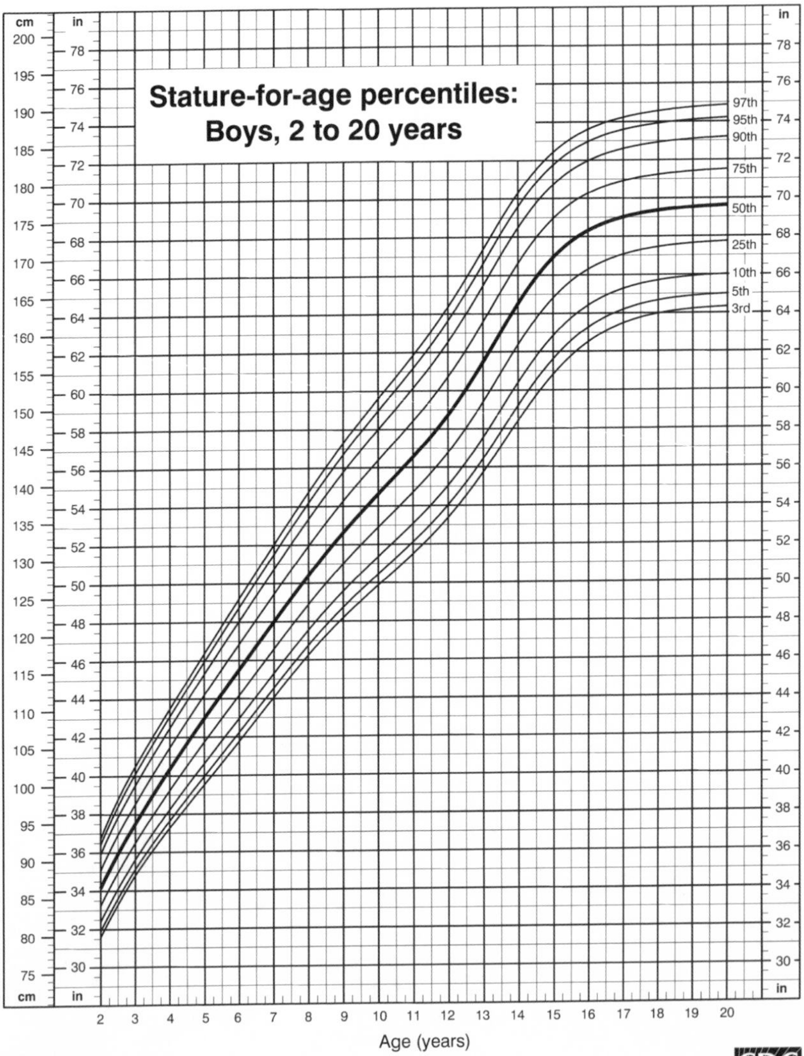

Stature-for-age percentiles: Boys, 2 to 20 years

Published May 30, 2000.
SOURCE: Developed by the National Center for Health Statistics in collaboration with the National Center for Chronic Disease Prevention and Health Promotion (2000).

CDC
SAFER · HEALTHIER · PEOPLE™

Figure 2.3. *Stature-for-Age Percentiles: Boys, 2 to 20 Years*

CDC Growth Charts: United States

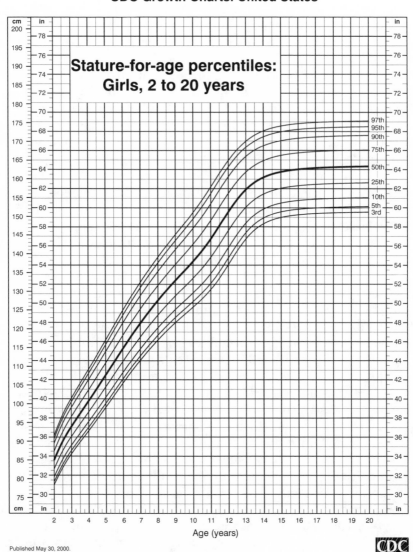

**Stature-for-age percentiles:
Girls, 2 to 20 years**

Age (years)

Published May 30, 2000.
SOURCE: Developed by the National Center for Health Statistics in collaboration with
the National Center for Chronic Disease Prevention and Health Promotion (2000).

Figure *2.4. Stature-for-Age Percentiles: Girls, 2 to 20 Years*

Changes in onset of markers correlate more strongly with the presence of secondary sex characteristics than they do with chronological age. Although recent studies suggest that differences appear to exist in the ordering of pubertal development across different racial groups, the order in which secondary sex characteristics appear and their subsequent stages of development had previously been considered to be relatively uniform.

On the basis of this earlier knowledge of pubertal development, Tanner (1962) developed a standard for assessing pubertal development (sexual maturity scale; SMS) that has been used widely in clinical practice for many years. In girls, this scale encompasses age at breast and pubic hair developmental stage and age at menarche. Other crude proxies of pubertal development in girls include presence/absence of axillary hair.

Although there is no direct analogy of age at menarche for boys, there is a Tanner scale for assessing pubertal stage in boys. In addition, some investigators have used proxy markers such as axillary hair, voice changes, testicular size, or age at ejaculation. It is important to note that these changes do not occur simultaneously but follow growth of the testes and penis at varying time intervals.

With respect to the Tanner method, a limitation for use in some populations or under certain circumstances is that it requires nude children and adolescents to be visually inspected by a trained clinician for the appearance of secondary sex characteristics.

Duke and colleagues (1980) were the first to develop a method to determine pubertal development via self-assessment (PDS). Adolescents were shown sex-specific sets of the SMS photographs (with accompanying descriptive phrases developed by the investigators) and were asked to indicate which photograph in each series (breast, penis, and pubic hair growth, as appropriate) most closely resembled their current stage of development.

In addition to the photograph and drawing-based methods of pubertal self-assessment, several teams of investigators developed verbal and written instruments. These assessment tools are thought to be more acceptable in a classroom setting, as school officials might find visual depictions to be inappropriate. Several years after the development of the PDS, Carskadon and Acebo (1993) adapted it for use on a written questionnaire. The investigators found the validity of the written adaptation of the PDS to be high.

In an attempt to simplify the assessment of pubertal development even further, Berg-Kelly and Erdes (1997) tested the use of a global question. Adolescents were asked, "Considering your bodily development, how do you rate yourself compared to your classmates: very late, some-what late, similar to most of your classmates, somewhat early, or very early?" Using this question, they reported a very high concordance with physician assessments: 95% for males and 93.5% among females.

Overall, many adolescents appear to be able to provide a reason-ably accurate assessment of their pubertal maturation based on the presence of secondary sex characteristics. Although the use of Tanner's SMS pictures with accompanying written explanations seems to per-form more favorably than other self-assessment methods, many of the methods yield correlations in the range of those reported for inter-rater agreement of pubertal assessments conducted by health profes-sionals.

Other Physical Biomarkers of Pubertal Development

Skeletal growth. Skeletal growth is one of the most striking char-acteristics of puberty. A commonly used marker of skeletal growth is linear growth velocity (height increase per year), and this correlates with the Tanner stages of sexual development. In females the puber-tal growth spurt starts at Tanner breast stage two (the start of pu-berty) and peaks at stage three. Linear-growth velocity begins to increase in males at genital stage three and pubic-hair stage two, but peak height velocity is not attained until Tanner stage four.

Body composition. Significant changes in body composition (body mass index and lean body mass) also occur during puberty and show distinct and important gender differences. Lean body mass, which primarily reflects muscle mass, begins to increase during early pu-berty in both boys and girls. As pubertal stage advances in boys, their body fat mass increases while the percentage of body fat decreases. Among girls both body fat mass and percentage of body fat increases with advancing pubertal stage.

The chief advantages of using height, weight, and fat mass as biomarkers of pubertal stage are that the methodology to obtain the data is noninvasive, socially acceptable, rapid, and simple to use. Equipment is relatively inexpensive in most cases, and there is a good selection of commercial products available for measuring height and body fat.

Fundamental voice frequency. Among males, the pitch of the voice, or the fundamental voice frequency, lowers substantially during puberty. Using laryngography, Harries and colleagues (1997) demon-strated that the most abrupt change in the adolescent male voice occurs during the transition from Tanner stage three to Tanner stage four in pubertal development. Recent advances in technology have made it possible to identify changes in fundamental voice frequency by recording adolescents reading standardized passages of text at regular intervals (for example, every three months). Although the technique appears to be less subjective than the various methods of pubertal self-assessment, additional work is needed to verify its reliability.

Molecular and Cellular Biomarkers of Puberty

Secondary sex characteristics determined using Tanner scales provide a relatively useful measure of pubertal stage and have formed the cornerstone of many studies into pubertal development. However, gross anatomical categorization is relatively limited in its applicability to a large and diverse population and is also limited in that it only informs on the physiological end point. That is, if puberty-associated problems exist, then these observational measurements of pubertal stage are usually of little use in diagnosis and prognosis.

If pubertal or other developmental problems are occurring or might be expected to occur (given, for example, a certain genetic makeup of an individual), then methods to observe and characterize such problems at an early (preclinical) stage are required. Such methods require monitoring molecular and cellular changes, and accessible tissues (urine or blood) are the normal source of material for such studies. Indeed, these specimens are used extensively to measure numerous indicators including chemical, hormone, and metabolite levels, the expression levels of genes and proteins, and the integrity of genetic material (DNA). Characterization of the normal molecular and cellular changes that occur in the prepubescent and pubescent body may offer the best approach to achieve this aim, and recent studies have uncovered a number of promising biomarkers of normal and abnormal pubertal development that may prove useful in longitudinal human studies.

Genetic markers. Our ability to identify the genetic factors primarily or partly responsible for developmental problems has increased. The identification of such biomarkers could facilitate the development of genetic screens capable of indicating the likelihood or cause of abnormal pubertal development.

Biomarkers of bone growth and mineralization. During puberty, bone growth and mineralization, as well as bone turnover, increase dramatically. Current data suggest biochemical markers of bone remodeling may be useful in the clinical investigation of bone turnover in children's health and disease.

Hormonal biomarkers of puberty. Increased secretion of adrenal androgens occurs in the earliest stages of puberty under the control of the hypothalamus-pituitary-adrenal axis. These hormones cause pubic and armpit hair to develop and sensitize the androgen receptors of the hypothalamus and the pituitary, eventually leading to the activation of the HPG (hypothalamus-pituitary-gonad) axis and the initiation of puberty.

The main hormone involved in the regulation of puberty is gonadotrophin-releasing hormone (GnRH). Produced in the hypothalamus, GnRH stimulates the production and release of both luteinizing hormone (LH) and follicle-stimulating hormone (FSH) from the pituitary. However, it is difficult to measure levels of GnRH, as it secreted into portal circulation and transported directly to the pituitary. Furthermore, it has a short half-life of only 4–8 minutes. Thus, the onset of pubertal development is usually measured through hormones regulated directly or indirectly by GnRH, including the gonadotrophins (LH, FSH) and sex steroid hormones (testosterone and estrogen).

The onset of puberty sees an increase in the levels of LH. At first this only occurs during the night and is associated with increases in testosterone (boys) and estrogen (girls) the following morning. Because all three of these hormones can be robustly and inexpensively measured in urine, these initial increases can be used as early biomarkers of pubertal onset.

In addition to the gonadotrophins and sex steroid hormones, there are a number of other hormones whose regulation and level of expression appear to be closely linked with pubertal development. These include:

- **Müllerian inhibiting substance** (MIS) (also known as antimüllerian hormone), a gonadal peptide hormone, is a member of the transforming growth factor-beta family and an important factor for male sex differentiation.

- **Inhibins** are peptides, mainly of gonadal origin, that suppress FSH production.

- **Leptin**, an adipocyte hormone important in regulating energy homeostasis, interacts with the reproductive axis at multiple sites, with stimulatory effects at the hypothalamus and pituitary, and inhibitory action on the gonads. Normal leptin secretion is necessary for normal reproductive function to proceed, and leptin may be a signal allowing for the point of initiation of and progression toward puberty.

Puberty is the most dramatic process in child development. Unfortunately, the multiple characteristics of puberty have made it difficult to determine an all-encompassing definition in terms of the biochemical and physiological changes that occur. Puberty also occurs at different rates and in different orders in different people, depending on genetic and environmental components. For example, in African-American girls, pubic hair, on average, seems to appear slightly ahead of breast development. In contrast, the first manifestation of puberty in Caucasian girls is usually breast development.

Chapter 3

Indicators of Adolescent Well-Being

Child and Family Statistics

The adolescent birth rate has reached another record low, according to a yearly compendium of statistics from federal agencies concerned with children. Also, youth are more likely to commit or be a victim of a violent crime, and reading scores of older children have declined slightly.

These findings are described in *America's Children: Key National Indicators of Well-Being 2005*, the U.S. government's 9th annual monitoring report on the well-being of the Nation's children and youth. The report was compiled by the Federal Interagency Forum on Child and Family Statistics and presents a comprehensive look at critical areas of child well-being, including health status, behavior and social environment, economic security, and education.

Health

The report said that the adolescent birth rate for 2003 was 22 for every 1,000 girls ages 15 to 17, down from 23 in 2002. Since 1991, the

This chapter includes: Excerpts from "Teen Birth Rate Continues Decline, Fewer Childhood Deaths," National Institute of Child Health and Human Development (NICHD), July 2005; and excerpts from "FASTATS–Adolescent Health," Centers for Disease Control and Prevention (CDC), February 2006. Also, reprinted with permission of the National Adolescent Health Information Center, 2003. Fact Sheet on Demographics: Adolescents, San Francisco, CA. Author, University of California, San Francisco.

adolescent birth rate dropped by more than two-fifths, from 39 births for every 1,000 girls. The decline followed a one-fourth increase in the teen birth rate from 1986 to 1991. "For the sixth consecutive year, the adolescent birth rate has reached a record low," said Duane Alexander, M.D., Director of the National Institute of Child Health and Human Development of the National Institutes of Health. "We welcome this trend and hope it continues."

Dr. Alexander noted that teen mothers face a number of problems unique to their age. Teen mothers are much less likely to finish high school or to graduate from college than are other girls their age. Infants born to teen mothers are more likely to be of low birthweight, which increases their chances for infant death and for blindness, deafness, mental retardation, mental illness, and cerebral palsy.

Adolescent birth rates varied by racial and ethnic group. The rate for Black, non-Hispanic adolescents dropped by more than half since the 1991 peak of 86 births for every 1,000 girls, to 39 for every 1,000 girls in 2003. The birth rate was at 9 for every 1,000 Asian/Pacific Islanders girls in 2003, 12 for White, non-Hispanics, 30 for American Indians/Alaska Natives, and 50 for Hispanics.

Behavior and Social Environment

The percentage of eighth graders who had used any illicit drugs in the past 30 days declined, from 10 percent in 2003 to 8 percent in 2004. The report noted that rates for illicit drug use in the past 30 days for tenth and twelfth graders had not changed during the same time period.

The rate at which youths were victims of serious violent crimes went up, from 10 per 1,000 youth ages 12 to 17 in 2002, to 18 per 1,000 in 2003. However, this rate was lower than the peak of 44 victims per 1,000 youth in 1993. The report noted that the rate of serious violent crime against youth decreased by 60 percent from 1993 to 2003.

In 2003, males were more likely to be victims of serious violent crime than were females, with 25 males per 1,000 male youth, compared with 10 females for every 1,000 female youth.

The rate at which youth committed serious violent crimes also increased, from 11 youth offenders of serious violent crimes per 1,000 youth ages 12 to 17 in 2002 to 15 per 1,000 in 2003. Although the 2003 rate is higher than the 2002 rate, the 2003 rate is 71 percent lower than the 1993 peak of 52 violent crimes committed per 1,000 youth.

Education

The average mathematics score for eighth graders rose from 273 to 278 in 2003, on the National Assessment of Educational Progress, the Nation's Report Card on elementary and secondary school performance. In 2003, the percentages of fourth and eighth graders scoring at or above the Proficient achievement level in math were higher than in all previous assessments. Twelfth-graders were not tested in reading or mathematics in 2003, but twelfth grade mathematics scores had not changed significantly from 1996 to 2000.

Eighth graders' reading score changed only from 264 in 2002 to 263 in 2003; the 2003 score was higher than in 1992. The reading score of twelfth graders was lower in 2002 than in 1992 or 1998.

Girls had higher reading scores than did boys in grades 4 and 8 in 2003 and in grade 12 in 2002. However, boys had higher math scores than did girls in grades 4 and 8 in 2003, and in grade 12 in 2000.

In 2003, 87 percent of young adults ages 18–24 had completed high school with a diploma or an alternative credential, such as a General Education Development (GED) certificate. The high school completion rate has increased slightly since 1980, when it was 84 percent.

The proportion of Black-alone, non-Hispanic youth (ages 16 to 19) who were neither in school nor working was 10 percent in 2004, down from 12 percent in 2003. More Black-alone, non-Hispanic youth moved from the category "not enrolled in school and not working" into the category of "enrolled in school and not working" in 2004. The report categorizes people who responded to a question on race by indicating only one race as a "race-alone" population. For example, those who indicated their race as only "Black" and no other race are referred to as "Black-alone."

U.S. Adolescent Health Statistics

Health Status

The *Summary Health Statistics for U.S. Children: National Health Interview Survey, 2004,* reported that for adolescents 12–17 years of age:

- 2.3% experience only fair or poor health.
- 6.7% missed 11 or more days of school in the past 12 months because of illness or injury.
- 10% are without health insurance.
- 6.8 % have no usual source of health care.

21

Health Risk Factors

Health United States, 2005 indicated that:

- 16% of 12–19 year-olds are overweight.
- 12% of 12–17 year-olds smoked cigarettes in the past month.
- 18% of 12–17 year-olds used alcohol in the past month.
- 67% of high school students participated in regular physical activity.

Mortality

In 2002, 15–19 year-olds deaths included:

- 13,812 total deaths
- 7,137 accidents (unintentional injuries)
- 1,892 homicides
- 1,513 suicides

National Adolescent Health Information Center Demographics Information on Adolescents

The U.S. Adolescent Population Is Growing

The number of adolescents in the U.S. began to increase in the 1990s and is expected to keep increasing through 2050. From 1990 to 2000, the adolescent population ages 10–19 increased by 16.6%, from 34.9 million to 40.7 million. Although the projected figures indicate substantial growth for the adolescent population, they represent a much smaller percentage increase than that projected for the overall population (2.2% between 2000 and 2010, versus an expected 6.6% increase for the total U.S. population) (Source: U.S. Census Bureau, 1992; U.S. Census Bureau, 2000; U.S. Census Bureau, 2003a; U.S. Census Bureau, 2003b; U.S. Census Bureau, 2003c).

Adolescent Population Is More Racially/Ethnically Diverse

The adolescent population (ages 10–19) is more racially/ethnically diverse than the overall population. While White, non-Hispanics (NH) comprise a majority of both populations, the adolescent population has a greater percentage of Black-NH, Hispanics, and American Indian (AI)/Alaskan Native (AN)-NH than the population as a whole (U.S.

Census Bureau, 2003b). Major factors underlying this diversity include the higher immigration of Hispanics and Asian/Pacific Islanders (A/PI), the decreased birth and fertility rates among Whites and Blacks, and an increase in birth and fertility rates among Hispanics (MacKay, Fingerhut, and Duran, 2000).

Racial/Ethnic Diversity Is Increasing in the Adolescent Population

The percentage of White-NH in the adolescent population is projected to drop from 62.9% in 2000 to 55.8% in 2020. The Hispanic adolescent population, the second most populous racial/ethnic group, will increase by 50%. Although small in numbers, the A/PI-NH population will experience the most rapid growth (83%). Relatively small growth is projected for the Black-NH and AI/AN-NH populations (2.5% and 6%, respectively) (Source: U.S. Census Bureau, 2000; U.S. Census Bureau, 2003b).

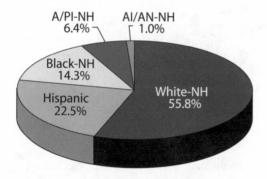

Figure 3.1. *Adolescents by Race/Ethnicity, Ages 10–19, 2020 (Projection)*

Racial/Ethnic Distribution of Adolescents Varies by Region

The racial/ethnic diversity of the adolescent population ages 10–19 varies by region.[1] The Northeast and Midwest have the highest percentages of White-NH adolescents, while the South has the highest percentage of Black-NH adolescents. The West has the highest percentage of Hispanic, AI/AN-NH, and A/PI-NH adolescents. The highest number of all adolescents lives in the South, followed by the Midwest, West, and Northeast (35.7%, 23.5%, 22.7%, and 18.1% of all adolescents, respectively) (Source: U.S. Census Bureau, 2003b).

More Adolescents Live in Suburbs Than in Rural Areas and Central Cities

Over half of all adolescents ages 12–17 live in suburban settings.[2] From 1990 to 2002, the percentage of adolescents ages 12–17 living in the suburbs increased from 46.6% to 53.8% (U.S. Census Bureau, 1992; U.S. Census Bureau, 2003a; Fields, 2003). In 2002, more than a quarter of adolescents lived in central city settings, while one in five lived in rural areas. White-NH and A/PI youth ages 12–17 are most likely to live in suburban settings (59.7% and 56.3%, respectively). Among same-age Black-NH, 50.4% live in central city settings and 36.6% live in suburban settings. Hispanic youths are about equally likely to live in central city or suburban settings (44.5% and 46.3%, respectively) (Fields, 2003).

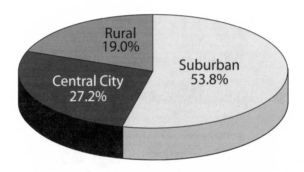

Figure 3.2. Location of Adolescents by Type of Setting, Ages 12–17, 2002

Two-Thirds of Adolescents Ages 12–17 Live with Both Parents

In 2002, two-thirds of adolescents ages 12–17 lived with both parents, a decrease from 73% in 1995 (Fields, 2003; Bryson, 1996). This parallels a trend for children ages 0–18: from 1980 to 2002, the number of children living with two parents decreased from 77% to 69% (FIFCFS, 2003). In 2002, about three-quarters of A/PI and White-NH youths ages 12–17 lived with both parents, as did 63.1% of same-age Hispanics. By contrast, about two-fifths of Black adolescents lived in two-parent families; of all racial/ethnic groups, they were most likely to live with mothers only (46%) or neither parent (10.3%) (Fields, 2003).

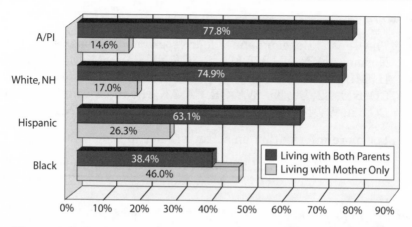

Figure 3.3. *Family Structure by Race/Ethnicity, Ages 12–17, 2002*

Black and Hispanic Youth Experience Poverty at a Higher Rate Than Their Peers

Black children and adolescents under age 18 experience poverty more than their same age peers in other racial/ethnic groups. Hispanic youths had the second highest poverty rate, followed by White and A/PI youth. In 2002, one out of six youths under age 18 lived below the Federal Poverty Line,[3] close to the lowest rate since data collection began in 1979 (Proctor and Dalaker, 2003).

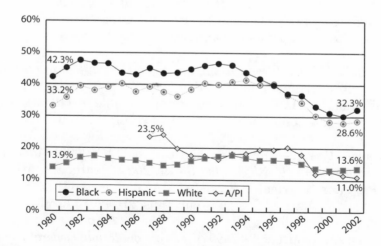

Figure 3.4. *Percent in Poverty by Race/Ethnicity, Under Age 18, 1980– 2002 (Note: Data collection for the A/PI population started in 1987.)*

References

1. The Census Bureau defines four geographic regions as 1)
   Northeast-MN, NH, VT, MA, RI, CT, NY, PA; 2) Midwest-OH, IN,
   IL, MI, WI, MN, IA, MO, ND, SD, NE, KS; 3) West-MT, ID, WY,
   CO, NM, AZ, UT, NV, WA, OR, CA, AK, HI; and 4) South-DE, MD,
   DC, VA, WV, NC, SC, GA, FL, AR, LA, OK, TX, KY, TN, AL, MO.

2. For more information on settings, refer to Fields, 2003.

3. The Federal Poverty Line was $18,392 for a family of four in
   2002.

Data Sources

Proctor, B. D., and Dalaker, J. (2003). *Poverty in the United States: 2002*
(Current Population Reports, Series P60-222). Washington, DC: U.S.
Government Printing Office. [Available at (12/03): http://www.census.gov/
hhes/www/poverty.html]

Bryson, K. (1996). *Household and family characteristics: March 1995*
(Current Population Reports, Series P20-488). Washington, DC: U.S.
Government Printing Office. [Available at (12/03): http://www.census.gov/
population/www/socdemo/hh-fam.html]

Federal Interagency Forum on Child and Family Statistics [FIFCFS].
(2003). *America's children: Key national indicators of well-being, 2003*.
Washington, DC: U.S. Government Printing Office. [Available at (12/
03): http://www.childstats.gov/americaschildren]

Fields, J. (2003). *Children's living arrangements and characteristics:
March 2002* (Current Population Reports, P20-547) [Detailed Tables].
Washington, DC: U.S. Census Bureau. [Available at (12/03): http://
www.census.gov/population/www/socdemo/hh-fam.html]

MacKay, A. P., Fingerhut, L. A., and Duran C. R. (2000). *Adolescent
health Chartbook. Health, United States, 2000*. Hyattsville, MD: National Center for Health Statistics. [Available at (12/03): http://
www.cdc.gov/nchs/products/pubs/pubd/hus/2010/2010.htm]

U.S. Census Bureau. (1992). *1990 census of population: General population characteristics, United States* (CP-1-1). Washington, DC: Author.
[Available at (12/03): http://www.census.gov/prod/www/abs/decenial.html]

U.S. Census Bureau. (2000). *Projections of the resident population by age, sex, race, and Hispanic origin: 1999 to 2100* (NP-D1-A Middle Series). Washington, DC: Author. [Available at (12/03): http://www.census .gov/population/www/projections/natdet-D1A.html]

U.S. Census Bureau. (2003a). *American FactFinder, Census 1990 summary tape file 1* [Tabulated Data]. Washington, DC: Author. [Available at (12/03): http://factfinder.census.gov/servlet/BasicFactsServlet]

U.S. Census Bureau. (2003b). *American FactFinder, Census 2000 summary file 1* [Tabulated Data]. Washington, DC: Author. [Available at (12/03): http://factfinder.census.gov/servlet/BasicFactsServlet]

U.S. Census Bureau. (2003c). *National estimates, 1980 to 1990* [Tabulated Data]. Washington, DC: Author. [Available at (12/03): http:// eire.census.gov/popest/archives/national/nat_80s_detail.php]

In all cases, the most recent available data were used. Some data are released one to three years after collection. For questions regarding data sources or availability, please contact the National Adolescent Health Information Center (NAHIC). For racial/ethnic data, the category names presented are those of the data sources used. Every attempt was made to standardize age ranges. When this was not possible, age ranges were those of the data sources used.

Additional Information

National Adolescent Health Information Center
School of Medicine
University of California, San Francisco
UCSF Box 0503
San Francisco, CA 94143-0503
Phone: 415-502-4856
Fax: 415-502-4858
Website: http://nahic.ucsf.edu
E-mail: nahic@ucsf.edu

Chapter 4

The Teenage Brain: A Work in Progress

Teenage Brain

New imaging studies are revealing—for the first time—patterns of brain development that extend into the teenage years. Although scientists do not know yet what accounts for the observed changes, they may parallel a pruning process that occurs early in life that appears to follow the principle of use-it-or-lose-it—neural connections, or synapses, that get exercised are retained, while those that do not are lost. At least, this is what studies of animals' developing visual systems suggest. While it is known that both genes and environment play major roles in shaping early brain development, science still has much to learn about the relative influence of experience versus genes on the later maturation of the brain. Animal studies support a role for experience in late development, but no animal species undergoes anything comparable to humans' protracted childhood and adolescence. Nor is it yet clear whether experience actually creates new neurons and synapses, or merely establishes transitory functional changes. Nonetheless, it is tempting to interpret the new findings as empowering teens to protect and nurture their brain as a work in progress.

This chapter includes: Excerpts from "Teenage Brain: A Work in Progress," National Institute of Mental Health (NIMH), February 2006; excerpts from "March 15 Through 21 Is Brain Awareness Week," Substance Abuse and Mental Health Services Administration (SAMHSA), March 2004; and "Adolescent Brains Show Reduced Reward Anticipation," National Institute on Alcohol Abuse and Alcoholism (NIAAA), March 2004.

The newfound appreciation of the dynamic nature of the teen brain is emerging from magnetic resonance imaging (MRI) studies that scan a child's brain every two years, as he or she grows up. Individual brains differ enough that only broad generalizations can be made from comparisons of different individuals at different ages. However, following the same brains as they mature allows scientists a much finer-grained view into developmental changes. In the first such longitudinal study of 145 children and adolescents, reported in 1999, National Institute of Mental Health (NIMH)'s Dr. Judith Rapoport and colleagues were surprised to discover a second wave of overproduction of gray matter, the thinking part of the brain—neurons and their branch-like extensions—just prior to puberty. Possibly related to the influence of surging sex hormones, this thickening peaks at around age 11 in girls, 12 in boys, after which the gray matter actually thins some.

Prior to this study, research had shown that the brain overproduced gray matter for a brief period in early development—in the womb and for about the first 18 months of life—and then underwent just one bout of pruning. Researchers are now confronted with structural changes that occur much later in adolescence. The teen's gray matter waxes and wanes in different functional brain areas at different times in development. For example, the gray matter growth spurt just prior to puberty predominates in the frontal lobe, the seat of executive functions—planning, impulse control, and reasoning. In teens affected by a rare, childhood-onset form of schizophrenia that impairs these functions, the MRI scans revealed four times as much gray matter loss in the frontal lobe as normally occurs. Unlike gray matter, the brain's white matter—wire-like fibers that establish neurons' long-distance connections between brain regions—thickens progressively from birth in humans. A layer of insulation called myelin progressively envelops these nerve fibers, making them more efficient, just like insulation on electric wires improves their conductivity.

Advancements in MRI image analyses are providing new insights into how the brain develops. Dr. Arthur Toga and colleagues of University of California, Los Angeles (UCLA) turned the NIMH team's MRI scan data into 4-D time-lapse animations of children's brains morphing as they grow up—the fourth dimension being rate-of-change. Researchers report a wave of white matter growth that begins at the front of the brain in early childhood, moves rearward, and then subsides after puberty. Striking growth spurts can be seen from ages six to thirteen in areas connecting brain regions specialized for language and understanding spatial relations, the temporal and parietal lobes. This growth drops off sharply after age twelve, coinciding with the end of a critical period for learning languages.

While this work suggests a wave of brain white matter development that flows from front to back, animal functional brain imaging, and postmortem studies have suggested that gray matter maturation flows in the opposite direction, with the frontal lobes not fully maturing until young adulthood. To confirm this in living humans, the UCLA researchers compared MRI scans of young adults, ages 23–30, with those of teens, ages 12–16. They looked for signs of myelin, which would imply more mature, efficient connections within gray matter. As expected, areas of the frontal lobe showed the largest differences between young adults and teens. This increased myelination in the adult frontal cortex likely relates to the maturation of cognitive processing and other executive functions. Parietal and temporal areas mediating spatial, sensory, auditory, and language functions appeared largely mature in the teen brain. The observed late maturation of the frontal lobe conspicuously coincides with the typical age-of-onset of schizophrenia—late teens, early twenties—which, as noted earlier, is characterized by impaired executive functioning.

Another series of MRI studies is shedding light on how teens may process emotions differently than adults. Using functional MRI (fMRI), a team led by Dr. Deborah Yurgelun-Todd at Harvard's McLean Hospital scanned subjects' brain activity while they identified emotions on pictures of faces displayed on a computer screen. Young teens, who characteristically perform poorly on the task, activated the amygdala, a brain center that mediates fear and other gut reactions, more than the frontal lobe. As teens grow older, their brain activity during this task tends to shift to the frontal lobe, leading to more reasoned perceptions and improved performance. Similarly, the researchers saw a shift in activation from the temporal lobe to the frontal lobe during a language skills task as teens got older. These functional changes paralleled structural changes in temporal lobe white matter.

While these studies have shown remarkable changes that occur in the brain during the teen years, they also demonstrate what every parent can confirm: the teenage brain is a very complicated and dynamic arena, one that is not easily understood.

Brain Awareness: How Your Brain Works

Your brain is involved in everything you do: how you think, how you feel, how you act, how you interact with others, and even what kind of person you are. It is the most complex structure in your body, much more complex than any computer. The brain is soft and fragile, almost like soft butter or a raw egg. Weighing about three pounds (or two percent of your body weight), your brain consumes about 20 to 30 percent of your body's energy. This means it uses about 20 to 30 percent of the calories you consume.

There are about 100 billion nerve cells (neurons) in your brain, and they can send signals to thousands of other cells at a rate of about 200 miles per hour. Each neuron is linked to other nerve cells in the brain. The number of connections in your brain, called dendrites, is greater than the number of stars in the sky.

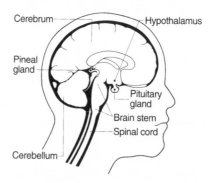

Figure 4.1. *Parts of the Brain (Source: National Cancer Institute).*

The Parts of Your Brain

Your brain contains many parts, including the cerebral cortex, also called the cerebrum, which includes the frontal lobe, parietal lobe, occipital lobes, and temporal lobes; along with the brain stem, cerebellum, the limbic system, and the hippocampus.

Cerebral cortex (cerebrum)—The largest part of your brain sits like a mushroom cap on the rest of your brain and takes up about two-thirds of its total mass. It includes the frontal lobe, parietal lobe, occipital lobes, and temporal lobes. Parts of the cerebral cortex control seeing, hearing, and touching. Your cerebral cortex is also where you create movements, like playing the piano or flipping your skateboard.

Frontal lobe—Part of your cerebral cortex, the frontal lobe is right under your forehead. It helps with reasoning, planning, parts of speech, movement (motor cortex), feelings, and problem-solving.

Parietal lobe—Part of your cerebral cortex, the parietal lobe is near the back and top of your head. This part of the brain is a processing center that makes sense of what you are feeling, smelling, and hearing. It also connects those sensations to memories and ideas. Its functions include visual attention, touch perception, voluntary movements, manipulation of objects, and integration of different senses that allow you to understand a single concept.

Occipital lobes—Part of your cerebral cortex, the occipital lobes are at the back of your head. They help you see.

Temporal lobes—Part of your cerebral cortex, the temporal lobes are on the side of your head, just above your ears. They help you hear, remember, and learn.

Brain stem—Located deep in your brain, the brain stem leads to your spinal cord. The brain stem tells your body to do all the things you need to do to live: breathe, pump blood, sleep, wake up, and digest food. Most of the time, you do not even know it is doing all that work.

Cerebellum—Located at the base of your skull, the cerebellum means "little brain." The cerebellum helps with daily tasks, the things you do over and over. Once you have learned, you do not really have to think about how to ride a bike, how to dribble a basketball, or how to comb your hair. The cerebellum and parts of the cerebral cortex constantly send messages to each other so you can adjust your actions when conditions change.

Limbic system—The limbic system is a bridge between your cerebral cortex and the parts of your brain that control your body's physical systems. It is responsible for emotions and also is involved in memory and memory storage. The limbic system is like a bridge between your thinking brain, the cerebral cortex, and the parts of your brain that control your body's physical systems. This makes it easy for strong feelings, such as pleasure, fear, or attraction to other people, to cause reactions in your stomach, muscles, and heart.

Hippocampus—This is the part of the limbic system that receives and stores your long-term memory. If you remember your teachers' names from last year, your hippocampus is working.

Adolescent Brains Show Reduced Reward Anticipation

Adolescents show less activity than adults in brain regions that motivate behavior to obtain rewards, according to results from the first magnetic resonance imaging (MRI) study to examine real-time adolescent response to incentives. The study also shows that adolescents and adults exhibit similar brain responses to having obtained rewards. Researchers in the Laboratory of Clinical Studies of the National Institute on Alcohol Abuse and Alcoholism (NIAAA), one of the National Institutes of Health, conducted the study, which appeared in the February 25, 2004 issue of the *Journal of Neuroscience* (Volume 24, Number 7).

"Understanding adolescent motivation is critical for understanding why so many young people drink alcohol and engage in associated behaviors such as drinking and driving and sexual risk-taking. That understanding also will be critical for shaping prevention messages that deter such behaviors," said Ting-Kai Li, M.D., Director, National Institute on Alcohol Abuse and Alcoholism.

In the MRI study, James Bjork, Ph.D., and others in the laboratory of Daniel Hommer, M.D., scanned the brains of twelve adolescents aged 12 to 17 years and twelve young adults aged 22 to 28 years. While being scanned, the subjects participated in a game-like scenario risking monetary gain or loss. The participants responded to targets on a screen by pressing a button to win or avoid losing 20 cents, $1.00, or $5.00.

For both age groups, the researchers found that the anticipation of potential gain activated portions of the ventral striatum, right insula, dorsal thalamus, and dorsal midbrain, with the magnitude of ventral striatum activation sensitive to gain amount. In adolescents, however, the researchers found lower activation of the right ventral striatum centered in the nucleus accumbens, a region at the base of the brain shown by earlier research to be crucial for motivating behavior toward the prospect of rewards.

"Our observations help to resolve a longstanding debate among researchers about whether adolescents experience enhanced reward from risky behaviors—or seek out alcohol and other stimuli because they require enhanced stimulation. They also may help to explain why so many young people have difficulty achieving long-term goals," according to James Bjork, Ph.D., first author on the study.

When the researchers examined brain activity following gain outcomes, they saw that in both adolescents and young adults monetary gain similarly activated a region of the mesial frontal cortex. "These results suggest that adolescents selectively show reduced recruitment of motivational but not consummatory components of reward-directed behavior," state the authors.

Chapter 5

Understanding Puberty

Your daughter's breasts are budding beneath what used to look like an innocent little tank top. Your son comes home from soccer practice smelling like a guy who's been digging on a road crew all day. What's going on here?

Welcome to puberty, that time in life when kids sprout up, fill out, and maybe even mouth off. Puberty was awkward enough when you were the one going through it. So how can you help your child through all the changes?

Stages of Puberty

Sure, most of us know the telltale signs of puberty—hair growth in new places, menstruation, body odor, lower voice in boys, breast growth in girls, etc. But we may not fully comprehend the science behind all of these changes. Here's a quick look at how it works.

At some point, usually not until after a girl's eighth birthday or after a boy turns nine or ten, puberty begins when an area of the brain called the hypothalamus starts to release gonadotropin-releasing hormone (GnRH). When GnRH travels to the pituitary gland (a small gland under the brain that produces hormones that control other

This information was provided by KidsHealth, one of the largest resources online for medically reviewed health information written for parents, kids, and teens. For more articles like this one, visit www.KidsHealth.org, or www.TeensHealth.org. © 2004 The Nemours Center for Children's Health Media, a division of The Nemours Foundation.

glands throughout the body), it releases two more puberty hormones—luteinizing hormone (LH) and follicle-stimulating hormone (FSH).

What happens next depends on a child's gender. For boys, the hormones travel through the bloodstream to the testes (testicles) and give the signal to begin production of sperm and the hormone testosterone. In girls, the hormones go to the ovaries (the two oval-shaped organs that lie to the right and left of the uterus) and trigger the maturation and release of eggs and the production of the hormone estrogen, which prepare a female's body for pregnancy.

For a Boy

The physical changes of puberty for a boy usually start with enlargement of the testicles and sprouting of pubic hair, followed by a growth spurt between ages ten and sixteen—on average one to two years later than when girls start. His arms, legs, hands, and feet also grow faster than the rest of his body. His body shape will begin to change as his shoulders broaden and he gains weight and muscle.

A boy may become concerned if he notices tenderness or swelling under his nipples. This temporary development of breast tissue is called gynecomastia and it happens to about 50% of boys during puberty. But it usually disappears within six months or so. And that first crack in the voice is a sign that his voice is changing and will become deeper.

Dark, coarse, curly hair will also sprout just above his penis and on his scrotum, and later under his arms and in the beard area. His penis and testes will get larger, and erections, which a boy begins experiencing as an infant, will become more frequent. Ejaculation—the release of sperm-containing semen—will also occur.

Many boys become concerned about their penis size. A boy may need reassurance, particularly if he tends to be a later developer and he compares himself to boys who are further along in puberty. If a boy is circumcised, he may also have questions about the skin that covers the tip of an uncircumcised penis.

For a Girl

Puberty generally starts earlier for a girl, sometime between eight and thirteen years of age. For most girls, the first evidence of puberty is breast development, but it may be the growth of pubic hair in some. As her breasts start to grow, a girl may have small, firm, tender lumps (called buds) under one or both nipples; the breast tissue will get larger and become less firm in texture over the next few years. Dark, coarse, curly hair will appear on her labia (the folds of skin surrounding the vagina), and later, similar hair will begin growing under her arms.

The first signs of puberty are followed one or two years later by a noticeable growth spurt. Her body will begin to build up fat, particularly in the breasts and around her hips and thighs, as she takes on the contours of a woman. Her arms, legs, hands, and feet will also get bigger.

The culminating event will be the arrival of menarche, her first period (also called menstruation). Depending on the age at which they begin their pubertal development, girls may get their first period between the ages of nine and sixteen.

Common Puberty Concerns

The term puberty is generally used to refer to the specific physical changes kids experience as they move toward adulthood, but that doesn't mean that these bodily changes are without emotional consequences. Some girls are excited about their budding breasts and new training bras; others may worry that all eyes are focused on their breasts. Some boys love the sight of themselves all lathered up with shaving cream; others may be uncomfortable with the attention they get for a few new shoots of hair.

Pimples are common for most teens. Acne is caused by glands in the skin that produce a natural oil called sebum. Puberty hormones make the glands produce extra sebum, which can clog the pores. Washing gently with water and mild soap can get rid of excess sebum and help reduce breakouts. In more severe cases of acne, there are several helpful over-the-counter and prescription medications available. Don't hesitate to talk to your child's doctor about recommending a dermatologist (a doctor specializing in skin).

Kids who once associated bath time with play need to learn to wash frequently enough and to apply deodorant or antiperspirant. A teen who is learning to use a razor will need instructions on how to keep it clean, to throw a disposable one away before it becomes dull and ineffective, and to not share it with others.

Boys, capable of having an erection since infancy, can now experience ejaculation. The first ejaculation usually occurs between the ages of eleven and fifteen, either spontaneously in connection with sexual fantasies, during masturbation, or as a nocturnal emission (also called a wet dream). If he doesn't know about wet dreams before he has one, a boy may think he has urinated accidentally or that something has gone wrong with his body.

As children mature physically and emotionally, they become increasingly curious about their sexuality and their own bodies. Although infants and younger children do touch their own genitals from time to time because they like the way it feels, masturbation is more common in older children from the preadolescent and teen years and beyond.

There are lots of myths and beliefs about masturbation. No, it won't cause your child to grow hair on his hands, become infertile, go blind, or develop new emotional problems. A small number of children and teens with already existing emotional problems may become preoccupied with masturbation—just as they may become overly occupied with other behaviors or thoughts. Constant or obsessive masturbation may be a sign of anxiety or other emotional problem. But, other than that, masturbation is generally considered by doctors to be a common form of normal sexual self-exploration. Although some preteens and teens may choose to masturbate, others may not.

Because masturbation is often considered a private topic, many children may feel too embarrassed to talk about it because they're concerned that their parents will be angry or disappointed with them. Some kids may prefer to talk to older siblings, friends, or their doctors than a parent. If you continue to be concerned or have questions about masturbation, talk with your child's doctor.

Talking to Your Child about Puberty

Boys and girls can see these changes happening to each other—in some cases, they can smell them. It's important to talk to your child about how bodies change—sooner, rather than later.

Be prepared to talk to a girl about the expected events of puberty, including menstruation, when you see the first signs of breast development, or earlier if she seems ready or has questions. A boy should know about normal penile development, erections, and nocturnal emissions before age twelve—sooner if he's an early developer. And it's also important to talk to your child about what's happening to members of the opposite sex.

It's best not to have "The Talk" but rather a series of talks, ideally beginning when your child is young and starting to ask questions about body parts. Each time you talk, offer more and more detail depending upon your child's maturity level and interest in the topic. And, if your child has a question, answer it right away. If you feel uncomfortable or uncertain about having these discussions with your child, ask your child's doctor for advice.

Chapter 6

Medical Care
of 13–18 Year Olds

By meeting yearly with your teen, the doctor can keep track of changes in his or her physical, mental, and social development and offer advice against unhealthy behaviors, such as smoking and drinking. The doctor can also help your child understand the importance of choosing a healthy lifestyle that includes good nutrition, proper exercise, and safety measures. The more teens understand about their physical growth and sexual development, the more they will recognize the importance of active involvement in their own health care.

What Happens at the Doctor's Office?

Teens should visit their doctors annually. At least three of these visits should include a complete physical examination: one performed during early adolescence (ages 11 to 14), one during middle adolescence (ages 15 to 17), and one during late adolescence (ages 18 to 21). If your child has a chronic medical condition or if certain clinical signs or symptoms are present, more frequent examinations may be indicated.

Medical care should include screenings for high blood pressure, obesity, and other eating disorders, and, if indicated, hyperlipidemia

This information was provided by KidsHealth, one of the largest resources online for medically reviewed health information written for parents, kids, and teens. For more articles like this one, visit www.KidsHealth.org, or www.TeensHealth.org. © 2005 The Nemours Center for Children's Health Media, a division of The Nemours Foundation.

(an excess of cholesterol and/or other fats in the blood). A tuberculin (PPD) test may be administered if your teen is at risk for tuberculosis.

Your teen's doctor will also check his or her teeth for tooth decay, abnormal tooth development, malocclusion (abnormal bite), dental injuries, and other problems. Your teen should also continue to have regular checkups with her dentist.

Vision and hearing will be checked. Teens will also be checked for scoliosis (curvature of the spine).

Teens should receive a diphtheria and tetanus booster (Td) ten years after their last childhood booster (usually at age four to six years) and every ten years thereafter. They should have already completed their other immunizations, including varicella (if they have not had chickenpox); measles, mumps, and rubella (MMR); and the hepatitis B series (Hep B). If your teen will be living in an institutional setting, such as a college dormitory, speak with his or her doctor about receiving the meningococcal meningitis vaccine.

As your child goes through puberty, issues of sexual health will be addressed. Your child's doctor will teach your daughter how to perform a monthly breast exam. The doctor may also perform (or refer her to a gynecologist for) a gynecologic exam and a Pap smear to check for cervical cancer. Males will be checked for hernias and testicular cancer and taught to perform a testicular self-examination.

Teens should be asked about behaviors or emotional problems that may indicate depression or the risk of suicide. The doctor should also provide counseling about risky behaviors and other issues, including:

- sexual activities that may result in unintended pregnancy and sexually transmitted diseases (STDs), including human immunodeficiency virus (HIV)

- emotional, physical, and sexual abuse

- use of alcohol and other substances, including anabolic steroids

- use of tobacco products, including cigarettes and smokeless tobacco

- use of alcohol while driving

- use of safety devices, including bicycle helmets, seat belts, and protective sports gear

- how to resolve conflicts without violence, including how to avoid the use of weapons

- learning problems or difficulties at school

- appropriate warm-ups before exercise and importance of regular physical activity

What Should I Do if I Suspect a Medical Problem?

Parents or other caregivers should receive health guidance at least once during early, middle, and late adolescence from their teen's doctor. During these sessions, the doctor will provide information about normal development, including signs and symptoms of illness or emotional distress and methods to monitor and manage potentially harmful behaviors. If you suspect that your teen has a physical disorder, a psychological problem, or a problem with drugs or alcohol, contact your child's doctor immediately.

Typical Medical Problems

Issues involving puberty and sexual development are typical concerns for this age group. Doctors who establish a policy of confidentiality can serve as a valuable resource for a teen by answering questions and providing guidance during this period of physical and emotional changes. Teens should be reassured that anything they discuss with their doctor will be kept confidential, unless their health or the health of others is endangered by the situation.

Sports injuries are common concerns. Osgood-Schlatter disease, a painful inflammation of the area just below the front of the knee, is particularly common in the early teen years. Knee pain is also a frequent complaint. Your teen's doctor should evaluate any severe or persistent pain of the joints, muscles, or other areas of the body.

Chapter 7

Sleep Deprivation Impacts Teen Health

How Much Sleep Do I Need?

Most teens need about 8.5 to more than 9 hours of sleep each night. The right amount of sleep is essential for anyone who wants to do well on a test or play sports without tripping over their feet. Unfortunately, though, many teens don't get enough sleep.

Why aren't teens getting enough sleep?

Until recently, teens were often given a bad rap for staying up late, oversleeping for school, and falling asleep in class. But recent studies show that adolescent sleep patterns actually differ from those of adults or kids.

These studies show that during the teen years, the body's circadian (pronounced: sur-kay-dee-un) rhythm (sort of like an internal biological clock) is reset, telling a person to fall asleep later and wake up later. Unlike kids and adults, whose bodies tell them to go to sleep and wake up earlier, most teens' bodies tell them go to sleep late at night and sleep into the late morning. This change in the circadian

This chapter includes: "Common Sleep Problems," and "How Much Sleep Do I Need?" This information was provided by KidsHealth, one of the largest resources online for medically reviewed health information written for parents, kids, and teens. For more articles like this one, visit www.KidsHealth.org, or www.TeensHealth.org. © 2004 The Nemours Center for Children's Health Media, a division of The Nemours Foundation.

rhythm seems to be due to the fact that melatonin, a hormone that regulates sleeping and waking patterns, is produced later at night for teens than it is for kids and adults. This can make it harder for teens to fall asleep early.

These changes in the body's circadian rhythm coincide with a time when we're busier than ever. For most teens, the pressure to do well in school is more intense than when they were kids, and it's harder to get by without studying hard. But teens also have other demands on their time—everything from sports and other extracurricular activities to fitting in a part-time job to save money for college.

Early start times in some schools also play a role in this sleep deficit. Teens who fall asleep after midnight may still have to get up early for school, meaning that they may only squeeze in six or seven hours of sleep a night. An hour or two of missed sleep a night may not seem like a big deal, but it can create a noticeable sleep deficit over time.

Why is sleep important?

This sleep deficit impacts everything from a teen's ability to pay attention in class to his or her mood. Research shows that 20% of high school students fall asleep in class, and experts have been able to tie lost sleep to poorer grades. Lack of sleep also damages people's ability to do their best in athletics.

Slowed responses and concentration from lack of sleep don't just affect school or sports performance. The fact that sleep deprivation slows reaction times can be life-threatening for teens who drive. The National Highway Safety Traffic Administration estimates that 1,500 people are killed every year in crashes caused by drivers between the ages of 15 and 24 who are simply tired. (More than half of the people who cause crashes because they fall asleep at the wheel are under the age of 26.)

Lack of sleep has also been linked to emotional troubles, such as feelings of sadness and depression. Sleep helps keep us physically healthy, too, by slowing our body's systems enough to re-energize us after everyday activities.

How do I know if I'm getting enough?

Even if you think you're getting enough sleep, you may not be. Here are some of the signs that you may need more sleep:

- difficulty waking up in the morning
- inability to concentrate

- falling asleep during classes

- feelings of moodiness and even depression

How can I get more sleep?

Recently, some researchers, parents, and teachers have suggested that middle and high school classes begin later in the morning to accommodate teens' need for more sleep. Some schools have already implemented later start times. You and your friends, parents, and teachers can lobby for later start times at your school, but in the meantime you'll have to make your own adjustments. Here are some things that may help you to sleep better:

- **Set a regular bedtime.** Going to bed at the same time each night signals to your body that it's time to sleep. Waking up at the same time every day can also help establish sleep patterns. So try to stick to your sleep schedule even on weekends. Don't go to sleep more than an hour later or wake up more than two to three hours later than you do during the week.

- **Exercise regularly.** Try not to exercise right before bed as it can raise your body temperature and wake you up. Sleep experts believe that exercising five or six hours before bedtime (in late afternoon) may actually help a person sleep.

- **Avoid stimulants.** Don't drink beverages with caffeine, such as soda and coffee, after 4:00 P.M. Nicotine is also a stimulant, so quitting smoking may help you sleep better. And drinking alcohol in the evening can also cause a person to be restless and wake up during the night.

- **Relax your mind.** Avoid violent, scary, or action movies or television shows right before bed—anything that might set your mind and heart racing. Reading books with involved or active plots may also keep you from falling or staying asleep.

- **Unwind by keeping the lights low.** Light signals the brain that it's time to wake up. Staying away from bright lights (including computer screens), as well as meditating or listening to soothing music, can help your body relax.

- **Don't nap too much.** Naps of more than 30 minutes during the day may keep you from falling asleep later.

- **Avoid all-nighters.** Don't wait until the night before a big test to study. Cutting back on sleep the night before a test may mean you perform worse than you would if you'd studied less but got more sleep.

- **Create the right sleeping environment.** Studies show that people sleep best in a dark room that is slightly on the cool side. Close your blinds or curtains (and make sure they're heavy enough to block out light) and turn down the thermostat in your room (pile on extra blankets or wear pajamas if you're cold). Lots of noise can be a sleep turnoff, too.

- **Wake up with bright light.** Bright light in the morning signals to your body that it's time to get going.

If you're drowsy, it's hard to look and feel your best, so schedule sleep as an item on your agenda to help you stay creative and healthy.

Common Sleep Problems

Garrett had a hard time waking up for school during his sophomore year. At first, he thought it was because he'd been going to bed late over summer vacation and then sleeping in the next day. He assumed he'd adjust to his school schedule after a couple of weeks. But as the school year progressed, Garrett found himself lying awake in bed until two or three in the morning, even though he got up at 6:30 A.M. every day. He began falling asleep in class and his grades started to suffer.

Most teens don't get enough sleep, but that's usually because they're overloaded and tend to skimp on sleep. But sleep problems can keep some teens, like Garrett, awake at night even when they want to sleep.

Over time, those nights of missed sleep (whether they're caused by a sleep disorder or simply not scheduling enough time for the necessary sleep) can build into a sleep deficit. People with a sleep deficit are unable to concentrate, study, and work effectively. They can also experience emotional problems, like depression.

What happens during sleep?

You don't notice it, of course, but while you're asleep, your brain is still active. As people sleep, their brains pass through five stages of sleep. Together, these stages—which doctors call one, two, three, four, and REM (rapid eye movement) sleep—make up a sleep cycle. One complete sleep cycle lasts about 90 to 100 minutes. So during an average night's sleep, a person will experience about four or five cycles of sleep.

Stages one and two are periods of light sleep from which a person can easily be awakened. During these stages, eye movements slow down and eventually stop, heart and breathing rates slow down, and body temperature decreases. Stages three and four are deep sleep stages. It's more difficult to awaken someone during these stages, and when awakened, a person will often feel groggy and disoriented for a few minutes. Stages three and four are the most refreshing of the sleep stages—it is this type of sleep that we crave when we are very tired.

The final stage of the sleep cycle is known as REM sleep because of the rapid eye movements that occur during this stage. During REM sleep, other physical changes take place—breathing becomes rapid, the heart beats faster, and the limb muscles don't move. This is the stage of sleep when a person has the most vivid dreams.

Why do teens have trouble sleeping?

Research shows that teens need 8.5 to more than 9 hours of sleep a night. You don't need to be a math whiz to figure out that if you wake up for school at 6:00 A.M., it means you have to go to bed at 9:00 P.M. to reach the nine-hour mark. Studies have found that many teens, like Garrett, have trouble falling asleep that early. It's not because they don't want to sleep. It's because their brains naturally work on later schedules and aren't ready for bed.

During adolescence, the body's circadian (pronounced: sur-kay-dee-un) rhythm (sort of like an internal biological clock) is reset, telling a teen to fall asleep later at night and wake up later in the morning. This change in the circadian rhythm seems to be due to the fact that melatonin, a hormone that regulates sleeping and waking patterns, is produced later at night in teens than it is for kids and adults, making it harder for teens to fall asleep. This phenomenon has a medical name: delayed sleep phase syndrome. Although it's common, delayed sleep phase syndrome doesn't affect every teen.

Changes in the body clock aren't the only reason teens lose sleep. Lots of people have insomnia—trouble falling or staying asleep. The most common cause of insomnia is stress. But all sorts of things can lead to insomnia, including physical discomfort (the stuffy nose of a cold or the pain of a headache, for example), emotional troubles (like family problems or relationship difficulties), and even sleeping environment (a room that's too hot, cold, or noisy).

It's common for everyone to have insomnia from time to time. But if insomnia lasts for a month or longer with no relief, then doctors consider it chronic. Chronic insomnia can be caused by problems like depression. People with chronic insomnia can often get help for their condition from a doctor, therapist, or other counselor.

For some people, insomnia can be made worse by worrying about the insomnia itself. A brief period of insomnia can build into something longer lasting when a person becomes anxious about not sleeping or worried about feeling tired the next day. Doctors call this psychophysiologic (pronounced: sye-ko-fih-zee-uh-lah-jik) insomnia.

There are a number of other conditions that can disrupt sleep in teens. They include:

Periodic limb movement disorder and restless legs syndrome. People with these conditions find their sleep is disrupted by leg (or, less frequently, arm) movements, leaving them tired or irritable from lack of sleep. In the case of periodic limb movement disorder (PLMD), these movements are involuntary twitches or jerks. They're called involuntary because the person isn't consciously controlling them and is often unaware of the movement. People with restless legs syndrome (RLS) actually feel physical sensations in their limbs, such as tingling, itching, cramping, or burning. The only way they can relieve these feelings is by moving their legs or arms to get rid of the discomfort. Doctors can treat PLMD and RLS. For some people, treating an iron deficiency makes RLS go away; other people may need to take other types of medication.

Obstructive sleep apnea. This sleep disorder causes a person to stop breathing temporarily during sleep. One common cause of obstructive sleep apnea is enlarged tonsils or adenoids (tissues located in the passage that connects the nose and throat). Being overweight or obese can also lead a person to develop obstructive sleep apnea. People with obstructive sleep apnea may snore, have difficulty breathing, and even sweat heavily during sleep. Because sleep apnea disrupts a person's sleep, people with the disorder may feel extremely sleepy or irritable during the day. People who show signs of obstructive sleep apnea, such as loud snoring or excessive daytime sleepiness, should be evaluated by a doctor.

Reflux. Some people have a condition called gastroesophageal reflux disease (GERD) that causes stomach acid to move backward up into the esophagus. This produces the uncomfortable, burning sensation we call heartburn. The symptoms of GERD can be worse when a person is lying down. So even if the person doesn't notice the feelings of heartburn because he or she is sleeping, the discomfort it causes can still interfere with the sleep cycle.

Nightmares. Most teens have nightmares on occasion, but frequent nightmares can disrupt a person's sleep patterns by waking him or her during the night. Some things can trigger more frequent nightmares, including certain medications, drugs, or alcohol. And, ironically, sleep deprivation can also be a cause. The most common triggers for more frequent nightmares, though, are emotional, such as stress or anxiety. If nightmares are interfering with your sleep, it's a good idea to talk to a doctor, therapist, or other counselor.

Sleepwalking. It's rare for teens to walk in their sleep; most sleepwalkers are children. Sleepwalking may run in families. It most often occurs when a person is sick, has a fever, is not getting enough sleep, or is feeling stress. Because most sleepwalkers don't sleepwalk often, it's not usually a serious problem. Sleepwalkers tend to go back to bed on their own and don't usually remember sleepwalking. (Sleepwalking often happens during the deeper sleep that takes place during stages three and four of the sleep cycle.) Sometimes, though, a sleepwalker will need help moving around obstacles and getting back to bed. It's also true that waking sleepwalkers can startle them (but it isn't harmful), so try to guide a sleepwalker back to bed gently.

What should I do?

If you're getting enough rest at night and you're still feeling tired during the day, it's a good idea to visit your doctor. Excessive tiredness can be caused by all sorts of health problems, not just difficulties with sleep.

If your doctor suspects a sleep problem, he or she will look at your overall health and sleep habits. In addition to doing a physical examination, the doctor will ask you about any concerns and symptoms you have, your past health, your family's health, any medications you're taking, any allergies you may have, and other issues. This is called the medical history. Your doctor may also do tests to find out whether any conditions—such as obstructive sleep apnea—might be interfering with your sleep.

Different sleep problems are treated differently. Some can be treated with medications, whereas others can be helped by special techniques such as light therapy (where a person sits in front of a light box for a certain amount of time each day) or other practices that can help reset a person's body clock.

Doctors also encourage teens to make lifestyle changes that promote good sleeping habits. You probably know that caffeine can make you stay awake, but did you know that playing video games or watching television before sleeping can do the same thing?

Chapter 8

Facts about Adolescent Mortality and Suicide

Facts about Mortality: Adolescents and Young Adults

Seven Out of Ten Deaths among Adolescents and Young Adults Are Preventable

In 2001, 71% of deaths among adolescents and young adults ages 10–24 were due to preventable causes of unintentional injury, homicide, and suicide.[1] There were 36,254 deaths in 2001 among a population of 60.9 million in this age group, which represents a mortality rate of 59.5/100,000.[2]

Mortality Rates Have Decreased during the Past Two Decades

During the past twenty years, mortality rates for adolescents and young adults ages 10–24 have decreased and are now at or near historical lows for all age groups. During two brief periods (1986 and 1991–93), the mortality rate increased slightly. Since 1993, the mortality rates for adolescents ages 10–19 have declined steadily. By contrast, the rates for young adults ages 20–24 declined until 1999, and increased between 1999 and 2001.[2, 3]

This chapter is reprinted with permission of the National Adolescent Health Information Center, 2004. It includes: "Fact Sheet on Mortality: Adolescents and Young Adults," and "Fact Sheet on Suicide: Adolescents and Young Adults," San Francisco, CA. University of California, San Francisco.

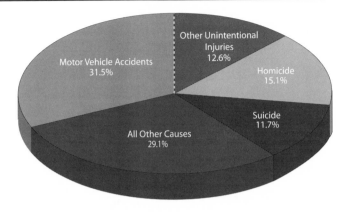

Figure 8.1. *Leading Causes of Death, Ages 10–24, 2001*[1]

Young Adults Have Five Times the Death Rate of Younger Adolescents

In 2001, young adults ages 20–24 were 4.9 times more likely to die than younger adolescents ages 10–14. Mortality rates continue to increase throughout the lifespan. Male adolescents have higher mortality rates than their female peers, a disparity that increases with age. For young adolescents ages 10–14, the death rate for males was 1.5 times that of females; this difference in rates increased to 2.4 for adolescents ages 15–19 and 3.0 for young adults ages 20–24.[2]

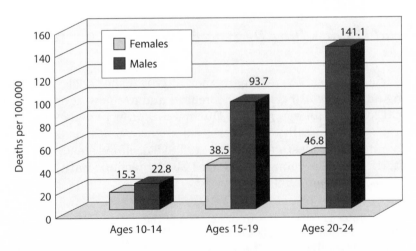

Figure 8.2. *Mortality Rates by Age and Gender, Ages 10–24, 2001*[2]

Black and American Indian Adolescent Males Have the Highest Mortality Rate

Black-non Hispanic and American Indian males ages 10–24 have the highest mortality rates among same-age racial/ethnic groups. In 2001, Black-non Hispanic male adolescents and young adults were 1.3 to 2.9 times more likely to die than their male peers, and were 2.7 to 7.4 times more likely to die than their female peers. Among same age females, American Indians have the highest mortality rate, followed by Black-non Hispanics, White-non Hispanics, Hispanics, and Asian/Pacific Islanders.[2]

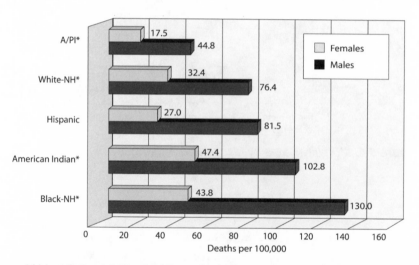

Abbreviations: NH=non Hispanic; AI/AN=American Indian/Alaskan Native; A/PI=Asian/Pacific Islander

Figure 8.3. *Mortality Rates by Race/Ethnicity* and Gender, Ages 10–24, 2001[2]*

Motor Vehicle Accidents Are the Leading Cause of Death for Adolescents

Adolescents and young adults ages 10–24 are most likely to die from motor vehicle accidents (MVA). The overall MVA mortality rate for adolescents and young adults ages 15–24 is 5.8 times higher than the rate for younger adolescents ages 10–14. This pattern is similar for homicide and suicide: the homicide rate for 15–24 year olds is 14.8 times the rate of 10–14 year olds; and, the suicide rate for 15–24 year olds is 7.6 times the rate for 10–14 year olds.

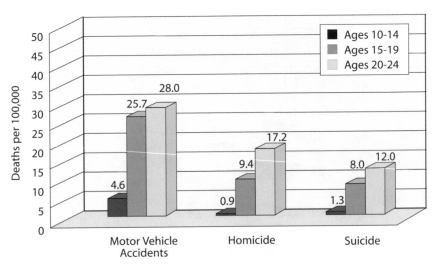

Figure 8.4. *Mortality Rates by Cause and Age, Ages 10–24, 2001[1]*

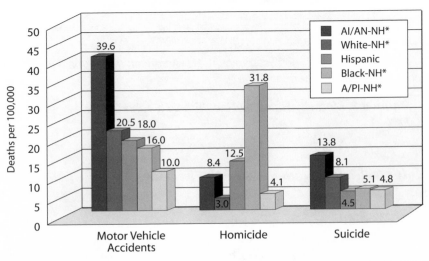

Figure 8.5. *Mortality Rates by Cause and Race/Ethnicity, Ages 10–24, 2001[1]*

Racial/Ethnic Disparities in Adolescent Mortality Rates Are Greatest for Homicide

Large racial/ethnic disparities exist for homicide, with rates for Black-non Hispanic adolescents and young adults 2.5 to 10.6 times that of other racial/ethnic groups in 2001. American Indian/Alaskan Native-non Hispanic adolescents have the highest mortality rates among all racial/ethnic groups for motor vehicle accidents and suicide.[1]

Malignant Neoplasms Are the Leading Cause of Other Mortality among Adolescents and Young Adults

Malignant neoplasms, such as leukemia and brain cancer, were responsible for the greatest number of deaths among other causes of mortality for adolescents and young adults. Heart disease and congenital anomalies were the next leading causes of death. Rates for other causes of mortality varied by age group and gender.[1]

Facts about Adolescent and Young Adult Suicide

Suicide Is the Third Leading Cause of Death for Adolescents and Young Adults

In 2001, the Centers for Disease Control and Prevention reported that 4,243 adolescents and young adults ages 10–24 took their own lives, resulting in a suicide rate of 7 per 100,000. In 2001, suicide accounted for 11.7% of all deaths for this age group. This makes

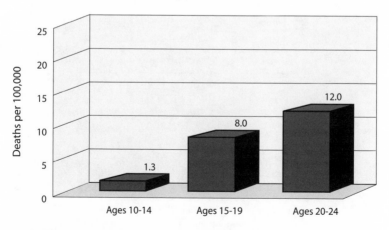

Figure 8.6. *Suicide Rates by Age, 10–24, 2001*[4]

55

suicide the third leading cause of death for adolescents and young adults after unintentional injury and homicide.[4]

Suicide Rates Increase Dramatically from Early Adolescence to Young Adulthood

Older adolescents are six times more likely to commit suicide than younger adolescents. The rate also increases for young adults, who are nine times more likely than younger adolescents to commit suicide. Suicide rates continue to increase in adulthood until age 50.[4] Between 1960 and 2000, the suicide rate among adolescents increased dramatically (128%) compared to the rate of the general population (2%).[4, 5]

Adolescent Males Are Much More Likely to Commit Suicide Than Adolescent Females

Adolescent and young adult males ages 10–24 have a consistently higher suicide rate than their female peers, averaging more than five times the rate of same-age females. This is a long-standing trend: from 1981 to 2001, 84% of 10–24 year olds who committed suicide were male. Males have higher suicide rates throughout the lifespan.[4]

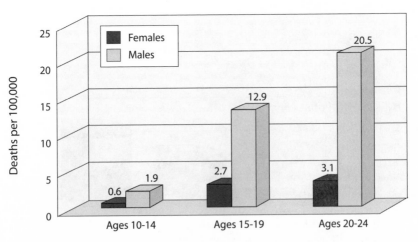

Figure 8.7. *Suicide Rates by Age and Gender, Ages 10–24, 2001*[4]

American Indian/Alaskan Native Male Adolescents Have the Highest Suicide Rates

Among adolescents and young adults ages 10–24, non Hispanic American Indians/Alaskan Natives have the highest suicide rate. In 2001, the suicide rate for American Indian/Alaskan Native-non Hispanic males was 1.5 to 3 times that of same-age males in other racial/ethnic groups and about ten times that of same-age females. Asian/Pacific Islander-non Hispanic and Hispanic youth are least likely to commit suicide. Suicide is the second leading cause of death for Asian/Pacific Islander and Alaskan Native-non Hispanic adolescent and young adult males.[4]

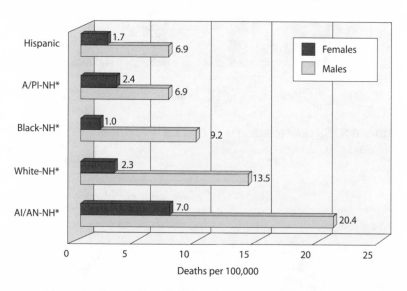

Figure 8.8. Suicide Rates by Gender and Race/Ethnicity,* Ages 10–24, 2001[4](*Abbreviations: NH=non Hispanic; AI/AN=American Indian/Alaskan Native; A/PI=Asian/Pacific Islander)

Female Adolescents Are More Likely to Attempt Suicide Than Their Male Peers

While adolescent males commit suicide at greater rates, adolescent females are more likely to exhibit non-lethal suicidal behavior and ideation. Among high school students in 2003, twice as many females attempted suicide as males (11.5% vs. 5.4%).[6] The percentage of students who reported an attempted suicide in the past year increased slightly from 7.3% in 1991 to 8.5% in 2003.[7] About one-fifth (21.3%) of female students seriously considered suicide in 2003, compared to 12.8% of same-age males.[6]

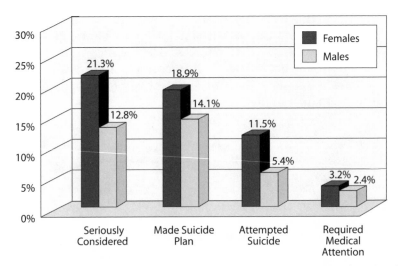

Figure 8.9. Suicidal Ideation and Non-Lethal Behavior by Gender, High School Students, 2003[6]

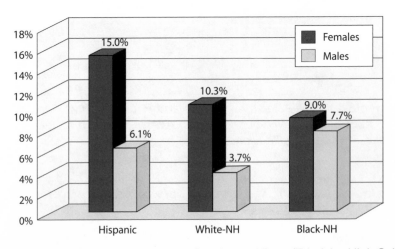

Figure 8.10. Suicide Attempts by Gender and Race/Ethnicity, High School Students, 2003[6]

Female Hispanic Adolescents Are More Likely to Attempt Suicide Than Their Black or White Peers

Female Hispanic students are more likely to attempt suicide than all other students. The suicide attempt rate varies by race/ethnicity: attempts are slightly higher for Hispanic students (10.6%) than for Black-non Hispanic and White-non Hispanic students (8.4% and 6.9%, respectively).[6] Hispanic students have reported higher rates of suicide attempts than Black-non Hispanic and White-non Hispanic students since data collection began in 1991.[7]

Since Peaking in the Early 1990s, Suicide Rates Have Fallen Sharply for Male Adolescents

Suicide rates for older adolescents and young adult males ages 15–24 have decreased since peaking in the early 1990s. By contrast, the rate (per 100,000) for adolescent males ages 10–14, while relatively low, increased from 1.2 in 1981 to 1.9 in 2001. Rates for all females ages 10–24 have decreased slightly over the same period.[4]

Data and Figure Sources

1. National Center for Injury Prevention and Control [NCIPC]. (2004). *Mortality reports database* [Online Database]. Atlanta, GA: Centers for Disease Control and Prevention, National Center for Injury Prevention and Control. [Available online at URL (9/04): http://www.cdc.gov/ncipc/wisqars/]

2. Anderson, R.N., and Smith, B.L. (2003). Deaths: Leading causes for 2001. *National Vital Statistics Reports*, 52(9), 1–86. [Available online at URL (9/04): http://www.cdc.gov/nchs/products/pubs/pubd/nvsr/nvsr52/nvsr52_09.pdf]

3. Centers for Disease Control and Prevention [CDC]. (2004). *CDC Wonder: Compressed mortality/population data* [Private Data Run]. Atlanta, GA: Author. [Available online at URL (9/04): http://wonder.cdc.gov/mortSQL.html]

4. National Center for Injury Prevention and Control [NCIPC]. (2004). *Mortality reports database* [Online Database]. Atlanta, GA: Centers for Disease Control and Prevention, National Center for Injury Prevention and Control. [Available online at URL (5/04): http://www.cdc.gov/ncipc/wisqars/]

5. Garland, A.F., & Zigler, E. (1993). Adolescent suicide prevention: Current research and social policy implications. *American Psychologist*, 48, 169–182.

6. Grunbaum, J.A., Kann, L., Kinchen, S.A., Ross, J., Hawkins, J., Lowry, R., et al. (2004). Youth Risk Behavior Surveillance-United States, 2003. In: Surveillance Summaries, May 21, 2004. *MMWR*, 53(No.SS-2), 1–100. [Available online at URL (5/04): http://www.cdc.gov/mmwr/PDF/ss/ss5302.pdf]

7. Youth Risk Behavior Surveillance System [YRBSS], Division of Adolescent and School Health, Centers for Disease Control and Prevention. (2004). *Youth Online* [Online Database]. [Available online at URL (5/04): http://apps.nccd.cdc.gov/yrbss/]

In all cases, the most recent available data were used. Some data are released 1–3 years after collection. In some cases, trend data with demographic breakdowns (for example, racial/ethnic) are relatively limited. For racial/ethnic data, the category names presented are those of the data sources used. Every attempt was made to standardize age ranges; when this was not possible, age ranges are those of the data sources used.

Additional Information

National Adolescent Health Information Center
School of Medicine
University of California, San Francisco
UCSF Box 0503
San Francisco, CA 94143-0503
Phone: 415-502-4856
Fax: 415-502-4858
Website: http://nahic.ucsf.edu
E-mail: nahic@ucsf.edu

Chapter 9

Disabilities That Qualify Youth for Services under the Individuals with Disabilities Education Act (IDEA)

Every year, under the federal law known as the Individuals with Disabilities Education Act (IDEA), millions of children with disabilities receive special services designed to meet their unique needs. For infants and toddlers with disabilities from birth through age two and their families, special services are provided through an early intervention system. For school-aged children and youth (aged 3–21), special education and related services are provided through the school system. These services can be very important in helping children and youth with disabilities develop, learn, and succeed in school and other settings.

Who Is Eligible for Services?

Under the IDEA, states are responsible for meeting the special needs of eligible children with disabilities. To find out if a child is eligible for services, he or she must first receive a full and individual initial evaluation. This evaluation is free. Two purposes of the evaluation are:

- to see if the child has a disability, as defined by IDEA
- to learn in more detail about his or her special needs

Excerpted from "General Information about Disabilities," National Dissemination Center for Children with Disabilities, 2002.

Children and Youth Aged 3 through 21

The IDEA lists thirteen different disability categories under which 3–21 year-olds may be eligible for services. For a child to be eligible for services, the disability must affect the child's educational performance. The disability categories listed in IDEA are:

- autism
- deaf-blindness
- emotional disturbance
- hearing impairment (including deafness)
- mental retardation
- multiple disabilities
- orthopedic impairment
- other health impairment
- specific learning disability
- speech or language impairment
- traumatic brain injury
- visual impairment (including blindness)

Under IDEA, a child may not be identified as a child with a disability just because he or she speaks a language other than English and does not speak or understand English well. A child may not be identified as having a disability just because he or she has not had enough instruction in math or reading.

How Does IDEA Define the Thirteen Disability Categories?

The IDEA provides definitions of the thirteen disability categories previously listed. These federal definitions guide how states define who is eligible for a free, appropriate, public education under IDEA. The definitions of disability terms are as follows:

Autism

A developmental disability significantly affecting verbal and nonverbal communication and social interaction, generally evident before age three that adversely affects educational performance.

Characteristics often associated with autism are engaging in repetitive activities and stereotyped movements, resistance to changes in daily routines or the environment, and unusual responses to sensory experiences. The term autism does not apply if the child's educational performance is adversely affected primarily because the child has emotional disturbance, as defined under the emotional disturbance definition. A child who shows the characteristics of autism after age three could be diagnosed as having autism if the criteria above are satisfied.

Deaf-Blindness

Concomitant [simultaneous] hearing and visual impairments, the combination of which causes such severe communication and other developmental and educational needs such that they cannot be accommodated in special education programs solely for children with deafness or children with blindness.

Deafness

A hearing problem so severe that a child is impaired in processing linguistic information through hearing—with or without amplification—that adversely affects a child's educational performance.

Emotional Disturbance

A condition exhibiting one or more of the following characteristics over a long period of time and to a marked degree that adversely affects a child's educational performance including:

- an inability to learn that cannot be explained by intellectual, sensory, or health factors
- an inability to build or maintain satisfactory interpersonal relationships with peers and teachers
- inappropriate types of behavior or feelings under normal circumstances
- a general pervasive mood of unhappiness or depression
- a tendency to develop physical symptoms or fears associated with personal or school problems

Emotional disturbance includes schizophrenia. The term does not apply to children who are socially maladjusted, unless it is determined that they have an emotional disturbance.

Hearing Impairment

A weakened or diminished reduction in hearing, whether permanent or fluctuating, that adversely affects a child's educational performance but is not included under the definition of deafness.

Mental Retardation

Significantly subaverage general intellectual functioning, existing concurrently [at the same time] with deficits in adaptive behavior and manifested during the developmental period, that adversely affects a child's educational performance.

Multiple Disabilities

Concomitant [simultaneous] impairments (such as mental retardation and blindness, mental retardation and orthopedic impairment, etc.), the combination of which causes such severe educational needs that cannot be accommodated in a special education program solely for one of the impairments. The term does not include deaf-blindness.

Orthopedic Impairment

A severe orthopedic impairment that adversely affects a child's educational performance. The term includes impairments caused by a congenital anomaly (for example, clubfoot, absence of some member), impairments caused by disease (for example, poliomyelitis, bone tuberculosis), and impairments from other causes (for example, cerebral palsy, amputations, and fractures or burns that cause contractures).

Other Health Impairment

Having limited strength, vitality, or alertness, including a heightened alertness to environmental stimuli, that results in limited alertness with respect to the educational environment that affects a child's educational performance. This may be due to chronic or acute health problems such as asthma, attention deficit disorder (ADD) or attention deficit hyperactivity disorder (ADHD), diabetes, epilepsy, a heart condition, hemophilia, lead poisoning, leukemia, nephritis, rheumatic fever, or sickle cell anemia.

Specific Learning Disability

A disorder in one or more of the basic psychological processes involved in understanding or in using language, spoken or written, that may manifest itself in an imperfect ability to listen, think, speak, read, write, spell, or to do mathematical calculations. The term includes such conditions as perceptual disabilities, brain injury, minimal brain dysfunction, dyslexia, and developmental aphasia. The term does not include learning problems that are primarily the result of visual, hearing, or motor disabilities; mental retardation; emotional disturbance; or environmental, cultural, or economic disadvantage.

Speech or Language Impairment

A communication disorder such as stuttering, impaired articulation, language impairment, or a voice impairment that adversely affects a child's educational performance.

Traumatic Brain Injury

Acquired injury to the brain caused by an external physical force, resulting in total or partial functional disability or psychosocial impairment, or both, that adversely affects a child's educational performance. The term applies to open or closed head injuries resulting in impairments in one or more areas, such as cognition, language, memory, attention, reasoning, abstract thinking, judgment, problem-solving, psychosocial behavior, physical functions, information processing, speech, and sensory, perceptual, and motor abilities. The term does not include brain injuries that are congenital or degenerative, or brain injuries induced by birth trauma.

Visual Impairment Including Blindness

Impairment in vision that, even with correction, adversely affects a child's educational performance. The term includes both partial sight and blindness.

Services Available to Eligible Youth with Disabilities

Special services are available to eligible children with disabilities and can do much to help children develop and learn. For children and youth ages 3 through 21, special education and related services are provided through the public school system. Probably the best way to find out about these services is to call your local public school. The school should be able to tell you about special education policies in your area or refer you to a district or county office for this information. If you are a parent who thinks your child may need special education and related services, be sure to ask how to have your child evaluated under IDEA for eligibility. Often there are materials available to tell parents and others more about local and state policies for special education and related services.

There are many sources of information about services for children with disabilities. Within your community, you may wish to contact the:

- Child Find coordinator for your district or county (IDEA requires that states conduct Child Find activities to identify, locate, and evaluate infants, toddlers, children, and youth with disabilities aged birth through 21);

- principal of your child's school; or

- special education director of your child's school district or local school.

Any of these individuals should be able to answer specific questions about how to obtain special education and related services, or early intervention services, for your child.

In addition, every state has a Parent Training and Information (PTI) center, which is an excellent source of information. The PTI can:

- help you learn about early intervention and special education services;

- tell you about what the IDEA requires; and

- connect you with disability groups and parent groups in the community or state.

Additional Information

National Dissemination Center for Children with Disabilities (NICHCY)
P.O. Box 1492
Washington, DC 20013
Toll-Free (Voice/TTY): 800-695-0285
Fax: 202-884-8441
Website: http://www.nichcy.org
E-mail: nichcy@aed.org

NICHCY offers a listing organizations and agencies within each state that address disability-related issues. It is available on the Internet at http://www.nichcy.org/states.htm.

Part Two

Adolescent Nutrition and Weight Management

Chapter 10

Nutrition and the Health of Young People

Nutrition Facts

Eating Behaviors of Young People

- Less than 40% of children and adolescents in the United States meet the U.S. dietary guidelines for saturated fat.

- Almost 80% of young people do not eat the recommended number of servings of fruits and vegetables.

- Only 39% of children ages 2–17 meet the USDA's dietary recommendation for fiber (found primarily in dried beans and peas, fruits, vegetables, and whole grains).

- Eighty-five percent of adolescent females do not consume enough calcium.

- A large number of high school students use unsafe methods to lose or maintain weight.

This chapter includes: An excerpt titled "Nutrition Facts," from "Nutrition and the Health of Young People," Centers for Disease Control and Prevention (CDC), July 2005; excerpts titled "The Adolescent Years," from "Adolescents Group, Section 6.1," from the *National Children's Study Dietary Assessment Literature Review*, National Cancer Institute (NCI); and "Food Intake Pattern Calorie Levels," and "Food Intake Patterns," from the U.S. Department of Agriculture (USDA), April 2005.

Diet and Academic Performance

- Research suggests that not having breakfast can affect children's intellectual performance.

- The percentage of young people who eat breakfast decreases with age; while 92% of children ages 6–11 eat breakfast, only 75–78% of adolescents ages 12–19 report eating breakfast.

The Adolescent Years

Adolescent needs for energy and all nutrients significantly increase to support the rapid rate of growth and development; as much as 50% of adult ideal body weight is gained in adolescence. Although appetite and food intake increase, the struggle for independence that characterizes adolescent psychosocial development often leads to the development of high-risk nutritional behaviors such as excessive dieting, meal skipping, use of unconventional nutritional and non-nutritional supplements, adoption of fad diets, and excessive alcohol consumption. The high prevalence of overweight and obesity, eating disorders, adolescent pregnancy, and the lack of consumption of five fruits and vegetables a day are among the challenging nutritional issues facing adolescents in the United States.

A number of factors contribute to the challenge of collecting valid dietary information from teenagers.

- **Rapidly changing eating habits.** The eating habits of adolescents are not static; they fluctuate throughout adolescence in relation to psychological and cognitive development and to growth and appetite changes.

- **Unstructured eating.** Snacking and meal skipping are routine. Grazing is commonplace and teens may combine snacks and meals.

- **Peer influence exceeds parental influence.** Eating away from home becomes commonplace, and fast-food accounts for 31% of food eaten away from home; only one-third of middle class U.S. 14 year-olds eat dinner with their family on most days.

- **Age-related compliance.** An overall trend toward an increase in energy underreporting with increasing age has been documented with studies in adolescents.

Table 10.1. Adolescent Development and Nutritional and Physical Needs

What's happening in your body	What your body needs	How to get what you need
Bones		
Getting larger	Calcium	Milk, cheese, calcium-enriched orange juice, calcium enriched tofu
Getting larger	Protein	Meat, fish, eggs, cheese, milk
Getting stronger	Exercise	Walking, running, sports
Muscles		
Increasing muscle size	Protein	Meat, fish, eggs, cheese, milk
Building muscle strength	Exercise	Walking, running, sports
Reproductive system		
Development of male/female systems	Protein	Meat, fish, eggs, cheese, milk
Females: beginning	Iron	Red meat, eggs, green vegetables, fortified bread and grain products
Brain		
Brain tissues changing	Protein	Meat, fish, eggs, cheese, milk
Developing new connections	Protein for neurotransmitters	Meat, fish, eggs, cheese, milk
Developing new connections	Mental activity	Learning new things
Energy for every day	Animal fats	Meat, seafood, butter, cheese, ice cream
Energy for every day	Vegetable fats	Nuts, peanut butter, olive oil
Energy for every day	Carbohydrates	Bread, pasta, cereal, apples, oranges, potatoes

Source: "Teacher Reference 1: Body Grid," Changing the Face of Medicine, National Library of Medicine, 2003.

71

Table 10.2. Calorie Levels for Males Ages 8–25 by Activity Level

Age	Sedentary[1]	Moderately active[2]	Active[3]
8	1400	1600	2000
9	1600	1800	2000
10	1600	1800	2200
11	1800	2000	2200
12	1800	2200	2400
13	2000	2200	2600
14	2000	2400	2800
15	2200	2600	3000
16	2400	2800	3200
17	2400	2800	3200
18	2400	2800	3200
19–20	2600	2800	3000
21–25	2400	2800	3000

[1]Sedentary equals less than 30 minutes a day of moderate physical activity in addition to daily activities.
[2]Moderately active equals at least 30 minutes and up to 60 minutes a day of moderate physical activity in addition to daily activities.
[3]Active equals 60 or more minutes a day of moderate physical activity in addition to daily activities.

- **High prevalence of restrained eating.** The well-documented high prevalence of dissatisfaction of many normal weight adolescents with their weight has implications for bias in dietary surveys; inclusion of measures of dietary restraint and body image is important in this age group.

- **Overweight and obesity may lead to underreporting of intake.** As with obese adults, obese adolescents underreport intake significantly more than their non-obese counterparts; up to 40% of energy intake in obese adolescents may not be reported.

- **Reporting format.** Dietary assessment probing, coding, and reporting formats designed for adults do not adequately reflect the eating patterns of teens. Dietary assessment methods should address the eating environments and patterns of teens as well as capabilities and motivation at different stages of adolescence.

- **Research in school settings is difficult.** Increasing time pressures on school curriculum limit time for recruitment and

Table 10.3. Calorie Levels for Females Ages 8–25 by Activity Level*

Age	Sedentary[1]	Moderately active[2]	Active[3]
8	1400	1600	1800
9	1400	1600	1800
10	1400	1800	2000
11	1600	1800	2000
12	1600	2000	2200
13	1600	2000	2200
14	1800	2000	2400
15	1800	2000	2400
16	1800	2000	2400
17	1800	2000	2400
18	1800	2000	2400
19–20	2000	2200	2400
21–25	2000	2200	2400

[1]Sedentary equals less than 30 minutes a day of moderate physical activity in addition to daily activities.
[2]Moderately active equals at least 30 minutes and up to 60 minutes a day of moderate physical activity in addition to daily activities.
[3]Active equals 60 or more minutes a day of moderate physical activity in addition to daily activities.

adequate explanation of study forms and procedures; alternative approaches and locations that appeal to young people are needed.

Food Intake Pattern Calorie Levels for Young People

Tables 10.2 and 10.3 identify the calorie levels required for males and females by age and activity level. Calorie levels are provided for ages 8–25.

Food Intake Patterns

Tables 10.4 and 10.5 identify the suggested amounts of food to consume from the basic food groups, subgroups, and oils to meet recommended nutrient intakes at 12 different calorie levels. Nutrient and energy contributions from each group are calculated according to the nutrient-dense forms of foods in each group (for example, lean meats and fat-free milk). Table 10.4 also shows the discretionary calorie allowance that can be accommodated within each calorie level, in addition to the suggested amounts of nutrient-dense forms of foods in each group.

Table 10.4. Daily Amount of Food from Each Group

Calorie Level[1]	1,000	1,200	1,400	1,600	1,800	2,000	2,200	2,400	2,600	2,800	3,000	3,200
Fruits[2]	1 cup	1 cup	1.5 cups	1.5 cups	1.5 cups	2 cups	2 cups	2 cups	2 cups	2.5 cups	2.5 cups	2.5 cups
Vegetables[3]	1 cup	1.5 cups	1.5 cups	2 cups	2.5 cups	2.5 cups	3 cups	3 cups	3.5 cups	3.5 cups	4 cups	4 cups
Grains[4]	3 oz-eq	4 oz-eq	5 oz-eq	5 oz-eq	6 oz-eq	6 oz-eq	7 oz-eq	8 oz-eq	9 oz-eq	10 oz-eq	10 oz-eq	10 oz-eq
Meat and Beans[5]	2 oz-eq	3 oz-eq	4 oz-eq	5 oz-eq	5 oz-eq	5.5 oz-eq	6 oz-eq	6.5 oz-eq	6.5 oz-eq	7 oz-eq	7 oz-eq	7 oz-eq
Milk[6]	2 cups	2 cups	2 cups	3 cups	3 cups	3 cups	3 cups	3 cups	3 cups	3 cups	3 cups	3 cups
Oils[7]	3 tsp	4 tsp	4 tsp	5 tsp	5 tsp	6 tsp	6 tsp	7 tsp	8 tsp	8 tsp	10 tsp	11 tsp
Discretionary calorie allowance[8]	165	171	171	132	195	267	290	362	410	426	512	648

Table 10.5. Vegetable Subgroup Amounts Per Week

Calorie Level	1,000	1,200	1,400	1,600	1,800	2,000	2,200	2,400	2,600	2,800	3,000	3,200
Dark green veg.	1 c/wk	1.5 c/wk	1.5 c/wk	2 c/wk	3 c/wk	3 c/wk	3 c/wk	3 c/wk	3 c/wk	3 c/wk	3 c/wk	3 c/wk
Orange veg.	.5 c/wk	1 c/wk	1 c/wk	1.5 c/wk	2 c/wk	2 c/wk	2 c/wk	2 c/wk	2.5 c/wk	2.5 c/wk	2.5 c/wk	2.5 c/wk
Legumes	.5 c/wk	1 c/wk	1 c/wk	2.5 c/wk	3 c/wk	3 c/wk	3 c/wk	3 c/wk	3.5 c/wk	3.5 c/wk	3.5 c/wk	3.5 c/wk
Starchy veg.	1.5 c/wk	2.5 c/wk	2.5 c/wk	2.5 c/wk	3 c/wk	3 c/wk	6 c/wk	6 c/wk	7 c/wk	7 c/wk	9 c/wk	9 c/wk
Other veg.	3.5 c/wk	4.5 c/wk	4.5 c/wk	5.5 c/wk	6.5 c/wk	6.5 c/wk	7 c/wk	7 c/wk	8.5 c/wk	8.5 c/wk	10 c/wk	10 c/wk

c/wk= cup/week

1. Calorie Levels are set across a wide range to accommodate the needs of different individuals.

2. Fruit Group includes all fresh, frozen, canned, and dried fruits and fruit juices. In general, 1 cup of fruit, 1 cup of 100% fruit juice, or 1/2 cup of dried fruit can be considered as 1 cup from the fruit group.

3. Vegetable Group includes all fresh, frozen, canned, and dried vegetables and vegetable juices. In general, 1 cup of raw or cooked vegetables or vegetable juice, or 2 cups of raw leafy greens can be considered as 1 cup from the vegetable group.

4. Grains Group includes all foods made from wheat, rice, oats, corn meal, barley, such as bread, pasta, oatmeal, breakfast cereals, tortillas, and grits. In general, 1 slice of bread, 1 cup of ready-to-eat cereal, or 1/2 cup of cooked rice, pasta, or cooked cereal can be considered as 1 ounce equivalent (oz-eq) from the grains group. At least half of all grains consumed should be whole grains.

5. Meat and Beans Group in general, 1 ounce of lean meat, poultry, or fish, 1 egg, 1 tablespoon peanut butter, 1/4 cup cooked dry beans, or 1/2 ounce of nuts or seeds can be considered as 1 ounce equivalent from the meat and beans group.

6. Milk Group includes all fluid milk products and foods made from milk that retain their calcium content, such as yogurt and cheese. Foods made from milk that have little to no calcium, such as cream cheese, cream, and butter, are not part of the group. Most milk group choices should be fat-free or low-fat. In general, 1 cup of milk or yogurt, 1.5 ounces of natural cheese, or 2 ounces of processed cheese can be considered as 1 cup from the milk group.

7. Oils include fats from many different plants and from fish that are liquid at room temperature, such as canola, corn, olive, soybean, and sunflower oil. Some foods are naturally high in oils, like nuts, olives, some fish, and avocados. Foods that are mainly oil include mayonnaise, certain salad dressings, and soft margarine.

8. Discretionary Calorie Allowance is the remaining amount of calories in a food intake pattern after accounting for the calories needed for all food groups—using forms of foods that are fat-free or low-fat and with no added sugars.

Chapter 11

Why Milk Matters for Teens

Tweens (Ages 9–12) and Teens Have Growing Needs for Milk

It takes calcium to build strong bones. And calcium is especially important during the tween and teen years, when bones are growing their fastest. Boys and girls in these age groups have calcium needs that they cannot make up for later in life. Tweens and teens can get most of their daily calcium from three cups of low-fat or fat-free milk (900 milligrams [mg] of calcium), but they also need additional servings of calcium-rich foods to get the 1,300 mg of calcium necessary to build strong bones for life.

Low-fat or fat-free milk is a great source of calcium because it also has other important nutrients that are good for bones and teeth. One especially important nutrient is vitamin D, which helps the body absorb more calcium.

Babies Are Not the Ones Who Need the Most Calcium

Starting around age nine, young people need almost twice as much calcium as younger children to help during the critical bone-building time between the ages of 11 and 15. Unfortunately, fewer than one in ten girls and only one in four boys ages 9 to 13 are at or above their adequate intake of calcium.

"Milk Matters: For Strong Bones, For Lifelong Health," National Institute of Child Health and Development (NICHD), NIH Publication No. 05–4521, September 2005.

Table 11.1. Daily Calcium Needs by Age

Age	Calcium Needs
Birth to 6 months	210 mg
6 to 12 months	270 mg
1 to 3 years	500 mg
4 to 8 years	800 mg
9 to 18 years	1,300 mg

Source: Dietary Reference Intakes for Calcium, National Academy of Sciences, 1997.

Building Strong Bones in the Tween and Teen Years Makes a Lifelong Difference

Having a calcium-rich diet when you are young makes a big difference in health, now and later. By getting the calcium they need now, tweens and teens will:

- **Strengthen bones now.** Our bodies continually remove and replace small amounts of calcium from our bones. If more calcium is removed than is replaced, bones will become weaker and have a greater chance of breaking. Some researchers suspect that the rise in forearm fractures in children is due to decreased bone mass, which may result because children are drinking less milk and more soda and are getting less physical activity.

- **Help prevent osteoporosis later in life.** Osteoporosis is a condition that makes bones weak so they break more easily. Although the effects of osteoporosis might not show up until adulthood, tweens and teens can help prevent it by building strong bones when they are young.

Weight-Bearing Physical Activity Also Builds Strong Bones

Bones are living tissue. Weight-bearing physical activity causes new bone tissue to form, which makes bones stronger. This kind of physical activity also makes muscles stronger. When muscles push and tug against bones during physical activity, bones and muscles become stronger.

Weight-bearing activities are those that keep you active and on your feet so that your legs carry your body weight. Activities such as walking, running, dancing, climbing stairs, and playing team sports like basketball, soccer, and volleyball help make bones stronger. Older teenagers can build even more bone strength through weight training, but they should check with a health care provider before starting any type of training.

Some activities, such as swimming, do not provide weight-bearing benefits. But they are good for cardiovascular fitness and overall good health.

Calcium Keeps Mouths Healthy

Calcium is important for a healthy mouth too. Even before they come in, baby teeth and adult teeth need calcium to develop fully. And after the teeth are in, calcium may also help protect them against decay. Calcium makes jawbones strong and healthy too.

Besides making sure your children get enough calcium, there are other things you can do to keep their teeth healthy:

- Make sure your children brush with a fluoride toothpaste. Fluoride protects teeth from decay and helps heal early decay.

- Ask your child's dental care or health care provider if there is fluoride in your town or city's drinking water. If there is not, ask about fluoride tablets or drops or prescription fluoride toothpaste for your child.

- Ask your child's dental care provider about proper brushing and flossing techniques and other ways your tween or teen can make sure teeth stay healthy.

Sources of Calcium

The foods listed in Tables 11.2 and 11.3 help tweens and teens reach the 1,300 mg of calcium they need every day.

There are lots of different calcium-rich foods to choose from, making it easy for tweens and teens to get the calcium they need every day. For example, just 1 cup of yogurt gives young people 25 percent of their daily calcium requirement. Low-fat and fat-free milk and milk products, such as low-fat or fat-free cheese and yogurt, are also excellent sources of calcium. Remember: Tweens and teens can get most of their daily calcium from 3 cups of low-fat or fat-free milk (900 mg of calcium), but they also need additional servings of calcium-rich foods to get the 1,300 mg of calcium necessary.

Food labels can tell you how much calcium is in one serving of food. Look at the % Daily Value (% DV) next to the calcium number on the food label.

Getting Enough Calcium when Teens Do Not Like Plain Milk

Even if your tweens or teens do not like the taste of plain milk, there are still plenty of ways to get calcium in their diet:

Table 11.2. Calcium-Rich Foods

Food	Serving Size	Calories	Amount of Calcium
Plain yogurt, fat-free	1 cup	127	452 mg
Orange juice with added calcium	8 fluid ounces (1 cup)	120	350 mg
Fruit yogurt, low-fat	1 cup	232	345 mg
Ricotta cheese, part skim	½ cup	170	334 mg
American cheese, low-fat and fat-free	2 ounces (about 3 slices)	Calories vary	312 mg
Milk (fat-free, low-fat, whole, or lactose-free)	8 fluid ounces (1 cup)	Calories vary	300 mg
Soybeans, cooked	1 cup	175	298 mg
Cheddar cheese, low-fat and fat-free	½ cup	Calories vary	204 mg
Tofu, firm, with added calcium sulfate	½ cup	97	204 mg
Soy beverage with added calcium	8 fluid ounces (1 cup)	100–130	200–300 mg
Cheese pizza	1 slice	240	200 mg

- Try a flavored low-fat or fat-free milk, such as chocolate, vanilla, or strawberry. Flavored milk has just as much calcium as plain.

- Serve foods that go with milk, such as fruit bars and fig bars.

- Drink milk or yogurt smoothies for breakfast or a snack. You can make these at home or try one of the ready-made versions now available at many grocery stores.

- Keep portable, calcium-rich foods on hand for snacks on the run, such as low-fat or fat-free string cheese or individual pudding cups with calcium added.

- In moderation, low-fat or fat-free ice cream and frozen yogurt are calcium-rich treats.

- Serve non-milk sources of calcium, such as calcium-fortified soy beverages or orange juice with added calcium.

- Try a spinach salad or have fresh or cooked broccoli.

Table 11.3. Other Foods with Calcium

Food	Serving Size	Calories	Amount of Calcium
Broccoli, raw	1 medium stalk	108	180 mg
Broccoli, cooked	1 cup	52	94 mg
Bok choy, boiled	1 cup	20	158 mg
Spinach, cooked from frozen	½ cup	27	139 mg
Frozen yogurt, soft serve vanilla	½ cup	114	103 mg
Macaroni and cheese	1 cup	230	100 mg
Almonds	1 ounce (22 nuts)	169	75 mg
Tortilla, flour (7–8 inches)	1 tortilla	150	58 mg
Tortilla, corn (6 inches)	1 tortilla	53	42 mg

Sources: USDA National Nutrient Database for Standard Reference, Release 17; Bowes and Church's Food Values of Portions Commonly Used, 2005. Some values have been rounded.

Choices in Milk Types

Today, tweens and teens have more milk choices than ever before. Most types of milk have approximately 300 mg of calcium per 8 fluid ounces (1 cup)—about 25 percent of the calcium that children and teenagers need every day. The best choices are low-fat or fat-free milk and milk products. Because these items contain little or no fat, it is easy to get enough calcium without adding extra fat to the diet. Children one to two years old should drink whole milk. After age two, low-fat or fat-free milk should become their regular drink.

Chocolate and other flavored milks have just as much calcium as plain milk, so it is fine for young people to drink these options if they prefer the taste. Remember to choose low-fat or fat-free which is best for tweens and teens.

Digestive Problems and Milk

Digestive problems may happen in some children (and adults) who have lactose intolerance. These people may have trouble digesting lactose, the natural sugar found in milk and milk products. Symptoms of lactose intolerance include stomach pain, diarrhea, bloating, and gas.

The best way for these people to get the health benefits of milk is to choose lactose-free milk and milk products. There are a variety of pills and drops, which are available without a prescription, that help people digest lactose.

In addition, most people who have problems digesting lactose can usually eat or drink:

- eight fluid ounces (1 cup) of low-fat or fat-free milk taken with meals
- low-fat or fat-free yogurt or cheese
- low-fat or fat-free milk poured on hot or cold cereal

People who have problems digesting lactose can also get some of their needed calcium from dark green vegetables, such as spinach, broccoli, and bok choy. Calcium supplements also provide an alternative way of getting calcium.

Foods with calcium added are also an option. Be sure to check the ingredient list for calcium in:

- tofu with added calcium sulfate
- orange juice with added calcium

- soy or rice beverages with added calcium
- calcium-fortified breakfast cereals or breads

Lactose intolerance is not common among children. However, if your children have problems with lactose, talk to their health care provider.

Lifelong Healthy Eating

The tween and teen years are an important time for young people to learn smart eating habits that will last a lifetime. Making low-fat or fat-free milk and other calcium-rich foods a part of the diet now teaches tweens and teens to make healthy choices. Also, learning to make healthy food choices at home will carry over into school and adulthood.

Put Calcium on the Menu at Every Meal

One way to make it easier for tweens and teens to get enough calcium is to serve low-fat or fat-free milk and other calcium-rich foods throughout the day. Putting calcium-rich foods on your family's menu at each meal is also a great way to make sure that everyone gets the calcium they need. When milk is the main beverage in the home, tweens and teens will choose it more often.

Ideas for Calcium-Rich Meals and Snacks

If you enjoy milk, chances are your children will, too. Tweens and teens look up to their parents and want to be like them. Young people make many food choices by watching their parents, so if you want your children to enjoy the bone-building benefits of at least three cups of low-fat or fat-free milk and milk products every day, show it. Drink milk yourself, and offer calcium-rich meals and snacks. This is the best way to show tweens and teens that milk matters.

Breakfast

- Pour low-fat or fat-free milk over your breakfast cereal.
- Have a cup of low-fat or fat-free yogurt.
- Drink a glass of orange juice with added calcium.
- Add low-fat or fat-free milk instead of water to oatmeal and hot cereal.

Lunch

- Add low-fat or fat-free cheese to a sandwich.
- Have a glass of low-fat or fat-free milk instead of soda.
- Have a pizza or macaroni and cheese.
- Add low-fat or fat-free milk instead of water to tomato soup.

Snack

- Make a smoothie with fruit, ice, and low-fat or fat-free milk.
- Try flavored low-fat or fat-free milk like chocolate or strawberry.
- Have a low-fat or fat-free frozen yogurt.
- Try some pudding made with low-fat or fat-free milk.
- Dip fruits and vegetables into low-fat or fat-free yogurt.
- Have some low-fat or fat-free string cheese.

Dinner

- Make a salad with dark green, leafy vegetables.
- Serve broccoli or cooked, dry beans as a side dish.
- Top salads, soups, and stews with low-fat or fat-free shredded cheese.
- Toss tofu with added calcium to stir fry and other dishes.

Source: American Dietetic Association's Complete Food and Nutrition Guide, 1996.

Additional Information

National Institute of Child Health and Human Development (NICHD)
Information Resource Center
P.O. Box 3006
Rockville, MD 20847
Toll-Free: 800-370-2943
Toll-Free TTY: 888-320-6942
Fax: 301-984-1473
Website: http://www.nichd.nih.gov/milk
E-mail: NICHDInformationResourceCenter@mail.nih.gov

Chapter 12

Food Marketing Influences Poor Nutrition in Teens

Food and beverage marketing targeted to children ages 12 and under leads them to request and consume high-calorie, low-nutrient products, says a new report from the Institute of Medicine of the National Academies. The report offers the most comprehensive review to date of the scientific evidence on the influence of food marketing on diets of children and youth.

Because dietary preferences and eating patterns form early in life and set the stage for an individual's long-term health prospects, significant changes are needed to reshape children's awareness of healthy dietary choices, the report says. Manufacturers and restaurants should direct more of their resources to developing and marketing child- and youth-oriented foods, drinks, and meals that are higher in nutrients and lower in calories, fat, salt, and added sugars.

Noting that many factors shape children's dietary habits and that leadership from both the public and the private sectors will be needed to redirect the nation's focus toward healthier products, the committee also called on the government to enhance nutritional standards, incentives, and public policies to promote the marketing of healthier foods and beverages. In addition, schools, parents, and the media should work with government and industry to pursue initiatives that support healthful diets for children and youth. If voluntary efforts by industry fail to successfully shift the emphasis of television advertising during children's programming away from high-calorie, low-nutrient products to healthier fare, Congress should enact legislation to mandate this change on both broadcast and cable television.

Concern has focused on food and beverage marketing practices because of the increase in new products targeted specifically to children and youth over the past decade and the media's increasing role in socializing young people. Companies spent an estimated $10 billion to market foods, beverages, and meals to U.S. children and youth in 2004, and four of the top ten items that children ages 8 to 12 say they can buy without parental permission are either foods or beverages.

"Current food and beverage marketing practices put kids' long-term health at risk," said committee chair J. Michael McGinnis, senior scholar, Institute of Medicine. "If America's children and youth are to develop eating habits that help them avoid early onset of diet-related chronic diseases, they have to reduce their intake of high-calorie, low-nutrient snacks, fast foods, and sweetened drinks, which make up a high proportion of the products marketed to kids. And this is an 'all hands on deck' issue. Parents have a central role in the turnaround required, but so do the food, beverage, and restaurant industries."

Findings about Marketing's Influence

The committee assessed hundreds of relevant studies and rigorously reviewed evidence from more than 120 of the best designed studies to determine what effects marketing may have on children's diets and health. Most of these studies focused only on television advertising, a shortcoming that should be addressed in future research, given that marketing strategies are rapidly evolving and now employ many tactics beyond television advertising, including Internet marketing, mobile phone ads, and product placements in video games and other media. For the most part, the committee did not have access to the substantial body of proprietary market research data held by marketing firms and food, beverage, and restaurant companies.

The committee found strong evidence that television advertising influences the food and beverage preferences and purchase requests of children ages two through eleven years old and affects their consumption habits, at least over the short-term. Most advertising geared toward children promotes high-calorie, low-nutrient foods, beverages, and meals, which, the committee concluded, influences children to request and choose these products. There is not enough evidence to determine the extent to which marketing influences the preferences and consumption habits of 12- to 18-year-olds; too few studies have focused on teens.

The evidence on whether television advertising directly affects children's long-term dietary patterns is limited and less conclusive. However, nutrition studies show that America's children and youth are consuming too many calories and too much added sugar, fat, and salt. Moreover, they are consuming less-than-recommended amounts of many key nutrients, including calcium, vitamin E, and fiber.

Available studies are too limited to determine whether television advertising is a direct cause of obesity among children. However, the statistical association between ad viewing and obesity is strong. Even a small influence would amount to a substantial impact when spread across the entire population, the report notes.

Recommendations to Promote Healthier Diets

Some companies and restaurants have recently taken steps to develop and promote healthier offerings, but overall the food, beverage, and restaurant industries spend the majority of their resources on products that contain high amounts of added sugar, fat, and salt, and that lack essential nutrients, the report says. These industries should shift their creativity and resources to develop a wider array of products that are nutritious, appealing, and affordable.

Food, beverage, and restaurant companies, as well as the entertainment and marketing industries, should expand, strengthen, and enforce their standards for marketing practices. For example, licensed characters, such as popular cartoon characters, should be used only to promote products that support healthful diets, the committee said. The industries should work with health officials and consumer groups to develop an industrywide rating system and labeling that conveys the nutritional quality of foods and beverages in a consistent and effective fashion. The Children's Advertising Review Unit—a group created and financed by the industry to monitor advertising directed toward children—should expand and apply its voluntary guidelines to newer forms of marketing, such as Internet and wireless phone advertising and product placement. The media and entertainment industries should incorporate story lines that promote healthful eating into programs, films, and games. The government should consider the use of awards and tax incentives that encourage companies to develop and promote healthier products for young people.

A long-term, multifaceted, national campaign should be initiated by the government in partnership with the private sector to educate families and children about making healthy food and beverage choices. This campaign should employ the full range of promotional and marketing tools and should be supported by both public funds and contributions from the food, beverage, and restaurant industries.

The committee called for governments and schools to develop and apply nutritional standards for all foods and beverages sold in schools that compete with federally reimbursed meals, including products sold in school stores and vending machines or for fundraising. School-based promotional efforts should focus on products that support healthful diets, the committee said.

The U.S. Department of Health and Human Services (HHS), in consultation with other federal agencies, should designate an agency to monitor the nation's progress in promoting more healthful diets. The HHS secretary should report to Congress within two years on the progress that has been made and additional actions that are needed.

Chapter 13

Adolescent Obesity

Chapter Contents

Section 13.1

Prevalence and Health Effects of Obesity in Youth

"Obesity in Youth," © 2005 American Obesity Association. Reprinted with permission.

Obesity in Youth

Note: Information for this section comes from various sources, some of which use different terminology for the 85th and 95th percentile of BMI. For consistency, the AOA refers to any use of the 85th percentile of BMI as overweight and the 95th percentile as obesity in children and adolescents. In general, childhood is defined as 6 to 11 years of age, and adolescence as 12 to 19 years of age.

Diabetes, hypertension, and other obesity-related chronic diseases that are prevalent among adults have now become more common in youngsters. The percentage of children and adolescents who are overweight and obese is now higher than ever before. Poor dietary habits and inactivity are reported to contribute to the increase of obesity in youth. Today's youth are considered the most inactive generation in history caused in part by reductions in school physical education programs and unavailable or unsafe community recreational facilities.

This section outlines many factors related to obesity in youth that make it the major health care challenge for the 21st century.

Overweight and Obesity Defined

- Overweight and obesity for children and adolescents are defined respectively in this section as being at or above the 85th and 95th percentile of Body Mass Index (BMI).

- Some researchers refer to the 95th percentile as overweight and other as obesity. The Centers for Disease Control and Prevention (CDC), which provides national statistical data for weight status of American youth, avoids using the word obesity, and identifies every child and adolescent above the 85th percentile as overweight.

- The American Obesity Association (AOA) uses the 95th percentile as criteria for obesity because it:

  - corresponds to a BMI of 30 which is obesity in adults. The 85th percentile corresponds to a BMI of 25 which is overweight in adults;

  - is recommended as a marker for when children and adolescents should have an in-depth medical assessment;

  - identifies children that are very likely to have obesity persist into adulthood;

  - is associated with elevated blood pressure and lipids in older adolescents, and increases their risk of diseases.

  - is a criteria for more aggressive treatment; and

  - is a criteria in clinical trials of childhood obesity treatments.

Prevalence and Trends

- Approximately 30.3 percent of children (ages 6 to 11) are overweight and 15.3 percent are obese. For adolescents (ages 12 to 19), 30.4 percent are overweight and 15.5 percent are obese.

- Excess weight in childhood and adolescence has been found to predict overweight in adults. Overweight children, aged 10 to 14, with at least one overweight or obese parent (BMI greater than 27.3 for women and greater than 27.8 for men in one study), were reported to have a 79 percent likelihood of overweight persisting into adulthood.

Gender

Overweight prevalence is higher in 6–11 year-old boys (32.7 percent) than girls (27.8 percent). In adolescents, overweight prevalence is about the same for females (30.2 percent) and males (30.5 percent). The prevalence of obesity quadrupled over the past 25 years among boys and girls, as shown in Table 13.1.

Obesity prevalence more than doubled over 25 years among adolescent males and females, as shown in Table 13.2.

Table 13.1. Increase in Obesity Prevalence (%) among U.S. Children (Ages 6 to 11)

Year	Boys	Girls
1999 to 2000	16	14.5
1988 to 1994	11.6	11
1971 to 1974	4.3	3.6

Source: CDC, National Center for Health Statistics, National Health and Nutrition Examination Survey. Ogden et. al. *JAMA.* 2002;288:1728–1732.

Table 13.2. Increase in Obesity Prevalence (%) among U.S. Adolescents (Ages 12 to 19)

Years	Males	Females
1999 to 2000	15.5	15.5
1988 to 1994	11.3	9.7
1971 to 1974	6.1	6.2

Source: CDC, National Center for Health Statistics, National Health and Nutrition Examination Survey. Ogden et. al. *JAMA.* 2002;288:1728–1732.

Race

African American, Hispanic American, and Native American children and adolescents have particularly high obesity prevalence. Overweight (85th percentile) and obesity (95th percentile) prevalence for children and adolescents is presented by racial group in Table 13.3.

- Among female youth, the highest overweight and obesity prevalence is found in black (non-Hispanic) girls (ages 6 to 11), 37.6 percent and 22.2 percent respectively, and black (non-Hispanic) adolescent females (ages 12 to 19), 45.5 percent and 26.6 percent respectively.

- Among male youth, the highest overweight and obesity prevalence is found in Mexican American boys (ages 6 to 11), 43 percent and 27.3 percent respectively, and Mexican American adolescent males (ages 12 to 19), 44.2 percent and 27.5 percent respectively.

- Overweight prevalence for Native American children and adolescents (ages 5 to 17) was reported in a 1999 study as 39 percent for males and 38 percent for females in the Aberdeen area Indian Health Service.

- Asian American adolescents (ages 13 to 18) were reported to have an overweight prevalence of 20.6 percent in the 1996 National Longitudinal Study of Adolescent Health.

- Asian American and Hispanic American adolescents born in the U.S. to immigrant parents are more than twice as likely to be overweight as foreign born adolescents who move to the U.S.

Table 13.3. Overweight and Obesity of Children and Adolescent by Race

Race	Children (Ages 6 to 11) Prevalence (%)		Adolescents (Ages 12 to 19) Prevalence (%)	
	Overweight	Obesity	Overweight	Obesity
Black (non-Hispanic)	35.9	19.5	40.4	23.6
Mexican American	39.3	23.7	43.8	23.4
White (non-Hispanic)	26.2	11.8	26.5	12.7

Source: CDC, National Center for Health Statistics, National Health and Nutrition Examination Survey. Ogden et. al. *JAMA*. 2002;288:1728–1732.

Health Effects

Many adverse health effects associated with overweight are observed in children and adolescents. Overweight during childhood and particularly adolescence is related to increased morbidity and mortality in later life.

Asthma

- Prevalence of overweight is reported to be significantly higher in children and adolescents with moderate to severe asthma compared to a peer group.

Diabetes (Type 2)

- Type 2 diabetes in children and adolescents has increased dramatically in a short period. The parallel increase of obesity in children and adolescents is reported to be the most significant factor for the rise in diabetes.

- Type 2 diabetes accounted for 2 to 4 percent of all childhood diabetes before 1992, but skyrocketed to 16 percent by 1994.

- Obese children and adolescents are reported to be 12.6 times more likely to have high fasting blood insulin levels, a risk factor for type 2 diabetes.

- Type 2 diabetes is predominant among African American and Hispanic youngsters, with a particularly high rate among those of Mexican descent.

Hypertension

- Persistently elevated blood pressure levels have been found to occur about 9 times more frequently among obese children and adolescents (ages 5 to 18).

- Obese children and adolescents are reported to be 2.4 times more likely to have high diastolic blood pressure and 4.5 times more likely to have high systolic blood pressure than their peers.

Orthopedic Complications

- Among growing youth, bone and cartilage in the process of development are not strong enough to bear excess weight. As a result, a variety of orthopedic complications occur in children and adolescents with obesity. In young children, excess weight can lead to bowing and overgrowth of leg bones.

- Increased weight on the growth plate of the hip can cause pain and limit range of motion. Between 30 to 50 percent of children with this condition are overweight.

Psychosocial Effects and Stigma

- Overweight children are often taller than other children.

- White girls, who develop a negative body image, are at a greater risk for the subsequent development of eating disorders.

- Adolescent females who are overweight have reported experiences with stigmatization such as direct and intentional weight-related teasing, jokes, and derogatory name calling, as well as less intentional, potentially hurtful comments by peers, family members, employers, and strangers.

- Overweight children and adolescents report negative assumptions made about them by others, including being inactive or lazy, being strong and tougher than others, not having feelings, and being unclean.

Sleep Apnea

- Sleep apnea, the absence of breathing during sleep, occurs in about 7 percent of children with obesity. Deficits in logical thinking are common in children with obesity and sleep apnea.

Section 13.2

Obesity Risk Assessment

"Aim for a Healthy Weight: Assess Your Risk," National Heart, Lung, and Blood Institute (NHLBI), December 2004.

Assessing Your Risk

According to the National Heart, Lung, and Blood Institute (NHLBI) guidelines, assessment of overweight involves using three key measures:

- body mass index (BMI),
- waist circumference, and
- risk factors for diseases and conditions associated with obesity.

The BMI is a measure of body weight relative to a person's height, and waist circumference measures abdominal fat. Combining these with information about additional risk factors yields an individual's risk for developing obesity-associated diseases.

What Is Your Risk?

Body Mass Index (BMI)

BMI is a reliable indicator of total body fat, which is related to the risk of disease and death. The score is valid for both men and women but it does have some limits. The limits are:

- It may overestimate body fat in athletes and others who have a muscular build.

- It may underestimate body fat in older persons and others who have lost muscle mass.

Use the BMI table to estimate total body fat. To use the table, find the appropriate height in the left-hand column labeled Height. Move across to a given weight (in pounds). The number at the top of the column is the BMI at that height and weight. Pounds have been rounded off.

Table 13.4. Body Mass Index Table

BMI	19	20	21	22	23	24	25	26	27	28	29	30	31	32	33	34	35
Height (inches)								Body Weight (pounds)									
58	91	96	100	105	110	115	119	124	129	134	138	143	148	153	158	162	167
59	94	99	104	109	114	119	124	128	133	138	143	148	153	158	163	168	173
60	97	102	107	112	118	123	128	133	138	143	148	153	158	163	168	174	179
61	100	106	111	116	122	127	132	137	143	148	153	158	164	169	174	180	185
62	104	109	115	120	126	131	136	142	147	153	158	164	169	175	180	186	191
63	107	113	118	124	130	135	141	146	152	158	163	169	175	180	186	191	197
64	110	116	122	128	134	140	145	151	157	163	169	174	180	186	192	197	204
65	114	120	126	132	138	144	150	156	162	168	174	180	186	192	198	204	210
66	118	124	130	136	142	148	155	161	167	173	179	186	192	198	204	210	216
67	121	127	134	140	146	153	159	166	172	178	185	191	198	204	211	217	223
68	125	131	138	144	151	158	164	171	177	184	190	197	203	210	216	223	230
69	128	135	142	149	155	162	169	176	182	189	196	203	209	216	223	230	236
70	132	139	146	153	160	167	174	180	188	195	203	209	216	222	229	236	243
71	136	143	150	157	165	172	179	186	193	200	208	215	222	229	236	243	250
72	140	147	153	162	169	177	184	191	199	206	213	221	228	235	242	250	258
73	144	151	159	166	174	182	189	197	204	212	219	227	235	242	250	257	265
74	148	155	163	171	179	186	194	202	210	218	225	233	241	249	256	264	272
75	152	160	168	176	184	192	200	208	216	224	232	240	248	256	264	272	279
76	156	164	172	180	189	197	205	213	221	230	238	246	254	263	271	279	287

The BMI score means the following:

- Underweight   BMI below 18.5
- Normal   BMI 18.5–24.9
- Overweight   BMI 25.0–29.9
- Obesity   BMI 30.0 and above

Waist Circumference

Determine your waist circumference by placing a measuring tape snugly around your waist. It is a good indicator of your abdominal fat which is another predictor of your risk for developing risk factors for heart disease and other diseases. This risk increases with a waist measurement of over 40 inches in men and over 35 inches in women.

Table 13.5 provides you with an idea of whether your BMI combined with your waist circumference increases your risk for developing obesity associated diseases or conditions.

Table 13.5. Overweight and Obesity Classification by BMI, Waist Circumference, and Associated Disease Risks

Classification	BMI (kg/m²)	Obesity Class	Men 102 cm (40 in) or less Women 88 cm (35 in) or less	Men greater than 102 cm (40 in) Women greater than 88 cm (35 in)
Underweight	less than 18.5			
Normal	18.5–24.9			
Overweight	25.0–29.9		Increased	High
Obesity	30.0–34.9	I	High	Very High
	35.0–39.9	II	Very High	Very High
Extreme Obesity	40.0 and over	III	Extremely High	Extremely High

*Disease risk for type 2 diabetes, hypertension, and cardiovascular disease (CVD).
Note: Increased waist circumference can also be a marker for increased risk even in persons of normal weight.

Other Risk Factors

Besides being overweight or obese, there are additional risk factors to consider including:

- high blood pressure (hypertension)

- high low density lipoprotein (LDL) cholesterol (bad cholesterol)
- low high density lipoprotein (HDL) cholesterol (good cholesterol)
- high triglycerides
- high blood glucose (sugar)
- family history of premature heart disease
- physical inactivity
- cigarette smoking

Assessment

For people who are considered obese (BMI greater than or equal to 30) or those who are overweight (BMI of 25 to 29.9) and have two or more risk factors, the guidelines recommend weight loss. Even a small weight loss (just 10 percent of your current weight) will help to lower your risk of developing diseases associated with obesity. Patients who are overweight, but do not have a high waist measurement, and have less than two risk factors may need to prevent further weight gain rather than lose weight.

Talk to your doctor to see if you are at an increased risk and if you should lose weight. Your doctor will evaluate your BMI, waist measurement, and others risk factors for heart disease. People who are overweight or obese have a greater chance of developing high blood pressure, high blood cholesterol or other lipid disorders, type 2 diabetes, heart disease, stroke, and certain cancers, and even a small weight loss (just 10 percent of your current weight) will help to lower your risk of developing those diseases.

Section 13.3

Teens, Fast Food, and Obesity

"Science in the News: New Study on Teens and Fast Food," *FDA and You*, Issue #5, Winter 2005, U.S. Food and Drug Administration (FDA).

Teens that frequently eat fast food gain more weight and have a greater increase of insulin resistance in early middle age, according to a large study funded by the National Heart, Lung, and Blood Institute (NHLBI).

After 15 years, those who ate fast food more than twice each week, compared to less than once a week, had gained an extra ten pounds and had a greater increase of insulin resistance, a risk factor for type 2 diabetes. Diabetes is a major risk factor for heart disease.

"Obesity and diabetes are on the rise in this country and this important study highlights the value of healthy eating habits," NHLBI Acting Director Barbara Alving, M.D. said. Fast food consumption has increased in the U.S. over the past three decades. "It's extremely difficult to eat in a healthy way at a fast food restaurant. Despite some of their recent healthful offerings, the menus still tend to include foods high in fat, sugar, and calories, and low in fiber and nutrients," said lead author Mark Pereira, Ph.D., assistant professor of epidemiology at the University of Minnesota. One reason for the weight gain may be that a single meal of fast food often contains enough calories to satisfy a person's caloric requirement for an entire day.

Participants were asked during the physical examinations given as part of the study how often they ate breakfast, lunch, or dinner at fast food restaurants. Researchers found that the adverse impact on participants' weight and insulin resistance was seen in both blacks and whites who often ate fast food, even after adjustment for other lifestyle habits. Study participants included 3,031 young black and white adults who were between the ages of 18 and 30 in 1985–1986. The participants, who were part of the Coronary Artery Risk Development in Young Adults (CARDIA) study, received dietary assessments over a 15-year period.

"It is important to watch carefully what you eat, especially at a fast food restaurant. Knowing the nutritional content is important. Consumers may want to ask for this information," NHLBI's Gina Wei, M.D., project officer for CARDIA said. Keep portion sizes small, and ask that high-fat sauces and condiments, such as salad dressing and mayonnaise, be on the side and use them sparingly to reduce calories, Wei said.

Section 13.4

Preventing Obesity and Chronic Diseases

This section includes excerpts from "Preventing Obesity and Chronic Diseases through Good Nutrition and Physical Activity," Centers for Disease Control and Prevention (CDC), November 2005. Also, excerpts from "Take Charge of Your Health," National Institute of Diabetes and Digestive and Kidney Diseases (NIDDK), December 2001; reviewed in April 2006 by Dr. David A. Cooke, M.D., Diplomate, American Board of Internal Medicine.

Chronic Disease Prevention

* More than a third of young people in grades 9–12 do not regularly engage in vigorous physical activity.

* Unhealthy diet and physical inactivity can cause or aggravate many chronic diseases and conditions, including type 2 diabetes, hypertension, heart disease, stroke, and some cancers.

The Cost of Obesity and Chronic Diseases

* Among children and adolescents, annual hospital costs related to obesity were $127 million during 1997–1999 (in 2001 constant U.S. dollars), up from $35 million during 1979–1981.

- In 2000, the total cost of obesity in the United States was estimated to be $117 billion. About $61 billion was for direct medical costs, and $56 billion was for indirect costs.

- In 1996, $31 billion of treatment costs (in year 2000 dollars) for cardiovascular disease among adults was related to overweight and obesity.

How Physical Activity and Weight Loss Save Money

- In 2000, health care costs associated with physical inactivity topped $76 billion.

- If 10% of adults began a regular walking program, $5.6 billion in heart disease costs could be saved.

- A sustained 10% weight loss will reduce an overweight person's lifetime medical costs by $2,200–$5,300 by lowering costs associated with hypertension, type 2 diabetes, heart disease, stroke, and high cholesterol.

Teenagers: Take Charge of Your Health

As a teenager, you are going through a lot of changes. Your body is changing and growing. Have you noticed that every year, you can't seem to fit into your old shoes anymore? Or that your favorite jeans are now tighter or three inches too short? Your body is on its way to becoming its adult size.

Along with your physical changes, you are also becoming more independent. You are starting to make more choices about your life. You are relying less on your parents and more on yourself and your friends when making decisions. Some of the biggest choices that you face are those about your health.

Why should you care about your health? Well, there are lots of reasons—like feeling good, looking good, and getting stronger. Doing well in school, work, or other activities (like sports) is another reason. Believe it or not, these can all be affected by your health.

Healthy eating and being active now may also help prevent diabetes, high blood pressure, heart disease, osteoporosis, stroke, and some forms of cancer when you are older. Some teenagers are not very physically active and some do not get the foods that their growing bodies need.

Now is the time to take charge of your health by eating better and being more physically active. Even small changes will help you look and feel your best.

Where Do I Start?

The road to better health starts with good eating and physical activity habits. Being aware of your habits will help you learn where you need to make changes.

Do you normally watch a lot of television or play a lot of video games? These activities can be relaxing, but you don't need to move much to do them. Spending too much time not moving around can make you feel tired and lazy and lead to poor muscle tone. You can be active every day and still have time to do other things you enjoy, like playing video games.

Physical Activity—It Doesn't Have to Be a Chore

Being active means moving more every day. You can choose activities that are fun and do them on your own or with your friends. Being more active will make you feel better and give you more energy. It can also help you think and concentrate better, which will help you in school or at work. Activity can help you feel less bored and depressed, and help you handle stress.

So don't wait—start today. Begin slowly and make small changes in your daily routine, like spending less time in front of the television, taking the stairs instead of the elevator, walking to school instead of taking the bus (or if you drive, parking further away on the school parking lot).

What you choose to do is up to you. Just pick something that you like to do and keep it up. Have fun while being active each day to stay healthy and fit. Remember, you don't have to give up the video games—just make sure that you also fit activity into your day.

You Are What You Eat

Take a look at your eating habits. What you eat, where you eat, and why you eat are important to your health. As a teen, you need to eat a variety of foods that give you the nutrients your growing body needs. Eating better and being more active can make you feel better and think more clearly.

The best reason to eat is because your body tells you that you are hungry. If you are eating when you are not hungry, try doing something else to get food off of your mind. Call a friend, exercise, read, or work on a craft. These activities can help you to cut back on eating when you are feeling bored, upset, or stressed.

Additional Information

Weight-Control Information Network (WIN)
1 WIN Way
Bethesda, MD 20892-3665
Toll-Free: 877-946-4627
Fax: 202-828-1028
Website: http://win.niddk.nih.gov
E-mail: win@info.niddk.nih.gov

American Obesity Association
1250 24th St. NW, Suite 300
Washington DC 20037
Phone: 202-776-7711
Fax: 202-776-7712
Website: http://www.obesity.org

Chapter 14

Diet Plans:
Is Yours Healthy and Safe?

Want to drop a few pounds before that big date on Friday? Feeling the need to lose weight to boost your athletic performance? Many people look for fast or easy ways to slim down at some point in their lives. And there are hundreds of diet plans out there to lure you. But before you choose between the all-juice diet and the no-carb diet, read on to find out exactly what these diets do—and don't do—for you.

What are popular weight-loss plans and how well do they work?

Commercial weight-loss plans typically fall into two categories: Those that drastically reduce a person's calorie intake or restrict the dieter to certain foods, and those that require a person to take dietary supplements. Dietary supplements are usually pills, but they sometimes include special food bars or drinks.

Most of the popular diets on the market today rely on a person's natural tendency to want to lose weight quickly. They play into a desire for fast results, which is what happened to Jamie, 16, who followed a 5-day juice diet. Although Jamie lost the weight she wanted, a week later the scale showed she was back to her original weight.

This information was provided by KidsHealth, one of the largest resources online for medically reviewed health information written for parents, kids, and teens. For more articles like this one, visit www.TeensHealth.org, or www.KidsHealth.org. © 2004 The Nemours Center for Children's Health Media, a division of The Nemours Foundation.

It's quite common for people to quickly gain back all the weight they lose after a few days on a highly restrictive diet. Here's a doctor's answer on why: "The first thing to be aware of with quick weight-loss diets is that our bodies simply aren't designed to drop pounds quickly," says Steven Dowshen, M.D., an expert in hormones and the endocrine system. In fact, doctors say that it's nearly impossible for a healthy, normally active teen or adult to lose more than about three pounds per week of actual fat from their bodies, even on a starvation diet.

So why does your scale tell you otherwise? "The trick these very low-calorie diets rely on is that your body's natural reaction to near-starvation is to dump water," Dr. Dowshen says. That means that most, if not all, of the weight you lose during the first few days on these diets is water, not fat. You may feel thinner, but you won't look it and you'll probably bounce back up to your original weight once you start eating normally again. "What these diet plans don't tell you is that your body will just suck this lost water back up like a sponge once you start eating more calories again," Dr. Dowshen says.

Losing water weight is also the key to the quick weight-loss claims of some of the diet pills on the market. Many of these pills contain laxatives or diuretics—ingredients that force a person's body to eliminate more water. Other diet pills rely on ingredients that claim to speed up a person's metabolism (the process by which the body turns food into energy and stores unused calories as fat); suppress appetite; or block the absorption of fat, sugars, or carbohydrates.

Do these types of supplements actually do what they say they will? Unfortunately, there's usually no reliable scientific research to back up the claims provided by the product's manufacturer. In addition, there are many unknowns about the substances used in diet supplements, so dietitians and doctors consider them risky. What research studies do show is that most of the people who try one of these "crash" diets regain all the weight they lost within a few weeks or months.

Do these diets put your health at risk?

Luckily, very few people stick to a highly restrictive diet for long periods of time and most people give up on them after a few days. But what happens if you keep following extremely low-calorie diets or taking weight-loss supplements? That's when things can get a little scary.

Radically cutting back on calories can make you tired, jittery, and moody. These symptoms usually go away when you resume healthy eating habits, but over the long term, a highly restrictive diet may cause other health problems. You may lose some of your hair, your fingernails may become brittle, dark circles may appear under your eyes, and your muscles may shrink and weaken. Sometimes staying on a highly restrictive diet for a long period of time can cause lasting damage to your body, especially to the heart and kidneys. Following extreme diets over the long term or a pattern of extreme dieting followed by binge eating are both signs that a person may have an eating disorder.

Drastically reducing your food intake depletes the body's access to the vitamins, minerals, and fiber that it needs to stay healthy. If a diet requires you to cut out all dairy products, for example, you are also losing valuable calcium. Over a prolonged period, a lack of calcium puts a person at increased risk for osteoporosis (pronounced: ahstee-oh-puh-ro-sis), a condition in which bones become brittle and more susceptible to injury as a person ages. Some diets—like those that omit all red meat—may leave the dieter lacking iron, which can lead to anemia, especially in teen girls. And trying to replace the foods you're cutting out with vitamin pills is a bad idea. Foods like fruits and vegetables contain more than just vitamins and minerals—they are some of the best sources of fiber. Fiber can help to prevent disease.

Restricting food intake over a long period during a person's teenage years can stunt growth. Following restrictive diets over a long period can also delay some of the changes associated with puberty, such as breast development in females and muscle bulk in males. Another side effect of restrictive diets in teenage girls is irregular menstrual periods—or even not getting a period at all.

Another effect of very low-calorie diets is a decrease in resting energy expenditure, or the amount of calories a person burns at rest. One reason for this "slower metabolism" is that people on restrictive diets often lose muscle mass, and muscle burns more calories than fat—even while a person is resting. This makes continuing to lose weight even more difficult and regaining weight easier.

What about the long-term effects of taking diet pills? Common ingredients in diet pills include caffeine, alcohol, 5-hydroxytryptophan (5-HTP), chromium (or chromium picolinate), phentermine, and vanadium. These ingredients may carry health risks for certain people. Ephedrine (also known as ephedra or ma huang), an ingredient in many diet and sports supplements during the late 1990s and early 2000s, was linked to heart problems and may have played a role in the death of at least one professional athlete. The U.S. Food and Drug Administration decided the health risks associated with ephedra were too great, and it banned the substance in December 2003.

If you have any health conditions or are taking medication, always check with your doctor before taking weight-loss supplements because the ingredients in some supplements may interact with specific drugs. For example, 5-HTP may cause adverse reactions in people who take certain medications for depression. Even ingredients that seem like a normal part of your diet can carry risks when used in weight-loss pills or other stimulants: For example, the average caffeine-based weight-loss pill contains as much caffeine as six cups of coffee. Imagine how wired you'd be if you took two or three of these pills each day. The side effects associated with these products include rapid heart rate, increased blood pressure, dizziness, sleeplessness, seizures, and even addiction.

Furthermore, it's important to know that most diet supplements have not been tested on teen users. Not only does this mean that the dosages prescribed may not be accurate, it could mean that taking certain supplements might carry unknown risks for teens.

How can you lose weight for the long term?

Regardless of concerns about the effectiveness and safety of restrictive diets, keeping the pounds off long term should be the major goal for anyone who wants to lose weight—and that can be more challenging than losing them in the first place. Weight loss is most likely to be successful and lasting when a person changes his or her habits to reduce the overall number of calories he or she eats while at the same time increasing the number of calories burned through exercise. Exercise not only burns calories, it also builds muscle. The more muscle you have, the more efficient your body becomes at burning calories, even when you aren't exercising. You don't have to become a gym rat, though: Walking the family dog, cycling to school, and doing other things that increase your daily level of activity can all make a difference. Research confirms that one reason people get less exercise these days is because of an increase in screen time—in other words, the amount of time spent watching television, looking at the computer, or playing video games. The American Academy of Pediatrics recommends limiting all screen time to one hour per day. If you're hanging with your friends at the mall instead of chatting to them on the computer, for example, you're getting more exercise.

A survey on health and nutrition conducted by the Centers for Disease Control and Prevention shows that serving sizes for both kids and adults have increased over the past ten years, and that this is a contributor to obesity. If you super-size your fries or always go for extra hot fudge on your sundae, you are probably taking in more calories than your body can use. Another key dietary factor in weight gain today is the increased consumption of flavored beverages, such as sodas, sweetened juice drinks, and sports drinks. Some people keep a food diary to track what they eat and drink. Writing everything you eat in a daily diary might help you identify those hidden foods that contribute to unwanted weight gain—like the candy bar you usually munch between third and fourth period.

The best way to build a weight-loss program that's right for you is to talk to your doctor or a registered dietitian. During your appointment, your doctor or dietitian may ask you what types of foods you eat, how much weight you want to lose, and the reasons why you want to lose weight. He or she will also help you figure out approximately where your weight should be based on your height and other factors and suggest a sound weight-loss plan that meets your individual needs. (Dietitians report that most guys and girls find weight-loss plans that take their daily schedule and food preferences into account are easier to follow.) The eating plan must include enough calories per day to keep your body working and developing properly. And if you're cutting calories to lose weight, your body will still need to get the same amount of nutrients to stay healthy.

Staying active is an important part of keeping off the weight you've lost. If you achieved your weight-loss goal by eating a variety of foods in smaller portions and exercising regularly, chances are better that you will stick with a healthier lifestyle and keep the pounds off in the long run. There's a lot of hype out there when it comes to dieting. "Trendy new diets sell books and magazines, so of course you're going to see a lot about the 'hot' new diet of the moment," says Neil Izenberg, M.D., an expert in adolescent medicine and the media. However, "the tried and true approach—cutting back on calories and increasing your level of exercise—is still the best way to lose weight and keep it off," Dr. Izenberg says.

Chapter 15

Physical Activity and Adolescent Health

Chapter Contents

Section 15.1

Fitness and Your 13–18 Year-Old

This section includes: "Children's Need for Physical Activity: Fact Sheet," reproduced with permission from www.americanheart.org. © 2004, American Heart Association. And, "Fitness and Your 13- to 18-Year-Old," this information was provided by KidsHealth, one of the largest resources online for medically reviewed health information written for parents, kids, and teens. For more articles like this one, visit www.kidsHealth.org, or www.TeensHealth.org. © 2005 The Nemours Center for Children's Health Media, a division of The Nemours Foundation. Also, excerpts from "Physical Activity and the Health of Young People," Centers for Disease Control and Prevention (CDC), July 2005.

Children's Need for Physical Activity

- Children in the United States today are less fit than they were a generation ago. Many are showing early signs of cardiovascular risk factors such as physical inactivity, excess weight, higher blood cholesterol and cigarette smoking.

- Inactive children, when compared with active children, weigh more, have higher blood pressure and lower levels of heart-protective high density lipoproteins (HDL cholesterol).

- Even though heart attack and stroke are rare in children, evidence shows that the process leading to those conditions begins in childhood.

- The *2003 Youth Risk Factor Surveillance Study* indicates that 33.4 percent of youth don't engage in physical activity that promotes long-term health.

- A fitness testing program sponsored by the Chrysler Fund Amateur Athletic Union, which tracks fitness among 9.7 million people between ages 6–17, shows that children are getting slower in endurance running and weaker.

- The National Health and Nutrition Examination Study (NHANES, 1999–2002) found that the prevalence of overweight

American adolescents ages 12–19 was 16.7 percent for males and 15.4 percent for females. There was an increase of 250 percent from 1970 to 2002.

- About 16 percent of adolescents ages 12–19 have total cholesterol levels exceeding 200 mg/dL.

- An estimated 22 percent of American children under age 18 are exposed to secondhand smoke in the home. An estimated 2,000 American young people become smokers every day.

- Children spend an average of three to four hours a day watching television.

- Inactive children are more likely to become inactive adults.

- Healthy lifestyle training should start in childhood to promote improved cardiovascular health in adult life. The following good health practices should be promoted among children:

  - regular physical activity

  - a low saturated fat, low cholesterol diet after age two

  - smoking prevention

  - appropriate weight for height

  - regular pediatric medical checkups

Fitness and Your 13- to 18-Year-Old

Kids who enjoy sports and exercise tend to stay active throughout their lives. The revised food guide pyramid emphasizes physical activity by showing a stick figure climbing steps to the top of the pyramid. The *2005 Dietary Guidelines* recommend that teens get at least one hour of physical activity on most, and preferably all days of the week.

Regular physical activity can help prevent heart disease, diabetes, and other medical problems down the road. But don't underestimate the immediate benefits of an active lifestyle: maintaining a healthy weight, feeling more energetic, and promoting a better outlook. Participating in team and individual sports can boost self-confidence, provide opportunities for social interaction, and offer a chance to have fun. Such benefits are not limited to competitive sports; noncompetitive activities can also help teens achieve these goals.

Fitness in the Teen Years

Physical activity tends to decline during the teen years. Many teens are dropping out of organized sports and participation in daily physical education classes is becoming a thing of the past.

But given the opportunity and interest, teens can pick up on almost any activity that they enjoy, from competitive to noncompetitive sports from exercise classes to playing with friends. Skateboarding, in-line skating, yoga, swimming, dancing, or kicking a footbag in the driveway all qualify as great fitness activities. Weight training, under supervision of a qualified adult, can improve strength and help prevent sports injuries. The possibilities to get physically fit are endless.

Teens can also incorporate activity into their everyday routine, such as walking to school, doing chores, or finding an active part-time job. Even younger teens can enjoy opportunities to take on new responsibilities and be in charge, so jobs as junior camp counselors, baby sitters, or assistant coaches for young sports teams can serve that need while also providing the child with a chance to be active.

Motivating Teens to Be Active

Teens face many new social and academic pressures in addition to dealing with emotional and physical changes. Recent studies have shown that teens on average are spending more than six hours a day on various media, including watching television, listening to music, going online, and playing video games. It is not surprising that teens cannot seem to find the time to exercise and many parents find it difficult to motivate their teens to get active.

It is a good idea to give your child control over how he or she decides to be physically active. Since teens are defining themselves as individuals and want the power to make their own decisions, they are reluctant to do yet another thing they are told to do. Emphasize that it's not what they do; they just need to physically active on a regular basis. There are plenty of options for physical activity, but to keep them motivated it has to be fun. Support your child's choices by providing equipment, transportation, and companionship. Peers can play an influential role in your child's life at this point, so create opportunities for them to be active with their friends. Once they get started, many teens enjoy the feeling of well-being, reduced stress, and increased strength and energy they get from exercise, so they often gravitate to exercise without nudging from a parent.

Help your teen stay active by finding an exercise regimen that fits with his or her schedule. Your teen may not have time to play a team sport at school or in a local league, but many gyms offer teen memberships, and your teen may be able to squeeze in a visit before or after school. Your teen might also feel more comfortable doing home exercise videos. If transportation is an obstacle, try coordinating your teen's exercise schedule with your own. And do not forget to talk with your teen about limiting the time he or she spends in sedentary activities, including watching television and using the computer.

When to Speak with Your Teen's Doctor about Fitness

If you are concerned about your teen's fitness, speak with your teen's doctor. Teens who are overweight or very sedentary may need to start slowly and your teen's doctor may be able to recommend programs or help you devise a fitness plan.

A teen with a chronic health condition or disability should not be excluded from fitness activities. Some activities may need to be modified or adapted, and some may be too risky depending on your child's condition. Consult your teen's doctor about which activities are safe.

On the other hand, some teens may overdo it when it comes to fitness. Young athletes, particularly those involved in gymnastics, wrestling, or dance, may face pressures to lose weight. If your teen refuses to eat certain food groups (such as fats), becomes overly concerned with body image, appears to be exercising compulsively, or experiences a sudden change in weight, seek help from your child's doctor.

Another dangerous issue that can arise is the use of steroids particularly in sports where size and strength are valued. Talk with your child's doctor if you suspect your child is using steroids or other performance-enhancing substances.

Finally, if your child complains of pain during sports and exercise, speak with your child's doctor.

Fitness for Everyone

Everyone can benefit from being physically fit. Staying fit can help improve your child's self-esteem and decrease the risk of serious illnesses (such as heart disease and stroke) later in life. In addition, regular physical activity can help your teen learn to meet physical and emotional challenges he or she faces every day.

Part of helping your teen commit to fitness may include becoming a positive role model by regularly exercising on your own and with your child. Try to spend time being active together. Take bike rides, hit a tennis ball around, go to a local swimming pool, or even play games like capture the flag and touch football together. Not only are you working together to reach your fitness goals, it's a great opportunity to stay connected with your teen.

Physical Activity and the Health of Young People

Regular physical activity has many benefits including:

* building and maintaining healthy bones and muscles

* reducing the risk of developing obesity and chronic diseases such as diabetes and cardiovascular disease

* reducing feelings of depression and anxiety and promotes psychological well-being

Long-term consequences of physical inactivity include:

* overweight and obesity, influenced by poor diet and inactivity, which are significantly associated with an increased risk of diabetes, high blood pressure, high cholesterol, asthma, arthritis, and poor health status

* increased risk of dying prematurely, dying of heart disease, and developing diabetes, colon cancer, and high blood pressure

Overweight among Youth

* The prevalence of overweight among children aged 6–11 has more than doubled in the past 20 years, increasing from 7% in 1980 to 16% in 2002.

* Children and adolescents who are overweight are more likely to be overweight or obese as adults; overweight adults are at increased risk for heart disease, high blood pressure, stroke, diabetes, some types of cancer, and gallbladder disease.

Participation in Physical Activity by Young People

* Seventy-seven percent of children aged 9–13 report participating in free-time physical activity, and 39% reported participating in organized physical activity.

* Sixty-three percent of high school students participate in sufficient vigorous physical activity, and 25% participate in sufficient moderate physical activity.

116

- Participation in physical activity declines as children get older.
- Sixty-seven percent of high school students met the national recommendations for both vigorous and moderate physical activity in 2003.

Table 15.1. Percentage of High School Students Participating in Different Types of Physical Activity, by Sex, 2003[9]

Type of Activity	Girls	Boys
Sufficient vigorous physical activity[a]	55%	70%
Sufficient moderate physical activity[b]	22%	27%
Sufficient strengthening exercises[c]	43%	60%
Played on a sports team[d]	51%	64%

[a] Physical activities that caused sweating and hard breathing, that were performed for 20 minutes or more on at least three of the seven days preceding the survey.
[b] Physical activities that did not cause sweating or hard breathing, that were performed for 30 minutes or more on at least five of the seven days preceding the survey.
[c] For example, push-ups, sit-ups, or weightlifting on at least three of the seven days preceding the survey to strengthen or tone their muscles.
[d] Run by their school or community groups during the twelve months preceding the survey.

Participation in Physical Education Classes

- Over half (56%) of U.S. high school students (71% of 9th graders but only 40% of 12th graders) were enrolled in a physical education class in 2003.

- The percentage of high school students who attended physical education classes daily decreased from 42% in 1991 to 25% in 1995, and has remained stable at that level until 2003 (28%). In 2003, 38% of 9th graders but only 18% of 12th graders attended a daily physical education class.

- Among the 56% of students who are enrolled in a physical education class, 80% exercised or played sports for 20 minutes or more during an average class.

Section 15.2

Tips to Reduce Teens' "Screen Time"

This section includes: "Limiting Screen Time—More Energy Out," and "Helpful Ways to Reduce Screen Time," National Heart, Lung, and Blood Institute (NHLBI), 2005.

Limiting Screen Time—More Energy Out

One of the biggest challenges to being more physically active for many Americans is the amount of sedentary time children and families spend in front of screens—television, computer, video games, DVDs, movies and such.

Did You Know?

According to the Henry J. Kaiser Foundation's survey, "Generation M: Media in the Lives of 8–18 Year Olds," March 2005:

- Every day, on average, 8 to 18-year-olds spend:
  - nearly four hours watching television, videos, DVDs, and prerecorded shows
  - just over one hour on the computer
  - about 50 minutes playing video games
- Two-thirds of 8 to 18-year-olds have a television in their bedroom and a video game player, and nearly one-third have a computer in their bedroom.
- Children and teens who have televisions in their rooms spend almost 1½ hours or more a day watching television than their peers without a set in their rooms.

It Is Time to Wean the Screen

Parents and caregivers not only set the example for their children in their levels of physical activity, but they also set the rules for use of the television and other screens, including DVDs, video games, and computer use.

The Henry J. Kaiser Foundation survey, "Generation M: Media in the Lives of 8–18 Year Olds," also found that:

- About half (53 percent) of all 8 to 18-year-olds said their parents gave them no rules about television watching.

- Nearly half (46 percent) said they do have rules but only 20 percent said the rules are enforced most of the time.

- Most important, youth with television rules that are enforced report two hours less daily media exposure than in homes without this supervision.

Setting and agreeing on a certain number of hours each day of "screen time" is important. Health experts recommend two hours or less a day that is not work- or homework-related time, such as watching documentary films or doing research or writing on a computer.

Helpful Ways to Reduce Screen Time

Here are a few simple tips to help your children reduce their screen time and increase physical activity in order to maintain a healthy weight.

- **Know how much screen time, active time your family is getting.** By knowing how much screen media, including television, DVD, video games, and non-school- or work-related computer and Internet use, your family spends and how much physical activity they get, you will be more aware of their needs for physical activity to maintain energy balance.

- **Talk to your family.** Explain to your children that it is important to sit less and move more to stay at a healthy weight. They will also be more energized, have a chance to practice certain skills (such as riding a bike or shooting hoops), and have fun with friends and peers. Tell them that you also are going to limit your screen time and increase your physical activity, so you will all be working toward this goal together.

- **Set limits on screen time.** Set a house rule that your children may spend no more than two hours a day of screen time. More importantly, enforce the rule once it's made.

- **Minimize the influence of television in the home.** Do not put a television or computer in your child's bedroom. This tends to physically isolate family members and decrease interaction. Also, children who have televisions in their room tend to spend almost 1½ hours more in a typical day watching television than their peers without a set in their room.

- **Make meal time, family time.** Turn off the television during family meal time. Better yet, remove the television from the eating area if you have one there. Family meals are a good time to talk to each other. Research has shown that families who eat together tend to eat more nutritious meals than families who eat separately. Make eating together a priority and schedule in family meals at least two to three times a week.

- **Provide other options and alternatives.** Watching television can become a habit for your child. Provide other alternatives for them to spend their time, such as playing outside, learning a hobby or sport, or spending time with family and friends.

- **Set a good example.** You need to be a good role model and also limit your screen time to no more than two hours per day. If your kids see you following your own rules, then they will be more likely to follow. Instead of watching television or surfing the Internet, spend time with your family doing something fun and active.

- **Don't use television to reward or punish a child.** Practices like this make television seem even more important to children.

- **Be a savvy media consumer.** Don't expect your child to ignore the influences of television advertising of snack foods, candy, soda, and fast food. Help your child develop healthy eating habits and become media savvy by teaching them to recognize a sales pitch. Ask your child why their favorite cartoon character is trying to get them to eat a certain brand of breakfast cereal. Explain to them that this is a way for advertisers to make the cereal more appealing to young people, so that they ask their parents to buy it for them and the company can make money.

- **Make screen time, active time.** Stretch, do yoga, lift hand weights while watching television; challenge the family to see who can do the most push-ups, jumping jacks or leg lifts during commercial breaks, or switch to an exercise tape during commercials.

Try a Screen Time Log

Prepare a simple log to determine how much time you are spending in front of a screen. Help your family do the same. Place the log in an easy location where everyone can see and use it, such as near the family television, by the computer, or on the refrigerator. If screen time for you or your family members is less than two hours a day, pat yourselves on the back. If it is two hours or more, then check out the other activities to help you reduce your screen time and switch to some physically active alternatives.

Part Three

Appearance, the Skin, and Related Issues during Adolescence

Chapter 16

Acne

What Is Acne?

Acne is a disease that affects the skin's oil glands. The small holes in your skin (pores) connect to oil glands under the skin. These glands make an oily substance called sebum. The pores connect to the glands by a canal called a follicle. Inside the follicles, oil carries dead skin cells to the surface of the skin. A thin hair also grows through the follicle and out to the skin. When the follicle of a skin gland clogs up, a pimple grows.

Most pimples are found on the face, neck, back, chest, and shoulders. Acne is not a serious health threat, but it can cause scars.

How Does Acne Develop?

Sometimes, the hair, sebum, and skin cells clump together into a plug. The bacteria in the plug cause swelling. Then when the plug starts to break down, a pimple grows.

There are many types of pimples. The most common types are:

- Whiteheads—pimples that stay under the surface of the skin.
- Blackheads—pimples rise to the skin's surface and look black. The black color is not from dirt.
- Papules—small pink bumps that can be tender.

"Fast Facts about Acne," National Institute of Arthritis and Musculoskeletal and Skin Diseases (NIAMS), March 2005.

- Pustules—pimples are red at the bottom and have pus on top.
- Nodules—large, painful, solid pimples that are deep in the skin.
- Cysts—deep, painful, pus-filled pimples can cause scars.

Who Gets Acne?

Acne is the most common skin disease. Nearly 17 million people in the United States have it. People of all races and ages get acne. But it is most common in teenagers and young adults. Nearly 85 percent of people between the ages of 12 and 24 get acne. For most people, acne goes away by age 30, but some people in their forties and fifties still get acne.

What Causes Acne?

The cause of acne is unknown. Doctors think certain factors might cause it:

- the hormone increase in teenage years (this can cause the oil glands to plug up more often)
- hormone changes during pregnancy
- starting or stopping birth control pills
- heredity (if your parents had acne, you might get it, too)
- some types of medicine
- greasy makeup

How Is Acne Treated?

Acne is treated by doctors who work with skin problems (dermatologists). Treatment goals include:

- healing pimples
- stopping new pimples from forming
- preventing scarring
- helping to reduce the embarrassment of having acne

Early treatment is the best way to prevent scars. Your doctor may suggest over-the-counter (OTC) or prescription drugs. Some acne medicines are put right on the skin. Other medicines are pills that you swallow. The doctor may tell you to use more than one medicine.

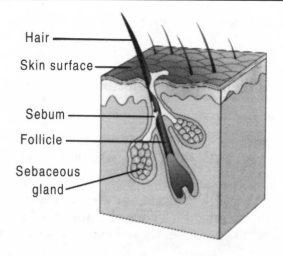

Figure 16.1. *Normal Pilosebaceous Unit (Source: "Q and A about Acne,"
NIAMS, NIH Publication No. 01–4998, October 2001.)*

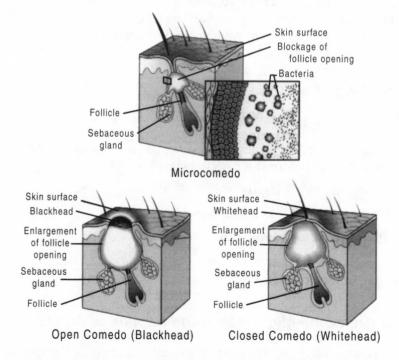

Figure 16.2. *Types of Acne Lesions (Source: "Q and A about Acne,"
NIAMS, NIH Publication No. 01–4998, October 2001.)*

127

How Should People with Acne Care for Their Skin?

Here are some ways to care for skin if you have acne:

- Clean skin gently. Use a mild cleanser in the morning, evening, and after heavy workouts. Scrubbing the skin does not stop acne. It can even make the problem worse.

- Try not to touch your skin. People who squeeze, pinch, or pick their pimples can get scars or dark spots on their skin.

- Shave carefully. If you shave, you can try both electric and safety razors. With safety razors, use a sharp blade. Also, it helps to soften your beard with soap and water before putting on shaving cream. Shave lightly and only when needed.

- Stay out of the sun. Many acne drugs can make people more likely to sunburn. Being in the sun a lot can also make skin wrinkle and raise the risk of skin cancer.

- Choose makeup carefully. All makeup should be oil free. Look for the word "noncomedogenic" on the label. This means that the makeup will not clog up your pores. But some people still get acne even if they use these products.

What Things Can Make Acne Worse?

Some things can make acne worse, such as:

- changing hormone levels in teenage girls and adult women two to seven days before their period starts

- leaning on or rubbing the skin

- pressure from bike helmets, backpacks, or tight collars

- pollution and high humidity

- squeezing or picking at pimples

- hard scrubbing of the skin

What Are Some Myths about the Causes of Acne?

There are many myths about what causes acne. Dirty skin and stress do not cause acne. Also, chocolate and greasy foods do not cause acne in most people.

What Research Is Being Done on Acne?

Scientists are looking at new ways to treat acne including:

- working on new drugs to treat acne
- looking at ways to prevent plugs
- looking at ways to stop the hormone testosterone from causing acne

Chapter 17

Cosmetics and Health

What are cosmetics? How are they different from over-the-counter (OTC) drugs?

Cosmetics are put on the body for a variety of reasons including:

- cleansing
- beautification
- making one attractive
- changing appearance or the way one looks

Cosmetic products include:

- skin creams
- lotions
- perfumes
- lipsticks
- fingernail polishes
- eye and face make-up products
- permanent waves
- hair dyes

Excerpted from "Cosmetics and Your Health," National Women's Health Information Center, November 2004.

- toothpastes
- deodorants

Unlike drugs, which are used to treat or prevent disease in the body, cosmetics do not change or affect the body's structure or functions.

What is in cosmetics?

Fragrances and preservatives are the main ingredients in cosmetics. Fragrances are the most common cause of skin problems. More than 5,000 different kinds are used in products. Products marked fragrance-free or without perfume mean that no fragrances have been added to make the product smell good.

Preservatives in cosmetics are the second most common cause of skin problems. They prevent bacteria and fungus from growing in the product and protect products from damage caused by air or light. But preservatives can also cause the skin to become irritated and infected. Some examples of preservatives are:

- paraben
- imidazolidinyl urea
- quaternium-15
- DMDM (1,3-dimethylol-5,5-dimethyl) hydantoin
- phenoxyethanol
- formaldehyde

The following ingredients cannot be used, or their use is limited, in cosmetics. They may cause cancer or other serious health problems.

- bithionol
- mercury compounds
- vinyl chloride
- halogenated salicylanilides
- zirconium complexes in aerosol sprays
- chloroform
- methylene chloride
- chlorofluorocarbon propellants
- hexachlorophene

Are cosmetics safe?

Yes, for the most part. Serious problems from cosmetics are rare. But sometimes problems can happen.

The most common injury from cosmetics is from scratching the eye with a mascara wand. Eye infections can result if the scratches go untreated. These infections can lead to ulcers on the cornea (clear covering of the eye), loss of lashes, or even blindness. To play it safe, never try to apply mascara while riding in a car, bus, train, or plane.

Sharing make-up can also lead to serious problems. Cosmetic brushes and sponges pick up bacteria from the skin. And if you moisten brushes with saliva, the problem can be worse. Washing your hands before using make-up will help prevent this problem.

Sleeping while wearing eye make-up can cause problems too. If mascara flakes into your eyes while you sleep, you might wake up with itching, bloodshot eyes, infections, or eye scratches. So be sure to remove all make-up before going to bed.

Cosmetic products that come in aerosol containers also can be a hazard. For example, it is dangerous to use aerosol hairspray near heat, fire, or while smoking. Until hairspray is fully dry, it can catch on fire and cause serious burns. Fires related to hairsprays have caused injuries and death. Aerosol sprays or powders also can cause lung damage if they are deeply inhaled into the lungs.

How can I protect myself?

- Never drive and put on make-up. Not only does this make driving a danger, hitting a bump in the road and scratching your eyeball can cause serious eye injury.

- Never share make-up. Always use a new sponge when trying products at a store. Insist that salespersons clean container openings with alcohol before applying to your skin.

- Keep make-up containers closed tight when not in use.

- Keep make-up out of the sun and heat. Light and heat can kill the preservatives that help to fight bacteria. Do not keep cosmetics in a hot car for a long time.

- Do not use cosmetics if you have an eye infection, such as pinkeye. Throw away any make-up you were using when you first found the problem.

- Never add liquid to a product unless the label tells you to do so.

- Throw away any make-up if color changes, or it starts to smell.

- Never use aerosol sprays near heat or while smoking, because they can catch on fire.

- Do not deeply inhale hairsprays or powders. This can cause lung damage.

- Avoid color additives that are not approved for use in the eye area, such as permanent eyelash tints and kohl (color additive that contains lead salts and is still used in eye cosmetics in other countries). Be sure to keep kohl away from children. It may cause lead poisoning.

What are cosmeceuticals?

Some products can be both cosmetics and drugs. This may happen when a product has two uses. For example, a shampoo is a cosmetic because it is used to clean the hair. But, an anti-dandruff treatment is a drug because it is used to treat dandruff. So an antidandruff shampoo is both a cosmetic and a drug.

Other examples include:

- toothpastes that contain fluoride

- deodorants that are also antiperspirants

- moisturizers and make-up that provide sun protection

These products must meet the standards for both cosmetics (color additives) and drugs.

Some cosmetic makers use the term cosmeceutical to refer to products that have drug-like benefits. The U.S. Food and Drug Administration (FDA) does not recognize this term. A product can be a drug, a cosmetic, or a combination of both. But the term cosmeceutical has no meaning under the law.

While drugs are reviewed and approved by FDA, FDA does not approve cosmetics. If a product acts like a drug, FDA must approve it as a drug.

How long do cosmetics last?

You may not be able to use eye make-up, such as mascara, eyeliner, and eye shadow for as long as other products. This is because of the risk of eye infection. Some experts recommend replacing mascara three months after purchase. If mascara becomes dry, throw it away.

Do not add water, or even worse, saliva to moisten it. That will bring bacteria into the product.

You may also need to watch certain all natural products that contain substances taken from plants. These products may be more at risk for bacteria. Since these products contain no preservatives or have non-traditional ones, your risk of infection may be greater.

If you do not store these products as directed, they may expire before the expiration date. For example, cosmetics stored in high heat may go bad faster than the expiration date. On the other hand, products stored the way they should be can be safely used until they expire.

What are hypoallergenic cosmetics?

Hypoallergenic cosmetics are products that makers claim cause fewer allergic reactions than other products. Women with sensitive skin, and even those with normal skin, may think these products will be gentler. But there are no federal standards for using the term hypoallergenic. The term can mean whatever a company wants it to mean. Cosmetic makers do not have to prove their claims to the FDA.

Some products that have natural ingredients can cause allergic reactions. If you have an allergy to certain plants or animals, you could have an allergic reaction to cosmetics with those things in them. For example, lanolin from sheep wool is found in many lotions. but it is a common cause of allergies too.

Can cosmetics cause acne?

Some skin and hair care products can cause acne. To help prevent and control acne flare-ups, take good care of your skin. For example, use a mild soap or cleanser to gently wash your face twice a day. Choose non-comedogenic make-up and hair care products. This means that they do not close up the pores.

Are hair dyes safe?

The decision to change your hair color may be a hard one. Some studies have linked hair dyes with a higher risk of certain cancers, while other studies have not found this link. Most hair dyes also do not have to go through safety testing that other cosmetic color additives do before hitting store shelves. Women are often on their own trying to figure out whether hair dyes are safe.

When hair dyes first came out, the main ingredient in coal-tar hair dye caused allergic reactions in some people. Most hair dyes are now made from petroleum sources. But FDA still considers them to be coal-tar dyes. This is because they have some of the same compounds found in these older dyes.

Cosmetic makers have stopped using things known to cause cancer in animals. For example, 4-methoxy-m-phenylenediamine (4MMPD) or 4-methoxy-m-phenylenediamine sulfate (4MMPD sulfate) are no longer used. But chemicals made almost the same way have replaced some of the cancer-causing compounds. Some experts feel that these newer ingredients are not very different from the things they are replacing.

Experts suggest that you may reduce your risk of cancer by using less hair dye over time. You may also reduce your risk by not dyeing your hair until it starts to gray.

What precautions should I take when I dye my hair?

You should follow these safety tips when dyeing your hair:

- Do not leave the dye on your head any longer than needed.

- Rinse your scalp thoroughly with water after use.

- Wear gloves when applying hair dye.

- Carefully follow the directions in the hair dye package.

- Never mix different hair dye products.

- Be sure to do a patch test for allergic reactions before applying they dye to your hair. It is important to do this each time you dye your hair.

- Never dye your eyebrows or eyelashes. An allergic reaction to dye could cause swelling or increase risk of infection in the eye area. This can harm the eye and even cause blindness. Spilling dye into the eye by accident could also cause permanent damage. FDA bans the use of hair dyes for eyelash and eyebrow tinting or dyeing even in beauty salons.

Chapter 18

Teen Tanning Hazards

The Truth about Tanning: What You Need to Know to Protect Your Skin

- There is no such thing as a safe tan.
- A tan is a sign of sun damage from ultraviolet (UV) rays and can cause premature aging and skin cancer.
- You can get sunburned on a cloudy day because UV rays can filter through the water droplets that make up clouds.
- Getting a tan does not protect your skin from further UV damage.
- The UVA rays emitted by a tanning lamp or bed are often much more intense than those produced by the sun. The aging and cancer risks associated with outdoor tanning are the same as tanning in a salon.
- Sunless tanning coats your skin with the chemical dihydroxy-acetone (DHA) which should not be inhaled, ingested, or in contact with eyes.
- Tanning pills are unsafe and none are approved by the FDA.

Excerpts from "The Truth about Tanning: What You Need to Know to Protect Your Skin," *FDA and You*, Issue #7, Summer 2005; and "Teen Tanning Hazards," by Carol Rados, *FDA Consumer*, March–April 2005, U.S. Food and Drug Administration (FDA).

- Protecting your skin now can help prevent the side effects caused by too much sun.

Protect Yourself with These Sun Safety Tips

- Avoid the sun, or seek shade, from 10:00 a.m. to 4:00 p.m. when the sun's rays are strongest.

- Apply a sun protection factor (SPF) 15 or higher sunscreen.

- Allow 30 minutes for skin to absorb sunscreen before going outside.

- Check the label and reapply sunscreen according to the instructions.

- Wear a wide-brimmed hat.

- Protect eyes with sunglasses that have a UV/UVB protection of at least 99%.

- Check with your doctor to find out if you are taking medications that will make you more sensitive to the sun.

Tanning Hazards for Teens

Parents of teenagers are strongly encouraged by public health experts and medical professionals to discuss with their children the dangers of indoor tanning equipment, and even to discourage its use. In fact, legislators in some states are proposing to make it illegal for a teen to tan in a commercial salon without parental consent.

According to the American Cancer Society (ACS), exposure to the sun's ultraviolet (UV) rays appears to be the most important environmental factor in developing skin cancer. Consequently, the dangers from exposure to UV rays from artificial sources of light, such as tanning beds and sunlamps, are similar to the dangers of exposure to sunlight. Moreover, some experts strongly believe that the sharp rise in the rates of the most serious type of skin cancer—malignant melanoma—may be due to increased exposure to UV radiation, whether from natural sunlight or artificial sources of light.

When exposed to UV radiation, the skin begins to produce a pigment called melanin to protect itself from burning. It is the production of melanin that causes the skin to darken and produce the tan. The production of new melanin takes three to five days.

Joshua L. Fox, M.D., a dermatologist in Fresh Meadows, N.Y., says, "Continued use of a tanning bed or sunlamp can be quite dangerous, particularly during the teenage years." Teens are at greater risk, he says, because they are still experiencing tremendous growth at the cellular level, and like other cells in the body, the skin cells are dividing more rapidly than they do during adulthood.

W. Howard Cyr, Ph.D., and Sharon A. Miller, both laboratory leaders in the Food and Drug Administration's Center for Devices and Radiological Health, say that the agency has regulated the manufacture of sunlamp products—sunlamps, tanning beds, tanning booths, and other related equipment—since 1979. Initially, there was a widespread acute risk from sunlamp products, as indicated by a large number of skin and eye injuries treated annually in hospital emergency rooms. Federal performance standards for sunlamp products were established to protect people from acute burns and exposure to hazardous shortwave UV radiation that was unnecessary for tanning.

In 1985, the agency decided to amend the standards to make the requirements more compatible with then-current products. When sunlamp technology changed and sunlamps emitting primarily UVA radiation—longer-wave, less efficient at producing sunburn—became prevalent, longer exposure times were allowed, Miller says.

In 1986, the FDA published a policy letter that described how the maximum timer limit should be determined and provided guidance on recommended exposure schedules. The manufacturers of sunlamp products are required to include a recommended exposure schedule in their labeling. This schedule should be clearly visible to users before they begin their exposure session.

"FDA does not recommend the use of indoor tanning equipment," Miller says. Fox agrees. "There is no such thing as a safe tan," he says. "Just one sunburn increases your risk for skin cancer."

However, Miller says that if people insist on using tanning devices, there are things they can do to reduce the potential dangers. "Start slowly, with short exposure times, and build up to a tan. If you get the maximum exposure the first time, you will probably get burned," Miller says. And, she adds, often people don't even know they are burned until it's too late. "Remember that a sunburn doesn't usually show up until several hours after the exposure," she says. In addition, the recommended exposure schedules do not allow for tanning more frequently than every other day. After a tan is developed, tanning frequency should be reduced to no more than twice a week.

Cyr and Miller warn that, in practice, tanning salon operators control the exposure time and that they may allow the customer to exceed exposure times written on the label. This is especially true for the beginning of the tanning course when users are advised to start off with very short exposures, usually five minutes or less. Fox says that people who use these products should always ask to see the information contained in the label. Be wary, he adds, if tanning salon operators cannot produce it.

Miller says that the use of FDA-compliant eyewear that blocks UV rays is absolutely essential for tanning bed users to protect their eyes from corneal burns and cataracts from long-term exposure.

A study done by researchers at Wake Forest University, published in the July 2004 issue of the *Journal of the American Academy of Dermatology*, found that participants thought UV exposure was not only desirable for improving appearances, but also was somewhat addictive. The study concluded that, "The relaxing and reinforcing effects of UV exposure contribute to tanning behavior in frequent tanners and should be explored in greater detail."

Fox advises parents to explore safer, alternative means for their children to acquire a tan. "Teens should know about the options," he says, which include self-tanners in the form of creams and gels. "Get the look you like without the damage that can occur with tanning equipment."

Additional Information

SunWise Program
U.S. Environmental Protection Agency
1200 Pennsylvania Ave. NW (6205J)
Washington, DC 20460
Phone: 202-343-9591
Fax: 202-343-2338
Website: http://www.epa.gov/sunwise
E-mail: sunwise@epa.gov

Chapter 19

Body Piercing

Over the past few years, body art has become popular, and it's hard to walk down the street, go to the mall, or watch television without seeing someone with a piercing or a tattoo. Whether it's ears, lips, nostrils, eyebrows, belly buttons, tongues, or even cheeks, you've probably seen piercing—maybe multiple piercing—on lots of people. You might think body piercing looks cool and you've thought about getting one. But are they safe? Are they a good idea? And what should you be aware of if you do decide to get one?

What Is a Body Piercing and What Can You Expect?

A body piercing is exactly that—a piercing or puncture made in your body by a needle. After that, a piece of jewelry is inserted into the puncture. The most popular pierced body parts seem to be the ears, the nostrils, and the belly button.

If the person performing the piercing provides a safe, clean, and professional environment, this is what you can expect from getting a body part pierced:

This chapter includes: "Body Piercing," provided by KidsHealth, one of the largest resources online for medically reviewed health information written for parents, kids, and teens. For more articles like this one, visit www.TeensHealth.org, or www.KidsHealth.org. © 2004 The Nemours Center for Children's Health Media, a division of The Nemours Foundation. And, "Body Piercing and Risky Behavior: Is There a Connection?" Substance Abuse and Mental Health Services Administration (SAMHSA), October 2004.

- The area you've chosen to be pierced (except for the tongue) is cleaned with a germicidal soap (a soap that kills disease-causing bacteria and microorganisms).

- Your skin is then punctured with a very sharp, clean needle.

- The piece of jewelry, which has already been sterilized, is attached to the area.

- The person performing the piercing disposes of the needle in a special container so that there is no risk of the needle or blood touching someone else.

- The pierced area is cleaned.

- The person performing the piercing checks and adjusts the jewelry.

- The person performing the piercing gives you instructions on how to make sure your new piercing heals correctly and what to do if there is a problem.

Before You Pierce That Part

If you're thinking about getting pierced, do your research first. If you're under 18, some places won't allow you to get a piercing without a parent's consent. It's a good idea to find out what risks are involved and how best to protect yourself from infections and other complications.

Certain sites on the body can cause more problems than others—infection is a common complication of mouth and nose piercing because of the millions of bacteria that live in those areas. Tongue piercing can damage teeth over time. And tongue, cheek, and lip piercing can cause gum problems.

Studies have shown that people with certain types of heart disease might have a higher risk of developing a heart infection after body piercing. If you have a medical problem such as allergies, diabetes, skin disorders, a condition that affects your immune system, or infections—or if you are pregnant—ask your doctor if there are any special concerns you should have or precautions you should take beforehand. Also, it's not a good idea to get a body piercing if you're prone to getting keloids (an overgrowth of scar tissue).

If you decide to get a body piercing:

- Make sure you're up to date with your immunizations (especially hepatitis and tetanus).

- Plan where you will get medical care if your piercing becomes infected (signs of infection include excessive redness/tenderness around the piercing site; prolonged bleeding; pus; or change in your skin color around the piercing area).

Also, if you plan to get a tongue or mouth piercing, make sure your teeth and gums are healthy.

Making Sure the Piercing Shop Is Safe and Sanitary

Body piercing is regulated in some states but not others. Although most piercing shops try to provide a clean and healthy environment, some shops might not take proper precautions against infections or other health hazards.

If you decide to get a body piercing, do a little investigative work about a shop's procedures and find out whether they provide a clean and safe environment for their customers. Every shop should have an autoclave (a sterilizing machine) and should keep instruments in sealed packets. Ask questions and make sure:

- the shop is clean

- the person doing the piercing washes his or her hands with a germicidal soap

- the person doing the piercing wears fresh disposable gloves (like those worn at a doctor's office)

- the person doing the piercing uses disposable or sterilized instruments

- the person doing the piercing does not use a piercing gun (they're not sterile)

- the needle being used is new and is being used for the first time

- the needle is disposed of in a special sealed container after the piercing

- there are procedures for the proper handling and disposal of waste (like needles or gauze with blood on it)

It's also a good idea to ask about the types of jewelry the shop offers because some people have allergic reactions to some types of metals. Before you get a piercing, make sure you know if you're allergic to certain metals or not. Only non-toxic metals such as the following should be used for body piercing:

- surgical steel

- solid 14-karat or 18-karat gold

- niobium

- titanium

- platinum

If you think the shop isn't clean enough, if all your questions aren't answered, or if you feel in any way uncomfortable, go somewhere else to get your piercing.

Some Health Risks

If all goes well, you should be fine after a body piercing except for some temporary symptoms, including some pain, swelling at the pierced area, and in the case of a tongue piercing, increased saliva. But be aware that several things, including the following, can go wrong in some cases:

- chronic infection

- uncontrollable or prolonged bleeding

- scarring

- hepatitis B and C

- tetanus

- skin allergies to the jewelry that's used

- abscesses or boils (collections of pus that can form under your skin at the site of the piercing)

- inflammation or nerve damage

Depending on the body part, healing times can take anywhere from a few weeks to more than a year. If you do get a piercing, make sure you take good care of it afterward—don't pick or tug at it, keep the area clean with soap (not alcohol), and don't touch it without washing your hands first. Never use hydrogen peroxide because it can break down newly formed tissue. If you have a mouth piercing, use an antibacterial mouthwash after eating.

If you're thinking of donating blood, keep in mind some organizations won't accept blood donations from anyone who has had a body piercing or tattoo within the last year because both procedures can transmit blood-borne diseases.

If your piercing doesn't heal correctly or you feel something might be wrong, it's important to have someone help you get medical attention. Most importantly—don't pierce yourself or have a friend do it—make sure it's done by a professional in a safe and clean environment.

Talk with Your Child: Body Piercing and Risky Behavior: Is There a Connection?

Body piercing has become more and more popular among teens and young adults. Pierced ears have been common for many years. But now, no part of the body seems to be off limits for rings, studs, and bars. Navels, tongues, eyebrows, and nostrils have become popular places for piercing.

Piercing has been around for a long time. It has been used in religious and cultural ceremonies and is common in some cultures around the world. For many of today's American youth, piercing is a fashion statement. Like tattoos, daring clothing, and extreme hair styles, piercing may be a badge of identity.

Adults may worry that piercing is unsafe, or just plain wrong. They may view it as a sign of delinquency and rejection of traditional values. While this may be true for some teens, others see body piercing as a form of self-expression.

So, which is it? Is body piercing a passing phase—part of a personal declaration of independence? Or, does it signal an urge to push social limits and to take risks? The answer is different for each teen. Risk-taking can be a growth experience; the key is to take the right kind of risk. This means taking part in activities that build ability, awareness, and character.

What to Say

If a young person wants a piercing or comes home with one; ask why he wants it and how it fits into his self-image and social life. Discussion will be more useful than anger or immediate rejection. You may learn something by listening to your teen's views on the subject and you may get a chance to share your own thoughts.

What to Know

Learn about piercing, including the proper procedures, risks (there's that word again), and safety issues. Having the facts will help you provide guidance and make it tougher for a child to dismiss your concerns. If a child gets a body piercing, remember, the industry is not well-regulated. However, there are professional standards for which some piercers are certified.

What to Do

Urging caution, keeping an eye on behavior, and enforcing rules can go a long way toward helping your teen make healthy choices. Prevention is about more than stopping problem behavior. Channeling a young person's search for adventure can yield great results. Exposing teens to people, places, and ideas can open them up to a world of opportunity, but that world is different for each teen. For many young people, body piercing is a decision to try something new and may satisfy their appetites for adventure.

Chapter 20

Tattoos and
Permanent Makeup

The inks used in tattoos and permanent makeup (also known as micropigmentation) and the pigments in these inks are subject to U.S. Food and Drug Administration (FDA) regulation as cosmetics and color additives. However, FDA has not attempted to regulate the use of tattoo inks or the pigments used in them, and it does not control the actual practice of tattooing. Rather, such matters have been handled through local laws and by local jurisdictions. But with the growth in popularity of tattooing and permanent makeup, FDA has begun taking a closer look at related safety questions. Among the issues under consideration are: tattoo removal, adverse reactions to tattoo colors, and infections that result from tattooing.

Another concern is the increasing variety of pigments and diluents being used in tattooing—more than fifty different pigments and shades with the list continuing to grow. Although a number of color additives are approved for use in cosmetics, none is approved for injection into the skin. Using an unapproved color additive in a tattoo ink makes the ink adulterated. Many pigments used in tattoo inks are not approved for skin contact at all. Some are industrial grade colors that are suitable for printers' ink or automobile paint.

This chapter includes: "Tattoos and Permanent Makeup," and "FDA Alerts Consumers about Adverse Events Associated with Permanent Makeup," U.S. Food and Drug Administration, July 2004. Also, "Can I Get HIV from Getting a Tattoo or through Body Piercing?" Centers for Disease Control and Prevention (CDC), December 2003.

Nevertheless, many individuals choose to undergo tattooing in its various forms. For some, it is an aesthetic choice or an initiation rite. Some choose permanent makeup as a time saver or because they have physical difficulty applying regular, temporary makeup. For others, tattooing is an adjunct to reconstructive surgery, particularly of the face or breast, to simulate natural pigmentation. People who have lost their eyebrows due to alopecia (a form of hair loss) may choose to have "eyebrows" tattooed on, while people with vitiligo (a lack of pigmentation in areas of the skin) may try tattooing to help camouflage the condition. Whatever their reason, consumers should be aware of the risks involved in order to make an informed decision.

What Risks Are Involved In Tattooing?

The following are the primary complications that can result from tattooing:

Infection. Unsterile tattooing equipment and needles can transmit infectious diseases, such as hepatitis. The risk of infection is the reason the American Association of Blood Banks requires a one-year wait between getting a tattoo and donating blood. It is extremely important to make sure that all tattooing equipment is clean and sterilized before use. Even if the needles are sterilized or never have been used, it is important to understand that in some cases the equipment that holds the needles cannot be sterilized reliably due to its design. In addition, the person who receives a tattoo must be sure to care for the tattooed area properly during the first week or so after the pigments are injected.

Removal problems. Despite advances in laser technology, removing a tattoo is a painstaking process, usually involving several treatments and considerable expense. Complete removal without scarring may be impossible.

Allergic reactions. Although allergic reactions to tattoo pigments are rare, when they happen they may be particularly troublesome because the pigments can be hard to remove. Occasionally, people may develop an allergic reaction to tattoos they have had for years.

Granulomas. These are nodules that may form around material that the body perceives as foreign, such as particles of tattoo pigment.

Keloid formation. If you are prone to developing keloids—scar tissue that grows beyond normal boundaries—you are at risk of keloid formation from a tattoo. Keloids may form any time you injure or traumatize your skin, and according to Office of Cosmetics and Colors (OCAC) dermatologist Ella Toombs, M.D., tattooing or micropigmentation is a form of trauma. *Micropigmentation: State of the Art*, a book written by Charles Zwerling, M.D., Annette Walker, R.N., and Norman Goldstein, M.D., states that keloids occur more frequently as a consequence of tattoo removal.

MRI complications. There have been reports of people with tattoos or permanent makeup who experienced swelling or burning in the affected areas when they underwent magnetic resonance imaging (MRI). This seems to occur only rarely and apparently without lasting effects.

There also have been reports of tattoo pigments interfering with the quality of the image. This seems to occur mainly when a person with permanent eyeliner undergoes MRI of the eyes. Mascara may produce a similar effect. The difference is that mascara is easily removable.

The cause of these complications is uncertain. Some have theorized that they result from an interaction with the metallic components of some pigments. However, the risks of avoiding an MRI when your doctor has recommended one are likely to be much greater than the risks of complications from an interaction between the MRI and tattoo or permanent makeup. Instead of avoiding an MRI, individuals who have tattoos or permanent makeup should inform the radiologist or technician of this fact in order to take appropriate precautions, avoid complications, and assure the best results.

The Most Common Problem: Dissatisfaction

According to Dr. Toombs, the most common problem that develops with tattoos is the desire to remove them. Removing tattoos and permanent makeup can be very difficult. Skill levels vary widely among people who perform tattooing. According to an article by J.K. Chiang, S. Barsky, and D.M. Bronson in the June 1999 issue of the *Journal of the American Academy of Dermatology*, the main complication with eyelid tattooing is improperly placed pigment. You may want to ask the person performing the procedure for references and ask yourself how willing you are to risk permanently wearing someone else's mistake.

149

Although tattoos may be satisfactory at first, they sometimes fade. Also, if the tattooist injects the pigments too deeply into the skin, the pigments may migrate beyond the original sites, resulting in a blurred appearance.

Another cause of dissatisfaction is that the human body changes over time, and styles change with the season. The permanent makeup that may have looked flattering when first injected may later clash with changing skin tones and facial or body contours. People who plan to have facial cosmetic surgery are advised that the appearance of their permanent makeup may become distorted. The tattoo that seemed stylish at first may become dated and embarrassing, and changing tattoos or permanent makeup is not as easy as changing your mind.

Removal Techniques

Methods for removing tattoos include laser treatments, abrasion, scarification, and surgery. Some people attempt to camouflage an objectionable tattoo with a new one. Each approach has drawbacks:

Laser treatments can lighten many tattoos, some more easily and effectively than others. Generally, several visits are necessary over a span or weeks or months, and the treatments can be expensive. Some individuals experience hypopigmentation—a lightening of the natural skin coloring—in the affected area. Laser treatments also can cause some tattoo pigments to change to a less desirable shade.

Unfortunately, knowing what pigments are in your tattoo or permanent makeup has always been difficult and has become more so as the variety of tattoo inks has multiplied. Inks are often sold by brand name only, not by chemical composition. Because the pigments are sold to tattoo parlors and salons, not on a retail basis to consumers, manufacturers are not required by law to list the ingredients on the labels. Furthermore, because manufacturers may consider the identity and grade of their pigments proprietary, neither the tattooist nor the customer may be able to obtain this information.

There also have been reports of individuals suffering allergic reactions after laser treatments to remove tattoos, apparently because the laser caused allergenic substances in the tattoo ink to be released into the body.

Dermabrasion involves abrading layers of skin with a wire brush or diamond fraise (a type of sanding disc). This process itself may leave a scar.

Salabrasion, in which a salt solution is used to remove the pigment, is sometimes used in conjunction with dermabrasion, but has become less common.

Scarification involves removing the tattoo with an acid solution and creating a scar in its place.

Surgical removal sometimes involves the use of tissue expanders (balloons inserted under the skin, so that when the tattoo is cut away, there is less scarring). Larger tattoos may require repeated surgery for complete removal.

Camouflaging a tattoo entails the injection of new pigments either to form a new pattern or cover a tattoo with skin-toned pigments. Dr. Toombs notes, however, that injected pigments tend not to look natural because they lack the skin's natural translucence.

What about temporary tattoos?

Temporary tattoos, such as those applied to the skin with a moistened wad of cotton, fade several days after application. Most contain color additives approved for cosmetic use on the skin. However, the FDA has issued an import alert for several foreign-made temporary tattoos.

According to Office of Cosmetics and Colors (OCAC) Consumer Safety Officer Allen Halper, the temporary tattoos subject to the import alert are not allowed into the United States because they do not carry the FDA-mandated ingredient labels or they contain colors not permitted by FDA for use in cosmetics applied to the skin. FDA has received reports of allergic reactions to temporary tattoos.

In a similar action, FDA has issued an import alert for henna intended for use on the skin. Henna is approved only for use as a hair dye, not for direct application to the skin. Also, henna typically produces a reddish brown tint, raising questions about what ingredients are added to produce the varieties of colors labeled as henna, such as black henna and blue henna.

Can I Get Human Immunodeficiency Virus (HIV) from Getting a Tattoo or through Body Piercing?

A risk of HIV transmission does exist if instruments contaminated with blood are either not sterilized or disinfected or are used inappropriately between clients. CDC recommends that instruments that are intended to penetrate the skin be used once, then disposed of or thoroughly cleaned and sterilized between clients.

Personal service workers who do tattooing or body piercing should be educated about how HIV is transmitted and take precautions to prevent transmission of HIV and other blood-borne infections in their settings.

If you are considering getting a tattoo or having your body pierced, ask staff at the establishment what procedures they use to prevent the spread of HIV and other blood-borne infections, such as the hepatitis B virus. You also may call the local health department to find out what sterilization procedures are in place in the local area for these types of establishments.

Adverse Events Associated with Permanent Makeup

The Food and Drug Administration (FDA) has alerted the public to a number of reported adverse events associated with individuals who have undergone certain micropigmentation procedures, a form of tattooing, used to apply permanent makeup for lip liner, eyeliner, or eyebrow color. The adverse events are associated with certain ink shades of the Premier Pigment brand of permanent makeup inks, which are manufactured by the American Institute of Intradermal Cosmetics, doing business as Premier Products, in Arlington, Texas. The FDA is currently investigating this matter.

The FDA has been made aware of more than 50 adverse events and is investigating additional reports sent to the manufacturer. Reactions that have been reported include swelling, cracking, peeling, blistering, and scarring as well as formation of granulomas (chronically inflamed tissue mass associated with an infection) in the areas of the eyes and lips. In some cases, the effects reported caused serious disfigurement, resulting in difficulty in eating and talking.

In July 2003, the manufacturer reported to the FDA its intent to remove five of its ink shades from the market, based on six adverse events that had been reported. However, the FDA has obtained additional reports of adverse events involving ink shades that were not included in the firm's removal effort.

The FDA considers intradermal tattoos (including permanent makeup) cosmetics and considers the pigments used in the inks to be color additives requiring pre-market approval under the Federal Food, Drug, and Cosmetic Act. However, the FDA has not traditionally regulated tattoo inks or the pigments used in them. The actual practice of tattooing is regulated by local jurisdictions.

Reporting Adverse Reactions

The FDA urges consumers and healthcare providers to report adverse reactions to tattoos and permanent makeup, problems with removal, or adverse reactions to temporary tattoos. Consumers and healthcare providers can register complaints by contacting their FDA district office (see the blue pages of your local phone directory) or by contacting:

FDA Center for Food Safety and Applied Nutrition (CFSAN)
Adverse Events Reporting System (CAERS)
Phone: 301-436-2405
E-mail: CAERS@cfsan.fda.gov.

FDA Emergency Operations Center
Phone: 301-443-1240

Chapter 21

Antiperspirant Awareness: It's Mostly No Sweat

The U.S. Food and Drug Administration (FDA) defines antiperspirant as a drug product applied topically that reduces the production of sweat (perspiration) at the site where it is applied. Antiperspirants, according to the FDA, can safely and effectively reduce sweat for up to 24 hours if formulated and tested properly, and for most, this means protection against both wetness and odor.

Why People Sweat

Sweating is the body's way of naturally regulating its temperature. During extended, vigorous activity, a person can lose several quarts of fluid through the evaporation of perspiration. A pea-sized bead of sweat can cool about one quart of blood one degree Fahrenheit, according to the Mayo Clinic, and only about one percent of the body's sweat is produced under the arms. Sweat itself is odorless. It is the bacteria that live on the skin and break down the sweat that cause the unpleasant odor. Antiperspirants, designed for both men and women, include aerosols, sprays, pumps, roll-ons, solid sticks, gels, and creams.

Given the amount of money people spend on personal hygiene products, it would seem that an offensive body odor should not be much of a problem. However, according to Gray's Anatomy, most people have

Excerpted from "Antiperspirant Awareness: It's Mostly No Sweat," by Carol Rados, *FDA Consumer*, July–August 2005, U.S. Food and Drug Administration (FDA).

several million sweat glands distributed over their bodies, providing plenty of opportunity for odors to develop.

There are two types of sweat glands. The eccrine glands, which we are born with and which are the most numerous, produce most of the sweat in the underarms. These glands open directly onto the surface of the skin. Apocrine glands, which are triggered by emotions, develop in areas abundant in hair follicles, such as the scalp, underarms, and genitals. These glands only begin to secrete sweat after puberty, and have little, if anything, to do with temperature regulation.

The sweat glands are located in the middle layer of skin called the dermis, which is also made up of nerve endings, hair follicles, and blood vessels. A sweat gland is a long, coiled, hollow tube of cells. Sweat is produced in the coiled part in the dermis, and the long part is a duct that connects the gland to the opening, or pore, on the skin's outer surface. When the sweat gland is stimulated, the cells secrete perspiration that travels from the coiled part of the gland up through the straight tube and out onto the skin's surface.

The American Academy of Dermatology (AAD) says that perspiration is 55 percent to 60 percent fluid, mainly water. Perspiration also contains salt (sodium chloride), as well as trace amounts of other substances, such as ammonia, calcium, chloride, copper, lactic acid, phosphorous, and potassium. These substances, called electrolytes, help to regulate the balance of fluids in the body. The most abundant electrolytes are phosphorous and sodium which cause sweat to sting the eyes and give sweat its salty taste.

The loss of excessive amounts of salt and water from the body can quickly dehydrate a person and can lead to circulatory problems, kidney failure, and heat stroke. So, although it's literally cool to sweat, it is also important that people drink fluids when exercising or when outside in high temperatures.

Antiperspirants 101

People tend to interchange the words antiperspirant and deodorant, but as regulated by the FDA, they are not the same. Antiperspirants have an aluminum-based compound as their main, active ingredient, which can be any number of compounds within an established concentration and dosage form. The active ingredient gives antiperspirants their sweat-blocking ability by forming a temporary plug within the sweat duct that stops the flow of sweat to the skin's surface.

The aluminum-based compound is always the first ingredient listed on the back of an antiperspirant container. A few common active ingredients are aluminum chloride, aluminum chlorohydrate, and aluminum zirconium. Some of the inactive ingredients in an antiperspirant include talc, fragrance, and butane—used as an aerosol propellant.

Many factors control how effective an antiperspirant is, such as the type and size of the active ingredient used in the formulation. The antiperspirant effectiveness test required by the FDA determines that a product is effective or ineffective in its final formulation. But, Matthew R. Holman, Ph.D., an FDA scientist in the Division of Over-the Counter Drug (OTC) Products says, "we do not have any data that suggest any dosage form is better than another." He also says there's a lot of variability between dosage forms. An antiperspirant in finished form may vary in degree of effectiveness because of minor variations in formulation, or in individual interpretation of the directions for its use.

For example, while a product label may instruct the user to hold a can of aerosol six inches from the underarm and then spray, Holman says, how long each person sprays, swipes, glides, wipes, or rolls will vary. Therefore, the directions don't directly reflect the conditions of effectiveness. But Holman adds that consumers can be assured that products are effective whether they are gels, sticks, aerosols, or others, if they pass the FDA's test.

Antiperspirants and the FDA

"People feel that those products on the shelf are a direct reflection of what we regulate," says Holman. "But mostly, it's based on what's selling." Like prescription drugs, the FDA oversees OTC drugs to ensure that they are properly labeled and that their benefits outweigh their risks. OTC drugs account for more than 100,000 products on the market that involve about 800 active ingredients. The FDA classifies these nonprescription drugs by treatment category, such as laxatives, antacids, and antiperspirants, and evaluates their ingredients. So, rather than review thousands of individual antiperspirant products, the FDA evaluates the far fewer active ingredients found in them.

Most OTC drugs are subject to rules called monographs, which state requirements for categories of nonprescription drugs, such as what ingredients may be used and for what intended use. If the standards of the OTC monograph are met, pre-market approval of a potentially new OTC product is not necessary.

The FDA is mainly concerned about claims being made for a product, Holman says. For example, in the familiar slogan, "strong enough for a man but made for a woman," the company had to prove that the product was tested in both men and women because there are physiological differences between them. Similarly, testing must confirm marketing statements such as "so effective you could skip a day."

By contrast, Holman says that if a company claimed that a new antiperspirant ingredient is effective, "it would require a new drug application because the ingredient is not already included in the antiperspirant monograph as generally recognized as safe and effective."

Holman also says that manufacturers tend to test antiperspirant products on more women than men. One reason seems to be underarm hair. Women are required to shave two days before testing to keep hair to a minimum and to minimize skin irritation. "With that said, skin irritation related to shaving is not a major safety concern because it is not serious or life-threatening," Holman says. "And common sense dictates women will not keep using a particular product if it causes irritation."

The important thing to remember, says Holman, "is that antiperspirants don't completely eliminate sweat." According to the FDA's testing standards, the most effective products—those that claim "extra strength" or "maximum strength"—are based on at least a 30 percent sweat reduction rate in most people. Regular strength products test at a 20 percent sweat reduction rate in most people.

Sweating Too Much, or Not Enough

If the complex biological mechanism of perspiration goes awry, it can result in either excessive perspiration (hyperhidrosis) or little or no perspiration (anhidrosis), a potentially life-threatening condition. Dermatologists at the American Academy of Dermatology (AAD) say that excessive sweating is normal when a person is anxious or has a fever. However, excessive sweating can be a chronic condition and may signal other medical conditions such as thyroid problems, low blood sugar levels, a nervous system disorder, or the onset of menopause.

Excessive sweating is more than a mild nuisance that some people experience. According to the AAD, hyperhidrosis affects about eight million Americans. Depending on where it occurs on the body, hyperhidrosis has several treatment options, including topical agents such as prescription antiperspirants, oral medications, and surgery. Prescription antiperspirants contain higher doses of the active ingredient aluminum chloride. Skin irritation is the main side effect with prescription antiperspirants such as Drysol (aluminum chloride hexahydrate).

In July 2004, the FDA approved Botox (botulinum toxin type A), a drug that is used to temporarily erase wrinkles for cosmetic purposes, to treat severe underarm sweating (primary axillary hyperhidrosis) that cannot be managed by topical agents. Available by prescription only, botulinum toxin type A is a protein produced by the bacterium *Clostridium botulinum*. This protein works by interrupting the chemical messages released by nerve endings that tell the sweat gland when to sweat. Administered into the armpit, small doses of an injectable form of the sterile purified botulinum toxin stop release of the chemical messenger acetylcholine that supplies nerves to the eccrine glands, thereby temporarily paralyzing the nerves in the underarm that stimulate sweat production.

To avoid the possibility that Botox treatments can mask a potentially serious disease, the FDA advises patients to be evaluated by a doctor for other possible causes of excessive sweating. Botox is approved for treatment of the underarms, but not for excessive sweating of other sites such as the feet and palms.

The Cancer Myth

One myth says that antiperspirants may cause breast cancer. According to the National Cancer Institute (NCI), the breast cancer-antiperspirant myth first appeared in the form of an e-mail in the 1990s, and continues to resurface and recirculate about every year or so. The false information suggests that antiperspirants contain harmful substances, which can be absorbed through the skin or can enter the body near the breasts through nicks in the skin caused by shaving. The e-mails also suggested that antiperspirants keep a person from sweating out toxins, resulting in the spread of cancer-causing toxins via the lymph nodes.

The NCI says that no existing scientific or medical evidence links the use of underarm antiperspirants or deodorants to the subsequent development of breast cancer. The FDA, the Mayo Clinic, the American Cancer Society (ACS), and the Cosmetic, Toiletry and Fragrance Association agree. Razor nicks may increase the risk of skin infection, but not cancer.

According to the ACS, sweat glands are not connected to the lymph nodes. Most cancer-causing substances are removed by the kidneys, are released through urine or by the liver, and are eliminated with feces. The ACS says that lymph nodes may help to clear some toxins from the body, but they do not release these toxins through sweating. Sweat is not a significant route for eliminating toxins from the body.

Some speculate that the myth could have been started by women being told not to wear antiperspirants or deodorants before a mammogram. They were told this, not for safety reasons, but because residue from these products appearing in the x-ray is often mistaken for an abnormality in the breast.

For More Information

American Academy of Dermatology
P.O. Box 4014
Schaumburg, IL 60618-4014
Toll-Free: 866-503-7546
Fax: 847-240-1859
Website: http://www.aad.org
E-mail: MCR@aad.org

International Hyperhidrosis Society
520 Walnut St., Suite 1160
Philadelphia, PA 19106
Website: http://www.sweathelp.org
E-mail: info@SweatHelp.org

Chapter 22

Tinea Infections: Athlete's Foot, Jock Itch, and Ringworm

What is tinea?

Tinea is a fungus that can grow on your skin, hair, or nails. As it grows, it spreads out in a circle, leaving normal-looking skin in the middle. This makes it look like a ring. At the edge of the ring, the skin is lifted up by the irritation and looks red and scaly. To some people, the infection looks like a worm is under the skin. Because of the way it looks, tinea infection is often called ringworm. However, there really is not a worm under the skin.

How did I get a fungal infection?

You can get a fungal infection by touching a person who has one. Some kinds of fungi live on damp surfaces, like the floors in public showers or locker rooms. You can easily pick up a fungus there. You can even catch a fungal infection from your pets. Dogs and cats, as well as farm animals, can be infected with a fungus. Often this infection looks like a patch of skin where fur is missing.

What areas of the body are affected by tinea infections?

Fungal infections are named for the part of the body they infect. Tinea corporis is a fungal infection of the skin on the body. (*Corporis* is the Latin word for body.) If you have this infection, you may see small, red spots that grow into large rings almost anywhere on your arms, legs, or chest.

Tinea pedis is usually called athlete's foot. (*Pedis* is the Latin word for foot.) The moist skin between your toes is a perfect place for a fungus to grow. The skin may become itchy and red, with a white, wet surface. The infection may spread to the toenails. (This is called tinea unguium—*unguium* comes from the Latin word for nail.) Here it causes the toenails to become thick and crumbly. It can also spread to your hands and fingernails.

When a fungus grows in the moist, warm area of the groin, the rash is called tinea cruris. (*Cruris* comes from the Latin for leg.) The common name for this infection is jock itch. Tinea cruris generally occurs in men, especially if they often wear athletic equipment.

Tinea capitis, which is called ringworm, causes itchy, red areas, usually on the head. (*Capitis* comes from the Latin for head.) The hair is destroyed, leaving bald patches. This tinea infection is most common in children.

How do I know if I have a fungal infection?

The best way to know for sure is to ask your doctor. Other skin problems can look just like a fungal infection but have very different treatments. To find out what is causing your rash, your doctor may scrape a small amount of the irritated skin onto a glass slide (or clip off a piece of nail or hair). Then he or she will look at the skin, nail, or hair under a microscope. After doing this, your doctor will usually be able to tell if your skin problem is caused by a fungus. Sometimes a piece of your skin, hair, or nail will be sent to a lab to grow the fungus in a test tube. This is another way the lab can tell if your skin problem is caused by a fungus. They can also find out the exact type of fungus. This process takes a while because a fungus grows slowly.

How do I get rid of a tinea infection?

Once your doctor decides that you have a tinea infection, medicine can be used to get rid of it. You may only need to put a special cream on the rash for a few weeks. This is especially true for jock itch. It can be harder to get rid of fungal infections on other parts of the body. Sometimes you have to take medicine by mouth. This medicine usually has to be taken for a long time, maybe even for months. Irritated skin takes time to heal. New hair or nails will have to grow back.

Some medicines can have unpleasant effects on the rest of your body, especially if you are also taking other medicines. There are some newer medicines that seem to work better with fewer side effects. You may need to have blood tests to make sure that your body is not having a bad reaction to the medicine.

What can I do to prevent tinea infections?

Skin that is kept clean and dry is your best defense. However, you are also less likely to get a tinea infection if you do the following things:

- When you are at home, take your shoes off and expose your feet to the air.

- Change your socks and underwear every day, especially in warm weather.

- Dry your feet carefully (especially between the toes) after using a locker room or public shower.

- Avoid walking barefoot in public areas. Instead, wear flip-flops, sandals, or water shoes.

- Do not wear thick clothing for long periods of time in warm weather. It will make you sweat more.

- Throw away worn-out exercise shoes. Never borrow other people's shoes.

- Check your pets for areas of hair loss. Ask your veterinarian to check them too. It is important to check pets carefully, because if you do not find out whether they are causing your fungal infection, you may get it again from them, even after treatment.

Can tinea cause serious illness?

A fungus rarely spreads below the surface of the body to cause serious illness. Your body usually prevents this. However, people with weak immune systems, such as people with acquired immune deficiency syndrome (AIDS), may have a hard time getting well from a fungal infection.

Tinea infections usually do not leave scars after the fungus is gone. Sometimes, people do not even know they have a fungal infection and get better without any treatment.

Source: Diagnosis and Management of Common Tinea Infections (*American Family Physician* July 1998, http://www.aafp.org/afp/980 700ap/noble.html).

Chapter 23

Identifying
and Treating Warts

Warts are simply areas of skin that grow faster than normal due to the presence of the wart virus. Warts are skin-colored and feel rough to the touch. The technical name is verruca vulgaris. They are most common on the hands, feet, and face, but they can grow almost anywhere in the body. They are infectious and some people, especially children, are more susceptible than others.

Flat warts are much smaller and are less rough than hand or foot warts. They tend to grow in great numbers—20 to 100 at any one time. They can occur anywhere, but in children they are most common on the face. In adults they are most often found in the beard area in men and on the legs in women. Skin irritation from shaving probably accounts for this.

A plantar wart is simply a wart growing on the weight-bearing surface of the foot that grows inward rather than outwards because it is pressed on when a person walks.

As warts are caused by a virus infection, the body will build up resistance over a period of time and eventually the body will cause the warts to disappear. This may take months or sometimes years but is the natural way the body deals with warts. If they are allowed to disappear in this way, it is less likely that a person will get any further ones as one will then be immune to that virus.

"Warts," reprinted with permission from the American Osteopathic College of Dermatology (AOCD). © 2004. All rights reserved. For additional information, visit the AOCD website at www.aocd.org.

The first treatment to try on warts is removal with a salicylic acid liquid or pad. Be patient as it takes up to twelve weeks to get rid of warts. One will need a bottle of wart medication like Occlusal-HP or Compound W, a roll of 1-inch surgical tape (Micropore or Blenderm are good) and a pumice stone or emery board. The wart should be soaked in warm water for 10 or 15 minutes. After soaking, rub away at the white, dead warty skin with the pumice stone. Apply the wart medication to the warts, getting as little as possible onto the surrounding skin and let dry. Put a piece of tape over the wart big enough to stop the medication from getting rubbed off.

One needs to keep going down until just below the level of the surrounding skin to eradicate a wart completely. Stop when the base of the wart looks exactly like normal skin (for example, no black dots or graininess). If they become sore or bleed a little, do not treat that night and carry on the following night. Special precautions are not needed if one goes swimming or walks barefoot to avoid infecting other people. The risk to others is very little.

Liquid nitrogen cryotherapy is what dermatologists use most often to cure warts. This method can cause pain, soreness, and blistering and usually cures 50% of warts after one treatment. Frequent applications of liquid nitrogen are needed to cure more stubborn warts.

Other Treatments

Warts around the fingers and nails are definitely a challenge. For finger and toe warts, there is a very good, but unusual treatment using duct tape. Apply the tape over the warts for 6½ days per week and give the finger ½ day off per week. In kids, the tape often has to be replaced every day, or every other day, etc. The tape needs to be occlusive—it cannot be tape that breathes such as cloth Band-Aids, etc. The tape probably works for two reasons. Warts are viruses, and thus susceptible to changes in temperature and decreased oxygen locally. The occlusive tape probably locally increases temperature. There is often a foul odor when the tape is removed.

There are special treatments such as contact hypersensitization and Bleomycin injections used for difficult warts that really need to be gone. These often work, but may have some side effects that must be understood before they are tried. Tagamet is an oral medication used for ulcers that may help boost the immune response. It is only effective in children, and not consistently so.

Burning warts off with a carbon dioxide (CO_2) laser or electric needle is often effective, but scars. The CO_2 laser is no better than burning with the needle. This can be used on one or two warts in difficult places. A more effective laser is the Pulsed dye laser, but this is not the laser most doctors have. The good thing about this laser is there is absolutely no downtime from pain, and scarring is rare. It is 60–75% effective (within 1–3 treatments spaced two weeks apart) for difficult warts.

Chapter 24

Teens and Plastic Surgery

Chapter Contents

Section 24.1

Facial Plastic Surgery during Adolescence

Reprinted with permission from the American Academy of Facial Plastic and Reconstructive Surgery, www.aafprs.org. Reviewed in April 2006 by Dr. David A. Cooke, M.D., Diplomate, American Board of Internal Medicine.

Teens Turn to Facial Plastic Surgery to Improve Self-Esteem

The teenage years are replete with rapid changes physically and mentally as a child tries to forge his or her own path into young adulthood. On top of issues of independence, there are concerns about acceptance by peers and anxiety about appearance. Why are teenagers seeking facial plastic surgery and is it right for my teen?

Giving a Good Reason

In a recent survey found on a Web site geared toward teens, nearly 15,000 teenagers were asked, "How do you feel about teens and cosmetic plastic surgery?" The majority, 54 percent (7,622), responded that it depends on the situation. If your child feels inadequate physically and this affects him socially or academically, you may want to look into treatment options. Congenital defects, scarring, loss of facial function, asymmetry, or imbalance can create extreme distress unnecessarily if it can be corrected with treatment or surgery.

Here are some questions for you and your teen to consider:

- Why do you want to change your appearance? Discuss with your teenager why he or she may feel insecure. Are the concerns well-founded? One teenager suffered years of acne and was left with extensive scarring. After he and his parents pursued scar revision surgery, the teen expressed that his biggest joy was not being teased about the scarring like he had been teased about the acne. Teens who pursue facial plastic or reconstructive surgery are looking to feel more confident and have a better self-image.

- What feature do you want to correct? Physicians will not recommend an invasive procedure just so the teenager may look prettier. Surgeries that produce subtle results with minimal benefits are not recommended. Rhinoplasty, including cosmetic and reconstructive (for example, correcting a nasal obstruction or cleft palate reconstruction), is the most popular procedure performed on teenagers. Other surgeries that may be appropriate include otoplasty (ear surgery), blepharoplasty (eyelid surgery), chin augmentation, and scar revision.

- What are your expectations for the results? Before deciding on a procedure or treatment option, discuss with your teenager what they hope to achieve by changing their appearance. Just because they alter their appearance does not mean that they will automatically become popular and get straight A's. Your physician will ensure that there is no pressure from family or friends to have surgery and that the teenager fully understands the procedure and results.

Making the Decision

As a parent, you want your child to feel secure and self-assured and help your child avoid any hardship. If your teenager approaches you regarding changing his or her physical appearance, be sensitive, ask questions, and be realistic. Make an appointment with a facial plastic surgeon who can screen your teen for maturity, motivations, and expectations, in addition to the physical examination. Then together, you can discuss the possibility of surgery or other treatments.

Section 24.2

Teens and Breast Implants

U.S. Food and Drug Administration (FDA), 2004.

Breast implant surgery is a growing trend among teenaged women. According to the American Society for Aesthetic Plastic Surgery (ASAPS), women 18 and under accounted for 11,326 breast implant surgeries performed in American women in 2003, compared to 3,872 in 2002.

Despite more than a decade of controversy over their safety, breast implants are more popular than ever among women who want to build upon what nature gave them or who want to restore what disease has taken away. Whatever the reason, opting for breast implants is a personal decision that should be made only after a woman fully understands and accepts the potential risks of the devices and the importance of follow-up evaluations with her doctor. Because it has not been well studied in young people, the Food and Drug Administration (FDA) discourages the use of any breast implant in a patient younger than 18.

Breast implants are designed to change the size and shape of the breast (augmentation), to rebuild the breast (reconstruction), and to replace existing implants (revision). There are two primary types of breast implants: saline-filled and silicone gel-filled. Depending on the type of implant, the shell is either pre-filled with a fixed volume of solution or filled through a valve during the surgery to the desired size. Some allow for adjustments of the filler volume after surgery. Breast implants vary in shape, size, and shell texture.

At this time, there are two manufacturers with approved saline-filled breast implants. No manufacturer has yet received FDA approval to market a silicone gel-filled breast implant for augmentation.

Health officials worry that teens and their parents may not realize the risks associated with breast implants. They also want to be sure that the teen's body has finished developing and that they are psychologically ready to handle the outcome of surgery. While every surgical procedure has potential risks, such as infection, bleeding, and

172

scarring, there are risks that are specific to breast implants. Learning about them is the key to being properly informed about the procedure.

"I didn't know my breasts were still growing when I signed up for the surgery," admits Kacey Long, who got saline-filled breast implants in July 2001, when she was 19. Prior to her surgery, the college student from Ennis, Texas, was a 34B, the breast size she thought she would be for life.

Teenagers who are dissatisfied with their bodies see breast implants as harmless and, according to Long, a fun thing to do to improve self-image. Following implantation, Long's breast size increased to a 34D. But complications convinced her to have the implants removed a short time later. Three years later, Long's breasts measure 36C—one size larger than before she was implanted—suggesting that her own breasts continued to develop even after the implants were removed.

Many of the changes to the breast that occur with an implant cannot be undone. If a teen chooses to have her implants removed, she may experience dimpling, puckering, wrinkling, or other cosmetic changes. "When you're making a decision that can impact your life at 19," Long advises other young women, "you need to research the subject like you're 50 years old."

Consider these breast implant facts:

- Breast implants will not last a lifetime. Either because of rupture or other complications, you will likely need to have the implants removed.

- Your breast may not be fully developed and could continue to grow larger, even after implant surgery.

- You are likely to need additional doctor visits and operations because of one or more complications over the course of your life.

- You are likely to have the implants removed, with or without replacement, because of one or more complications over the course of your life.

- Many of the changes to your breast following implantation may be cosmetically undesirable and cannot be undone.

- If you choose to have your implants removed, you may experience unacceptable dimpling, puckering, wrinkling, loss of breast tissue, or other undesirable cosmetic changes of the breast.

Additional Information

FDA Breast Implants
Website: http://www.fda.gov/cdrh/breastimplants

Part Four

Reproductive and Sexual Health during Adolescence

Chapter 25

Female Reproductive Development

Chapter Contents

Section 25.1

Menstruation and the Menstrual Cycle

Excerpts from "Menstruation and the Menstrual Cycle," National Women's Health Information Center, November 2002.

What is menstruation?

Menstruation is a woman's monthly bleeding. It is also called menses, menstrual period, or period. When a woman has her period, she is menstruating. The menstrual blood is partly blood and partly tissue from the inside of the uterus (womb). It flows from the uterus through the small opening in the cervix, and passes out of the body through the vagina. Most menstrual periods last from three to five days.

What is the menstrual cycle?

Menstruation is part of the menstrual cycle, which helps a woman's body prepare for the possibility of pregnancy each month. A cycle starts on the first day of a period. The average menstrual cycle is 28 days long. However, a cycle can range anywhere from 23 days to 35 days.

The parts of the body involved in the menstrual cycle include the brain, pituitary gland, uterus, cervix, ovaries, fallopian tubes, and vagina. Body chemicals called hormones rise and fall during the month and make the menstrual cycle happen. The ovaries make two important female hormones, estrogen and progesterone. Other hormones involved in the menstrual cycle include follicle-stimulating hormone (FSH) and luteinizing hormone (LH), made by the pituitary gland.

What happens during the menstrual cycle?

In the first half of the menstrual cycle, levels of estrogen rise and make the lining of the uterus grow and thicken. In response to follicle-stimulating hormone, an egg (ovum) in one of the ovaries starts to mature. At about day 14 of a typical 28-day cycle, in response to a surge of luteinizing hormone, the egg leaves the ovary. This is called ovulation.

In the second half of the menstrual cycle, the egg begins to travel through the fallopian tube to the uterus. Progesterone levels rise and help prepare the uterine lining for pregnancy. If the egg becomes fertilized by a sperm cell and attaches itself to the uterine wall, the woman becomes pregnant. If the egg is not fertilized, it either dissolves or is absorbed into the body. If pregnancy does not occur, estrogen and progesterone levels drop, and the thickened lining of the uterus is shed during the menstrual period.

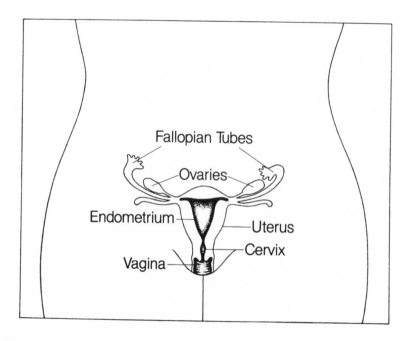

Figure 25.1. *Female Reproductive Anatomy (Source: NCI Visuals Online, National Cancer Institute)*

What is a typical menstrual period like?

During the menstrual period, the thickened uterine lining and extra blood are shed through the vaginal canal. A woman's period may not be the same every month, and it may not be the same as other women's periods. Periods can be light, moderate, or heavy, and the length of the period also varies. While most menstrual periods last from three to five days, anywhere from two to seven days is considered normal. For the first few years after menstruation begins, periods may be very irregular. They may also become irregular in women approaching menopause. Sometimes birth control pills are prescribed to help with irregular periods or other problems with the menstrual cycle.

Sanitary pads or tampons, which are made of cotton or another absorbent material, are worn to absorb the blood flow. Sanitary pads are placed inside the panties; tampons are inserted into the vagina.

At what age does a girl get her first period?

Menarche is another name for the beginning of menstruation. In the United States, the average age at which a girl starts menstruating is twelve. However, this does not mean that all girls start at the same age. A girl can begin menstruating anytime between the ages of eight and sixteen. Menstruation will not occur until all parts of a girl's reproductive system have matured and are working together.

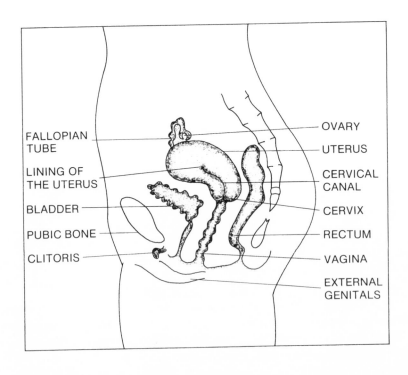

Figure 25.2. *Lateral View of Female Pelvis (Source: NCI Visuals Online, National Cancer Institute)*

How long does a woman have periods?

Women usually continue having periods until menopause. On average, menopause occurs around the age of 51. Menopause means that a woman is no longer ovulating (producing eggs) and therefore can no longer become pregnant. Like menstruation, menopause can vary from woman to woman and may take several years to occur. Some women have early menopause because of surgery or other treatment, illness, or other reasons.

When should I see a health care provider about my period?

You should consult your health care provider for the following:

- You have not started menstruating by the age of sixteen.
- Your period has suddenly stopped.
- You are bleeding for more days than usual.
- You are bleeding excessively.
- You suddenly feel sick after using tampons.
- You bleed between periods (more than just a few drops).
- You have severe pain during your period.

How often should I change my pad or tampon?

Sanitary napkins (pads) should be changed as often as necessary, before the pad is soaked with menstrual flow. Each woman decides for herself what is comfortable. Tampons should be changed often (at least every 4–8 hours). Make sure that you use the lowest absorbency of tampon needed for your flow. For example, do not use super absorbency on the lightest day of your period. This can put you at risk for toxic shock syndrome (TSS). TSS is a rare but potentially deadly disease. Women under 30, especially teenagers, are at a higher risk for TSS. Using any kind of tampon—cotton or rayon of any absorbency—puts a woman at greater risk for TSS than using menstrual pads. The risk of TSS can be lessened or avoided by not using tampons, or by alternating between tampons and pads during your period.

The Food and Drug Administration (FDA) recommends the following tips to help avoid tampon problems:

- Follow package directions for insertion.
- Choose the lowest absorbency for your flow.

- Change your tampon at least every 4 to 8 hours.
- Consider alternating pads with tampons.
- Know the warning signs of toxic shock syndrome.
- Do not use tampons between periods.

If you experience any of the following symptoms while you are menstruating and using tampons, you should contact your health care provider immediately:

- high fever that appears suddenly
- muscle aches
- diarrhea
- dizziness and/or fainting
- sunburn-like rash
- sore throat
- bloodshot eyes

Section 25.2

Premenstrual Syndrome

National Women's Health Information Center, July 2002.

What is premenstrual syndrome (PMS)?

Premenstrual syndrome (PMS) is a group of symptoms related to the menstrual cycle. PMS symptoms occur in the week or two weeks before your period (menstruation or monthly bleeding). The symptoms usually go away after your period starts. PMS may interfere with your normal activities at home, school, or work. Menopause, when monthly periods stop, brings an end to PMS.

The causes of PMS are not yet clear. Some women may be more sensitive than others to changing hormone levels during the menstrual cycle. Stress does not seem to cause PMS, but may make it worse. PMS can affect menstruating women of any age.

PMS often includes both physical and emotional symptoms. Diagnosis of PMS is usually based on your symptoms, when they occur, and how much they affect your life.

What are the symptoms of PMS?

PMS often includes both physical and emotional symptoms. Common symptoms are:

- breast swelling and tenderness
- fatigue and trouble sleeping
- upset stomach, bloating, constipation, or diarrhea
- headache
- appetite changes or food cravings
- joint or muscle pain
- tension, irritability, mood swings, or crying spells
- anxiety or depression
- trouble concentrating or remembering

Symptoms vary from one woman to another. If you think you have PMS, try keeping track of your symptoms for several menstrual cycles. You can use a calendar to note which symptoms you are having on which days of your cycle, and how bad the symptoms are. If you seek medical care for your PMS, having this kind of record is helpful.

How common is PMS?

Estimates of the percentage of women affected by PMS vary widely. According to the American College of Obstetricians and Gynecologists, up to 40 percent of menstruating women report some symptoms of PMS. Most of these women have symptoms that are fairly mild and do not need treatment. Some women (perhaps five to ten percent of menstruating women) have a more severe form of PMS.

What treatment is available for PMS?

Many treatments have been tried for easing the symptoms of PMS. However, no treatment has been found that works for everyone. A combination of lifestyle changes and other treatment may be needed. If your PMS is not so bad that you need medical help, a healthier lifestyle may help you feel better and cope with symptoms.

- Adopt a healthier way of life. Exercise regularly, get enough sleep, choose healthy foods, do not smoke, and find ways to manage stress in your life.

- Try avoiding excess salt, sugary foods, caffeine, and alcohol, especially when you are having PMS symptoms.

- Be sure that you are getting enough vitamins and minerals. Take a multivitamin every day that includes 400 micrograms of folic acid. A calcium supplement with vitamin D can help keep bones strong and may help with PMS symptoms.

- In more severe cases, drugs such as diuretics, ibuprofen, birth control pills, or antidepressants may be used.

Although PMS does not seem to be related to abnormal hormone levels, some women respond to hormonal treatment. For example, one approach has been to use drugs such as birth control pills to stop ovulation from occurring. There is evidence that a brain chemical, serotonin, plays a role in severe forms of PMS. Antidepressants that alter serotonin in the body have been shown to help many women with severe PMS.

What is premenstrual dysphoric disorder (PMDD)?

PMDD is a severe, disabling form of PMS. In PMDD, the main symptoms are mood disorders such as depression, anxiety, tension, and persistent anger or irritability. These severe symptoms lead to problems with relationships and carrying out normal activities. Women with PMDD usually also have physical symptoms, such as headache, joint and muscle pain, lack of energy, bloating, and breast tenderness. According to the American Psychiatric Association, a woman must have at least five of the typical symptoms to be diagnosed with PMDD. The symptoms must occur during the two weeks before her period and go away when bleeding begins.

Research has shown that antidepressants called selective serotonin reuptake inhibitors (SSRIs) can help many women with PMDD. The Food and Drug Administration (FDA) has approved two such medications to date for treatment of PMDD—sertraline (Zoloft) and fluoxetine (Sarafem).

For More Information about Premenstrual Syndrome

National Women's Health Information Center (NWHIC)
Office on Women's Health, DHHS
200 Independence Ave. SW, Room 712E
Washington, DC 20201
Toll-Free: 800-994-9662
Toll-Free TDD: 888-220-5446
Website: http://womenshealth.gov

National Institute of Mental Health
NIMH Public Inquiries
6001 Executive Blvd.
Room 8184, MSC 9663
Bethesda, MD 20892-9663
Toll-Free: 866-615-6464
Toll-Free TTY: 866-415-8051
Fax: 301-443-4279
Website: http://www.nimh.nih.gov
E-mail: nimhinfo@nih.gov

American College of Obstetricians and Gynecologists (ACOG)
409 12th St. SW
Washington, DC 20024-2188
Phone: 202-863-2518
Website: http://www.acog.org

Hormone Foundation
8401 Connecticut Ave., Suite 900
Chevy Chase, MD 20815-5817
Toll-Free: 800-467-6663
Website: http://www.hormone.org

Section 25.3

Menstrual Problems

This information was provided by KidsHealth, one of the largest resources online for medically reviewed health information written for parents, kids, and teens. For more articles like this one, visit www.KidsHealth.org, or www.TeensHealth.org. © 2005 The Nemours Center for Children's Health Media, a division of The Nemours Foundation.

Everyone knows the teen years can be difficult—for both teens and parents. All those physical changes during puberty can make adolescents feel awkward and unsure of themselves. This is particularly true for girls when it comes to menstruation. For a girl, getting her first period is a physical milestone and a sign of becoming a woman. But it can also be confusing, particularly if she encounters certain problems like irregular periods or premenstrual syndrome (PMS).

What Are Some Common Menstrual Problems?

Most issues teens confront when they start menstruating are completely normal. In fact, many girls and women have had to deal with one or more of them at one time or another:

Premenstrual Syndrome (PMS)

PMS includes both physical and emotional symptoms that many girls and women get right before their periods, such as:

- acne
- bloating
- fatigue
- backaches
- sore breasts
- headaches
- constipation
- diarrhea
- food cravings
- depression or feeling blue
- irritability
- difficulty concentrating
- difficulty handling stress

Different girls may have some or all of these symptoms in varying combinations. PMS is usually at its worst during the seven days before the period starts and disappears once it begins. But girls usually don't develop symptoms associated with PMS until several years after menstruation starts—if ever.

Although the exact cause of PMS is unknown, it seems to occur because of changing hormone levels. During the second half of the menstrual cycle, the amount of progesterone in the body increases. Then, about seven days before the period starts and right around when PMS occurs, levels of both progesterone and estrogen drop.

Cramps

Many girls experience abdominal cramps during the first few days of their periods. They're caused by prostaglandin, a chemical in the body that makes the smooth muscle in the uterus contract. These involuntary contractions can be either dull or sharp and intense.

The good news is that cramps usually become less severe as girls get older and they don't usually last long. But call your daughter's doctor if she has severe cramps that keep her home from school or from activities with her friends.

Irregular Periods

It can take up to two years from a girl's first period for her body to develop a regular cycle. During that time, the body is essentially adjusting to the influx of hormones unleashed by puberty. And what's regular varies from person to person. The typical cycle of an adult female is 28 days, although some are as short as 22 days and others are as long as 45.

Changing hormone levels might make a girl's period short one month (just a few days) and long the next (up to a week). She can skip months, get two periods almost right after each other, or alternate between heavy and light bleeding from one month to another.

But any girl who's sexually active and skips a period should see a doctor to make sure she's not pregnant. And if your daughter's period still hasn't settled into a relatively predictable pattern after three years, or if she has four or five regular periods and then skips her period for a couple of months, make an appointment with her doctor to check for possible problems.

Delayed Menarche

All girls go through puberty at different rates. Some reach menarche (the medical term for the first period or the beginning of menstruation) as early as nine or ten years old and others don't have their first periods until they're well into their teen years. So, if your daughter is a late bloomer, it doesn't necessarily mean there's something wrong with her.

When girls get their periods actually depends a lot on genetics. Girls often start menstruating at approximately the same age their mothers or grandmothers did. Also, certain ethnic groups, on average, go through puberty earlier than others. For instance, African-American girls, on average, start puberty and get their periods before Caucasian girls do. If your daughter hasn't started her period by the time she's 16 or you're concerned, see the section, "When Should You Call Your Child's Doctor?"

What Are Some Menstrual Problems That May Be Cause for Concern?

Although most period problems are harmless, a few conditions can be more serious and require medical attention.

Amenorrhea (the Absence of Periods)

Girls who haven't started their periods by the time they're 16 years old or three years after they've shown the first signs of puberty have primary amenorrhea, which is usually caused by a hormone imbalance or developmental problem. Hormones are also often responsible for secondary amenorrhea, which is when a girl who had normal periods suddenly stops menstruating for more than six months.

Of course, pregnancy is the first possible cause to rule out when a girl skips periods. But some other things that can cause both primary and secondary amenorrhea include:

- low levels of gonadotropin-releasing hormone (GnRH), which controls ovulation and the menstrual cycle

- stress

- significant weight loss or gain

- anorexia (In fact, amenorrhea can be an initial sign that a teen is losing too much weight and may have anorexia.)

- stopping birth control pills

- thyroid conditions

- ovarian cysts

- other conditions that can affect hormone levels

Something that can also cause primary and secondary amenorrhea is excessive exercising (usually distance running, ballet, or gymnastics) combined with a poor diet, which usually results in inappropriate weight loss or failure to gain weight during growth. But this doesn't include the usual gym class or school sports team, even those that practice often. To exercise so much that she delays her period, a girl would have to train vigorously for several hours a day, most days of the week, and not get enough calories, vitamins, and minerals.

Menorrhagia (Extremely Heavy, Prolonged Periods)

It's normal for a girl's period to be heavier on some days than others. But menorrhagia usually leads to soaking through at least one sanitary napkin (pad) an hour for several hours in a row or periods that last longer than seven days. Girls with menorrhagia sometimes stay home from school or social functions because they're worried they won't be able to control the bleeding in public.

The most frequent cause of menorrhagia is an imbalance between the levels of estrogen and progesterone in the body, which allows the endometrium (the lining of the uterus) to keep building up. When the endometrium is finally shed during menstruation, the resulting bleeding is particularly heavy.

Because many adolescents have slight hormone imbalances during puberty, menorrhagia isn't uncommon in teens. In some cases, heavy menstrual bleeding is caused by:

- fibroids (benign growths) or polyps in the uterus
- thyroid conditions
- clotting disorders
- inflammation or infection in the vagina or cervix

Dysmenorrhea (Painful Periods)

There are two types of dysmenorrhea, which is severely painful menstruation that can interfere with a girl's ability to attend school, study, or sleep:

- Primary dysmenorrhea is more common in teens and is not caused by a disease or other condition. Instead, the culprit is prostaglandin, the same chemical behind cramps. Large amounts of prostaglandin can lead to nausea, vomiting, headaches, backaches, diarrhea, and severe cramps. Fortunately, these symptoms usually last for only a day or two.

- Secondary dysmenorrhea is pain caused by some physical condition like polyps or fibroids in the uterus, endometriosis, pelvic inflammatory disease (PID), or adenomyosis (uterine tissue growing into the muscular wall of the uterus).

Having cramps for a day or two each month is common, but signs of dysmenorrhea should be discussed with your child's doctor.

Endometriosis

In this condition, tissue normally found only in the uterus starts to grow outside the uterus—in the ovaries, fallopian tubes, or other parts of the pelvic cavity. It can cause abnormal bleeding, dysmenorrhea, and general pelvic pain.

How Are Menstrual Problems Treated?

To determine whether a problem requires treatment, your child's doctor or gynecologist will likely do a thorough pelvic exam, a Pap smear, blood tests (to check hormone levels), and sometimes even urine and stool tests. If he or she thinks there's some sort of growth in the uterus or fallopian tubes, an ultrasound or computerized axial tomography (CAT) scan may be performed. Together, those tests can reveal how a condition should be handled.

Growths such as polyps or fibroids can often be removed and endometriosis can often be treated with medications or surgery. If a hormone imbalance is to blame, the doctor will likely suggest hormone therapy with birth control pills or other estrogen and/or progesterone-containing medications.

And for severe menstrual pain with no underlying medical cause, anti-inflammatory medicines are the most effective treatment. Conditions like clotting disorders or thyroid problems may require treatment with medications as well.

When Should You Call Your Child's Doctor?

Although most period problems aren't cause for alarm, certain symptoms do call for a trip to the doctor. This is particularly true if a girl's normal cycle changes. So take your daughter to her doctor if she:

- hasn't started her period by the time she's 16 or her period hasn't become regular after three years of menstruating. Although the most likely cause is a hormone imbalance (which may need treatment), this might also point to a problem with her diet, possibly even an eating disorder. If she doesn't consume enough vitamins, minerals, and calories, it could harm her growth and development.

- stops getting her period or it becomes irregular after it has been regular for about six months or longer. Again, this might signal a problem with nutrition, maybe even anorexia, which can be dangerous if left untreated. Sometimes girls who are developing anorexia will stop having periods months before significant weight loss has occurred.

- has extremely heavy or long periods, especially if her cycle is short and she gets her period frequently. In some cases, significant blood loss can cause iron-deficiency anemia. Also, heavy bleeding could be a sign of a growth in the uterus, a thyroid condition, an infection, or a blood clotting problem.

- has very painful periods. She might have endometriosis or benign (noncancerous) growths that should be removed. Or, if she's sexually active, she could have pelvic inflammatory disease.

191

What Can You Do to Help Your Daughter?

When your daughter is experiencing a particularly bad bout of PMS or cramps, there are several things you can do at home to make her more comfortable. Suggest that she:

- eat a balanced diet with lots of fresh fruit and vegetables
- reduce her intake of salt (which can cause water retention) and caffeine (which can make her jumpy and anxious)
- take magnesium, B-complex vitamins, and calcium, which may reduce the severity of her PMS symptoms
- try over-the-counter pain relievers like acetaminophen or ibuprofen for cramps, headaches, or back pain
- take a brisk walk or bike ride to relieve stress and aches (because exercise releases endorphins—chemicals in the body that make you feel good)
- soak in a warm bath or put a hot water bottle on her abdomen, which may help her relax

If you notice that your daughter's usual periods are causing her great discomfort and interfering with her life, check with her doctor about hormone treatment, usually in the form of birth control pills, which can help ease many symptoms associated with uncomfortable periods.

But the most important way you can help your daughter feel more at ease about her period is to talk to her and explain that most annoying or uncomfortable conditions that accompany menstruation are normal and may improve over time. And be understanding when she's cranky and unhappy. After all, no one's at her best all the time—including you.

Section 25.4

First Ob-Gyn Visit

This information was provided by KidsHealth, one of the largest resources online for medically reviewed health information written for parents, kids, and teens. For more articles like this one, visit www.kidsHealth.org, or www.TeensHealth.org. © 2005 The Nemours Center for Children's Health Media, a division of The Nemours Foundation.

Your Daughter's First Gynecological Exam

Most doctors recommend that a young woman have her first gynecologic exam when she turns 18 or becomes sexually active, whichever comes first. However, if your daughter is complaining of missed or painful periods, unusual vaginal secretions, or any other problems that may be associated with her sexual organs, she should have an exam as soon as possible.

The idea of having a pelvic exam may make your daughter feel nervous, embarrassed, or scared. By explaining why the visit is necessary, giving your daughter a sense of what to expect, and addressing any questions or fears she might have, you can help her feel more comfortable about taking this step.

Explaining the Importance of the Exam

Chances are, your daughter has associated visits to the doctor with health problems. She may not understand why she would go to the doctor when she feels perfectly fine. Explain that the visit serves at least three main purposes:

1. **Information.** She can get accurate information and confidential answers to any questions she may have concerning sex, sexuality, and her changing body.

2. **Prevention.** The doctor checks the reproductive organs to make sure they are developing as they should, and to head off any health problems that may be developing.

3. **Treatment.** For those who experience missed periods, pain, and other reproductive problems, the doctor can find out why the problems are occurring and offer treatment.

Also, you may want to reassure your daughter that even though there are a lot of different parts of the gynecological exam, the entire exam—and the part she might feel most uncomfortable about—doesn't take long.

Selecting a Health Practitioner

The doctor or nurse that your daughter sees should be someone who takes the time to make her feel as comfortable as possible during the visit. Though you have probably been the dominant force in making your daughter's health decisions up until now, it's a good idea to involve her in this one. Here are some ways to gauge your daughter's preferences:

- Ask your daughter what type of health professional she would prefer. A male or female? Someone who is younger or older? In some cases, your daughter might be able to stick with the pediatrician or family physician she has seen before. If either of you would like to move on, though, you have a variety of health professionals to choose from: nurse practitioners, general practitioners, or gynecologists.

- Before sending your daughter to the health professional that you use, check to see if she is comfortable with that. Some girls might be hesitant to confide in someone who has a connection to their mother.

- Ask her if she would like you to be in the exam room with her. Whatever your daughter decides, allow her some time alone with the doctor or nurse practitioner. You want your daughter to be completely honest with the doctor, not withhold information that she is too embarrassed to share in your presence. In addition, alone time will allow her to recognize the physician as an objective and knowledgeable person to talk to about any concerns she may have in the future.

Your needs are important, too—you should trust this person with providing your daughter appropriate information about important decisions in her life. Once you have your daughter's input, use these suggestions to find a doctor who best fits your family's needs.

- **Get a referral.** Ask your family doctor for recommendations. If you have close friends who have recently taken a daughter to her first exam, ask them if they liked their health professional. If there is a particular hospital or practice you prefer, see a physician or nurse practitioner associated with that facility.

- **Ask questions.** It's a good idea to ask about the health professional's confidentiality policy. The answer to this question may affect how open your daughter is during the exam. Most offices will not share the details of the exam with the parent unless the patient indicates that it is okay or if the physician feels that your child may be engaged in an activity that can be imminently harmful. Also, different states have different rules with regard to confidentiality and notifying parents about contraceptive use.

Other questions you may want to ask:

- Do you accept my insurance?
- Are you board certified?
- What is your approach toward a teen's level of sexual activity?
- Do you have experience with first-time patients and teens?
- Will a different health professional examine my daughter every time she goes?
- How many people will be in the examining room?

Share the answers to these questions with your daughter. And don't hesitate to interview several health practitioners before deciding on the best fit.

Remember: ultimately, it's your daughter's feet that are in those stirrups. Try to select a doctor who will make her as safe, informed, and comfortable as possible.

About the Exam

Before the appointment, it's a good idea to give your daughter a sense of what will happen in the exam room. Most gynecological exams include certain procedures, though they may not occur in the same order in every office. It's important for your daughter not only to know what to expect, but why the doctor is doing it and how any discomfort she is feeling can be minimized. If applicable—and both of you are comfortable with the idea—consider letting your daughter see these steps firsthand by sitting in on one of your exams.

The Talk

Your daughter should be prepared to answer questions the doctor asks relating to her medical and reproductive history, including:

- When was your last period?
- Are you sexually active? If so, are you using birth control?
- Are you having any problems with your period, such as discharge or pain?
- Do you think you are pregnant?

Through this discussion, the doctor will be able to get a sense of which tests to run and what issues to discuss. Stress to your daughter the importance of answering these questions truthfully, even though she might feel uncomfortable about it. For example, the health professional can help determine, based on your daughter's sexual history, whether she is at risk for a getting a sexually transmitted disease (STD). If she is, the doctor will know to test for it.

Encourage your daughter to ask any and all questions she has—no matter how stupid or embarrassing she fears they may be. Let her know that nothing she says will be something that the doctor or nurse hasn't heard before or will share with anyone else. Remind her that this information is confidential.

The Physical

Your daughter has probably experienced a physical before, so most of this will be familiar territory for her.

One of the health care workers, probably an assistant or nurse rather than the doctor, will measure your daughter's blood pressure, weight, height, and other factors. Her head, neck, breasts, heart, lungs, and abdomen will also be examined. Your daughter may also provide a urine sample. This examination gives the doctor background on your daughter's general health, and also gives her a baseline to use for comparisons in future exams.

The Breast Exam

During this part of the exam, the doctor or practitioner will do a breast exam to make sure that your child is developing normally, and to detect cysts or other benign (noncancerous) breast problems. The doctor also will show your daughter how to do a breast self-exam, which helps your child become familiar with how her breasts feel so that she knows which lumps are normal and which may indicate that something is wrong.

The External Vaginal Examination

If she hasn't already, your daughter will undress and put on an examination gown. She will lie on the table with her knees bent and spread apart. In this position, the doctor will check the vulva (outer lips of the vagina). Her pelvis and thighs will be draped with a sheet. To make the position more comfortable, she will place her feet in stirrups.

The purpose of this part of the exam is to make sure there are no sores, swelling, or any other problems with the outside of the vagina.

The Internal Vaginal Examination

The doctor will place one hand on the outside of your daughter's abdomen and two fingers inside the body. The doctor will also insert a speculum (a slender plastic or metal instrument) into the vagina.

The clinician's hands are used to make sure that the ovaries and uterus are in the correct location, the correct size and shape, and free of pain or discomfort. The speculum allows the doctor to visually examine the walls of the vagina and the cervix and to perform screening tests, such as a Pap smear and tests for STDs.

Let your daughter know that she may feel some pressure, but this shouldn't hurt. She may be able to decrease any discomfort by taking slow, deep breaths and relaxing her stomach and vaginal muscles. In addition, the clinician will likely make efforts to make her feel more comfortable by starting up a conversation or having interesting posters in the room to stare at.

The Pap Smear

While your daughter is lying on the exam table, the doctor or nurse will gently touch a cotton swab and then a small cylindrical brush to the surface of the cervix. The cells that are collected on the brush are sent to a lab to check for abnormalities, which might be a sign of infection or other health problems, such as cervical cancer. The Pap smear will likely not hurt your daughter. At most, some women notice a slight, quick twinge.

Sexually Transmitted Disease Test (Optional)

Testing for an STD is not automatically included in a gynecological exam. Usually, a patient has to request this service. The clinician obtains the sample with a cotton swab (just like during the Pap smear).

The sample is sent to a lab, where it is tested for STDs like gonorrhea, genital warts, and chlamydia. When talking to your daughter about whether she should get tested, it's important that she know that intercourse isn't the only way to contract these infections.

The office staff can let you know different options for getting the results confidentially. For instance, instead of calling the patient or sending a letter with the results, some offices require the patient to call in.

Once you and your daughter have gone to the first exam, encourage her to talk about the experience (as much as she is comfortable). If she indicates that the doctor or nurse practitioner made her feel uncomfortable, discuss finding a new one. Once she starts, your daughter should continue to go for gynecologic exams every year to keep her informed and healthy.

Chapter 26

Male Reproductive Development

Chapter Contents

Section 26.1

Reproductive System

This information was provided by TeensHealth, one of the largest resources online for medically reviewed health information written for parents, kids, and teens. For more articles like this one, visit www.Teens Health.org, or www.KidsHealth.org. © 2004 The Nemours Center for Children's Health Media, a division of The Nemours Foundation.

Ever wonder how the universe could allow the existence of someone as annoying as your bratty little brother or sister? The answer lies in reproduction. If people—like your parents—didn't reproduce, families would die out and the human race would cease to exist.

All living things reproduce. Reproduction—the process by which organisms make more organisms like themselves—is one of the things that sets living things apart from nonliving matter. But even though the reproductive system is essential to keeping a species alive, unlike other body systems it's not essential to keeping an individual alive.

In the human reproductive process, two kinds of sex cells, or gametes (pronounced: gah-meetz), are involved. The male gamete, or sperm, and the female gamete, the egg or ovum, meet in the female's reproductive system to create a new individual. Both the male and female reproductive systems are essential for reproduction.

Humans, like other organisms, pass certain characteristics of themselves to the next generation through their genes, the special carriers of human traits. The genes parents pass along to their children are what make children similar to others in their family, but they are also what make each child unique. These genes come from the father's sperm and the mother's egg, which are produced by the male and female reproductive systems.

What Is the Male Reproductive System?

Most species have two sexes: male and female. Each sex has its own unique reproductive system. They are different in shape and structure, but both are specifically designed to produce, nourish, and transport either the egg or sperm. Unlike the female, whose sex organs are located entirely within the pelvis, the male has reproductive organs, or genitals (pronounced: jeh-nuh-tulz), that are both inside and outside the pelvis. The male genitals include:

- the testicles

- the duct system, which is made up of the epididymis and the vas deferens

- the accessory glands, which include the seminal vesicles and prostate gland

- the penis

In a guy who's reached sexual maturity, the two testicles (pronounced: tes-tih-kulz), or testes (pronounced: tes-teez), produce and store millions of tiny sperm cells. The testicles are oval-shaped and grow to be about two inches (five centimeters) in length and one inch (three centimeters) in diameter. The testicles are also part of the endocrine system because they produce hormones, including testosterone (pronounced: teh-stass-tuh-rone). Testosterone is a major part of puberty in guys, and as a guy makes his way through puberty, his testicles produce more and more of it. Testosterone is the hormone that causes guys to develop deeper voices, bigger muscles, and body and facial hair, and it also stimulates the production of sperm.

Alongside the testicles are the epididymis (pronounced: eh-puh-dih-duh-mus) and the vas deferens (pronounced: vass de-fuh-runz), which make up the duct system of the male reproductive organs. The vas deferens is a muscular tube that passes upward alongside the testicles and transports the sperm-containing fluid called semen (pronounced: see-mun). The epididymis is a set of coiled tubes (one for each testicle) that connects to the vas deferens.

The epididymis and the testicles hang in a pouch-like structure outside the pelvis called the scrotum. This bag of skin helps to regulate the temperature of testicles, which need to be kept cooler than body temperature to produce sperm. The scrotum changes size to maintain the right temperature. When the body is cold, the scrotum shrinks and becomes tighter to hold in body heat. When it's warm, the scrotum becomes larger and more floppy to get rid of extra heat. This happens without a guy ever having to think about it. The brain and the nervous system give the scrotum the cue to change size.

The accessory glands, including the seminal vesicles and the prostate gland, provide fluids that lubricate the duct system and nourish the sperm. The seminal vesicles (pronounced: seh-muh-nul veh-sih-kulz) are sac-like structures attached to the vas deferens to the side of the bladder. The prostate gland, which produces some of the parts of semen, surrounds the ejaculatory ducts at the base of the urethra (pronounced: yoo-ree-thruh), just below the bladder. The urethra is the channel that carries the semen to the outside of the body through the penis. The urethra is also part of the urinary system because it is also the channel through which urine passes as it leaves the bladder and exits the body.

The penis is actually made up of two parts: the shaft and the glans (pronounced: glanz). The shaft is the main part of the penis and the glans is the tip (sometimes called the head). At the end of the glans is a small slit or opening, which is where semen and urine exit the body through the urethra. The inside of the penis is made of a spongy tissue that can expand and contract.

All boys are born with a foreskin, a fold of skin at the end of the penis covering the glans. Some boys have a circumcision (pronounced: sur-kum-sih-zhun), which means that a doctor or clergy member cuts away the foreskin. Circumcision is usually performed during a baby boy's first few days of life. Although circumcision is not medically necessary, parents who choose to have their children circumcised often do so based on religious beliefs, concerns about hygiene, or cultural or social reasons. Boys who have circumcised penises and those who don't are no different: All penises work and feel the same, regardless of whether the foreskin has been removed.

What Does the Male Reproductive System Do?

The male sex organs work together to produce and release semen into the reproductive system of the female during sexual intercourse. The male reproductive system also produces sex hormones, which help a boy develop into a sexually mature man during puberty (pronounced: pyoo-bur-tee).

When a baby boy is born, he has all the parts of his reproductive system in place, but it isn't until puberty that he is able to reproduce. When puberty begins, usually between the ages of 10 and 14, the pituitary (pronounced: puh-too-uh-ter-ee) gland—which is located in the brain—secretes hormones that stimulate the testicles to produce testosterone. The production of testosterone brings about many physical changes. Although the timing of these changes is different for every guy, the stages of puberty generally follow a set sequence.

- During the first stage of male puberty, the scrotum and testes grow larger.

- Next, the penis becomes longer, and the seminal vesicles and prostate gland grow.

- Hair begins to appear in the pubic area and later it grows on the face and underarms. During this time, a male's voice also deepens.

- Boys also undergo a growth spurt during puberty as they reach their adult height and weight.

Once a guy has reached puberty, he will produce millions of sperm cells every day. Each sperm is extremely small: only 1/600 of an inch (0.05 millimeters long). Sperm develop in the testicles within a system of tiny tubes called the seminiferous tubules (pronounced: seh-muh-nih-fuh-rus too-byoolz). At birth, these tubules contain simple round cells, but during puberty, testosterone and other hormones cause these cells to transform into sperm cells. The cells divide and change until they have a head and short tail, like tadpoles. The head contains genetic material (genes). The sperm use their tails to push themselves into the epididymis, where they complete their development. It takes sperm about four to six weeks to travel through the epididymis.

The sperm then move to the vas deferens, or sperm duct. The seminal vesicles and prostate gland produce a whitish fluid called seminal fluid, which mixes with sperm to form semen when a male is sexually stimulated. The penis, which usually hangs limp, becomes hard when a male is sexually excited. Tissues in the penis fill with blood and it becomes stiff and erect (an erection). The rigidity of the erect penis makes it easier to insert into the female's vagina during sexual intercourse. When the erect penis is stimulated, muscles around the reproductive organs contract and force the semen through the duct system and urethra. Semen is pushed out of the male's body through his urethra—this process is called ejaculation (pronounced: ih-jah-kyuh-lay-shun). Each time a guy ejaculates, it can contain up to 500 million sperm.

When the male ejaculates during intercourse, semen is deposited into the female's vagina. From the vagina the sperm make their way up through the cervix and move through the uterus with help from uterine contractions. If a mature egg is in one of the female's fallopian tubes, a single sperm may penetrate it, and fertilization, or conception, occurs.

This fertilized egg is now called a zygote (pronounced: zy-goat) and contains 46 chromosomes—half from the egg and half from the sperm. The genetic material from the male and female has combined so that a new individual can be created. The zygote divides again and again as it grows in the female's uterus, maturing over the course of the pregnancy into an embryo, a fetus, and finally a newborn baby.

Things That Can Go Wrong with the Male Reproductive System

Guys may sometimes experience reproductive system problems. Following are some examples of disorders that affect the male reproductive system.

Disorders of the Scrotum, Testicles, or Epididymis

Conditions affecting the scrotal contents may involve the testicles, epididymis, or the scrotum itself.

- Testicular injury. Even a mild injury to the testicles can cause severe pain, bruising, or swelling. Most testicular injuries occur when the testicles are struck, hit, kicked, or crushed, usually during sports or due to other trauma. Testicular torsion (pronounced: tor-zhun), when one of the testicles twists around, cutting off the blood supply, is also a problem that some teen guys experience—although it's not common.

- Varicocele (pronounced: var-uh-koh-seal). This is a varicose vein (an abnormally swollen vein) in the network of veins that run from the testicles. Varicoceles commonly develop while a guy is going through puberty. A varicocele is usually not harmful, although in some people it may damage the testicle or decrease sperm production, so it helps for a guy to see his doctor if he's concerned about changes in his testicles.

- Testicular cancer. This is one of the most common cancers in men younger than 40. It occurs when cells in the testicle divide abnormally and form a tumor. Testicular cancer can spread to other parts of the body, but if it's detected early, the cure rate is excellent. All guys should perform testicular self-examinations regularly to help with early detection.

- Epididymitis (pronounced: eh-puh-dih-duh-my-tus) is inflammation of the epididymis, the coiled tubes that connect the testes with the vas deferens. It is usually caused by an infection, such as the sexually transmitted disease chlamydia, and results in pain and swelling next to one of the testicles.

- Hydrocele. A hydrocele (pronounced: high-druh-seel) occurs when fluid collects in the membranes surrounding the testes. Hydroceles may cause swelling of the testicle but are generally painless. In some cases, surgery may be needed to correct the condition.

- Inguinal hernia. When a portion of the intestines pushes through an abnormal opening or weakening of the abdominal wall and into the groin or scrotum, it is known as an inguinal hernia (pronounced: in-gwuh-nul her-nee-uh). The hernia may look like a bulge or swelling in the groin area. It can be corrected with surgery.

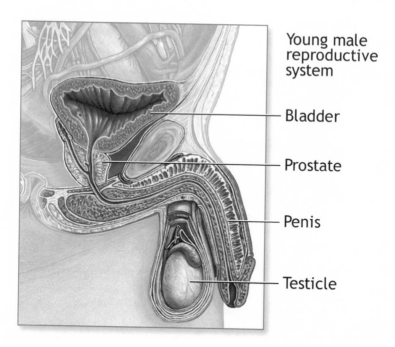

Young male reproductive system

Bladder

Prostate

Penis

Testicle

Figure 26.1. *Young Male Reproductive System (Source: Copyright 2006 A.D.A.M., Inc. Reprinted with permission.)*

Disorders of the Penis

Disorders affecting the penis include the following:

- Inflammation of the penis. Symptoms of penile inflammation include redness, itching, swelling, and pain. Balanitis occurs when the glans (the head of the penis) becomes inflamed. Posthitis is foreskin inflammation, which is usually due to a yeast or bacterial infection.

- Hypospadias is a disorder in which the urethra opens on the underside of the penis, not at the tip.

- Sexually transmitted diseases (STDs) that can affect guys include human immunodeficiency virus/acquired immunodeficiency syndrome (HIV/AIDS), human papilloma virus (HPV, or genital warts), syphilis, chlamydia, gonorrhea, herpes genitalis, and hepatitis B. They are spread from one person to another mainly through sexual intercourse.

If you think you have symptoms of a problem with your reproductive system or if you have questions about your growth and development, talk to your parent or doctor—many problems with the male reproductive system can be treated.

Section 26.2

Testicular Exams

This information was provided by TeensHealth, one of the largest resources online for medically reviewed health information written for parents, kids, and teens. For more articles like this one, visit www.teens Health.org, or www.kidshealth.org. © 2004 The Nemours Center for Children's Health Media, a division of The Nemours Foundation.

Why Do I Need Testicular Exams?

Medical exams, whether they're for school, a sport, or camp, are usually pretty straightforward. Many parts of the exam make sense to most guys: The scale is used to weigh you, the stethoscope is used to listen to your heartbeat. But why does the doctor need to touch and feel your testicles? What could be going on down there—and isn't there a better, less embarrassing way for him or her to check things out?

When you are healthy and going for a physical exam, the doctor is interested in finding out specific things about your body and your health. He or she will check your height and weight and take your blood pressure. You'll have your heart listened to, and you may be asked to breathe deeply or cough, so the doctor can hear sounds or problems with your lungs. He or she will examine your eyes, ears, nose, and throat; test your reflexes by tapping your knees and ankles; and take your temperature. For all these parts of the exam, the doctor relies on tools and equipment to get the information that's needed.

However, for other parts of your body, the doctor must rely on his or her sense of touch and training in knowing how things should feel. During the physical, the doctor will touch your belly to feel for any problems with your liver or spleen. He or she will feel the lymph nodes in your neck, armpits, and groin to detect if there is any swelling, which can indicate an infection or other problem. And he or she will also need to feel the testicles and the area around them to detect two important things: a hernia or a tumor.

Hernias

A hernia can occur when a part of the intestine pushes out from the abdomen and into the groin or scrotum (the sac of skin that the testicles hang in). Some people believe that this can only happen when a person lifts something heavy, but usually this isn't the case. Most hernias occur because of a weakness in the abdominal wall that the person was born with. If a piece of intestine becomes trapped in the scrotum, it can cut off the blood supply to the intestine and cause serious problems if the situation isn't quickly corrected.

A doctor is able to feel for a hernia by using his or her fingers to examine the area around the groin and testicles. The doctor may ask you to cough while he or she is pressing on or feeling the area. Sometimes, the hernia causes a bulge that the doctor can detect; if this happens, surgery almost always repairs the hernia completely.

Cross Section of Testicle

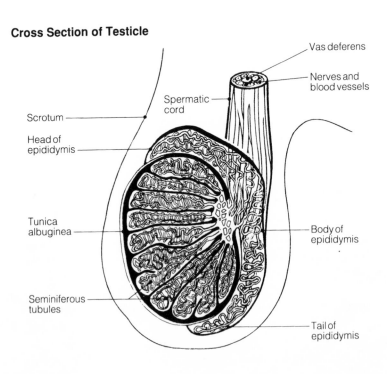

Figure 26.2. *Lateral View of a Testicle (Source: NCI Visuals Online, National Cancer Institute)*

Testicular Cancer

Although testicular cancer is unusual in teen guys (it occurs in 3 out of 100,000 guys between the ages of 15 and 19 in the United States), it is the second most common cancer seen during the teen years. It is the most common cancer in guys 20 to 34 years of age. Comedian Tom Green and Tour de France champion bicyclist Lance Armstrong have both successfully won battles with testicular cancer.

It's very important that your doctor examines your testicles at least once a year. When examining your testicles, your doctor will grasp one testicle at a time, rolling it gently between his or her thumb and first finger. He or she will feel for lumps and also pay attention to whether the testicle is hardened or enlarged. The doctor will explain how to do testicular self-exams.

If you're a teen guy, learning how to examine yourself at least once a month for any lumps or bumps on your testicles is very important. A tumor (growth or bump) on the testicles could be cancer. Knowing how your testicles feel when they're healthy will help you know when something feels different and possibly abnormal down there. Noticing any new testicular lumps or bumps as soon as possible gives the best chances for survival and total cure if it turns out to be cancer.

Finally, keep in mind that even though it might feel weird to have a doctor checking out your testicles, it's no big deal to him or her. Sometimes when a doctor is examining that area, you might get an erection, something you can't control. This is a normal reaction that happens frequently during genital exams on guys. If it happens, it won't upset or bother the doctor, so there's no need to feel embarrassed.

Section 26.3

Prostate Disorders of Young Men

"Prostatitis: Disorders of the Prostate," National Institute of Diabetes
and Digestive and Kidney Diseases (NIDDK), NIH Publication No. 04–
4553, December 2003.

Prostatitis may account for up to 25 percent of all office visits by young
and middle-aged men for complaints involving the genital and urinary
systems. The term prostatitis actually encompasses four disorders.

1. **Acute bacterial prostatitis** is the least common of the four
    types but also the easiest to diagnose and treat effectively.
    Men with this disease often have chills, fever, pain in the
    lower back and genital area, urinary frequency and urgency
    often at night, burning or painful urination, body aches, and a
    demonstrable infection of the urinary tract as evidenced by
    white blood cells and bacteria in the urine. The treatment is
    an appropriate antibiotic.

2. **Chronic bacterial prostatitis,** also relatively uncommon, is
    acute prostatitis associated with an underlying defect in the
    prostate, which becomes a focal point for bacterial persistence
    in the urinary tract. Effective treatment usually requires
    identifying and removing the defect and then treating the in-
    fection with antibiotics. However, antibiotics often do not cure
    this condition.

3. **Chronic prostatitis/chronic pelvic pain syndrome** is
    the most common but least understood form of prostatitis. It
    is found in men of any age, its symptoms go away and then
    return without warning, and it may be inflammatory or non-
    inflammatory. In the inflammatory form, urine, semen, and
    other fluids from the prostate show no evidence of a known in-
    fecting organism but do contain the kinds of cells the body
    usually produces to fight infection. In the noninflammatory
    form, no evidence of inflammation, including infection-fighting
    cells, is present.

4. **Asymptomatic inflammatory prostatitis** is the diagnosis when the patient does not complain of pain or discomfort but has infection-fighting cells in his semen. Doctors usually find this form of prostatitis when looking for causes of infertility or testing for prostate cancer.

Antibiotics will not help nonbacterial prostatitis. You may have to work with your doctor to find a treatment that's good for you. Changing your diet or taking warm baths may help. Your doctor may give you a medicine called an alpha blocker to relax the muscle tissue in the prostate. No single solution works for everyone with this condition.

Additional Information

American Urological Association
1000 Corporate Blvd., Suite 410
Linthicum, MD 21090
Toll-Free: 866-746-4282
Phone: 410-689-3700
Fax: 410-689-3800
Website: http://www.urologyhealth.org

National Kidney and Urologic Diseases Information Clearinghouse
3 Information Way
Bethesda, MD 20892–3580
Toll-Free: 800-891-5390
Fax: 703-738-4929
Website: http://kidney.niddk.nih.gov
E-mail: nkudic@info.niddk.nih.gov

Chapter 27

Reproductive Health Trends among Adolescents

Adolescent Pregnancy Rates Have Decreased to Record Lows

There has been a substantial decline in adolescent pregnancy over the last decade. The 1999 pregnancy rate is the lowest since data collection for ages 15–19 began in 1972 (Henshaw, 2003). About one in five sexually active adolescents becomes pregnant each year (Darroch and Singh, 1999). About 846,000 teenagers aged 15–19 became pregnant in 1999, a decrease from more than 1,000,000 in 1990. Birth rates also decreased in the 1990s, while abortion rates declined significantly (Ventura et al., 2003).

Adolescents' Initiation of Sexual Activity Has Declined during the Past Decade

The percentage of high school students who reported initiation of sexual activity decreased from 54.1% in 1991 to 45.6% in 2001. Rates declined for all racial/ethnic groups: between 1991 and 2001, the percentage of Black non-Hispanic high school students who

Reprinted with permission of the National Adolescent Health Information Center 2003. Fact Sheet on Reproductive Health of Adolescents and Young Adults, San Francisco, CA. University of California, San Francisco. Also, "Trends in the Prevalence of Sexual Behaviors," Centers for Disease Control and Prevention (CDC), 2003.

reported being sexually experienced declined from 81.4% to 60.8%. For Hispanic and White non-Hispanic students, these figures were 53.1% to 48.4%, and 50.0% to 43.2%, respectively (Brener et al., 2002).

Male and Black Students Report Sexual Activity at an Earlier Age Than Their Peers

Male students report sexual activity at an earlier age, with females reporting similar rates by their senior year. Black non-Hispanic students report first sexual intercourse at earlier ages. Almost two-thirds of 9th grade Black non-Hispanic males have had sexual intercourse, compared to about half of their Hispanic and one-third of their White non-Hispanic peers. Black non-Hispanic female students are also more likely to have had sexual intercourse than their peers. By 12th grade the overall gender and race/ethnicity gaps decrease significantly (YRBSS, 2003a).

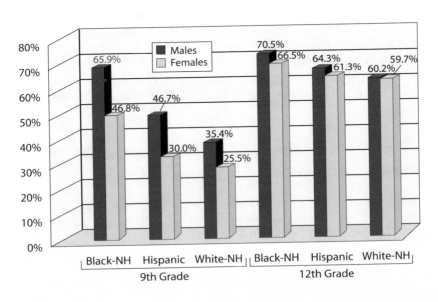

Figure 27.1. Sexual Intercourse Experience by Race/Ethnicity, Gender, and Grade Level, 2001* (*NH=non Hispanic; AI/AN=American Indian/Alaskan Native; A/PI=Asian/Pacific Islander)

214

Almost Three-Fifths of Sexually Active Students Use Condoms

Among sexually active high school students, condom use at last intercourse rose from 46.2% in 1991 to 57.9% in 2001. Black non-Hispanic students were more likely to report condom use than White non-Hispanic and Hispanic students. By contrast, sexually active White non-Hispanic students are two to three times more likely to report using oral contraceptive pills than their Black non-Hispanic and Hispanic peers (Grunbaum et al., 2002). Data from 1995 show that Black non-Hispanic female teenagers were over three times more likely to use implant or injectable contraception than their White non-Hispanic peers (16% vs. 5%) (Abma and Sonenstein, 2001).

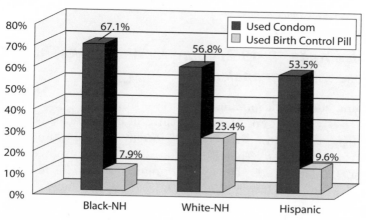

Figure 27.2. *Use of Condoms and Birth Control Pills by Race/Ethnicity, High School Students, 2001*

White Adolescent Females Have a Lower Rate of Pregnancy Than Their Black and Hispanic Peers

White non-Hispanic females ages 15–19 have lower rates of pregnancy than their Hispanic and Black non-Hispanic peers. Between 1991 and 1999, pregnancy rates declined most markedly for Black non-Hispanic and White non-Hispanic adolescents, while declines were more modest for Hispanic adolescents. As figures in the graph indicate, Black non-Hispanic and Hispanic adolescents continue to become pregnant at a rate greater than two times that of White non-Hispanic adolescents (Ventura et al., 2003).

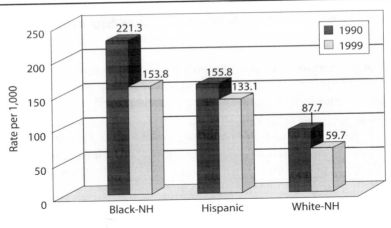

Figure 27.3. *Pregnancy Rates by Race/Ethnicity, Ages 15–19, 1990 and 1999*

Females Ages 18–19 Account for about Two-Thirds of Adolescent Pregnancies

Among adolescent females, about two-thirds of pregnancies occur in the 18–19 age group. About one-third of pregnancies occur in the 15–17 age group and a little over 2% occur in the 14 and under age group. Pregnancy rates (per 1,000) for all three age groups decreased between 1990 and 1999. The overall pregnancy rate for females ages 15–19 fell from 116.9 in 1990 to 85.6 in 1999, the lowest level since data collection began in 1972 (Henshaw, 2003). Similarly, the percentage of high school males who reported they got someone pregnant decreased from 5.3% in 1991 to 4.0% in 2001 (YRBSS, 2003b).

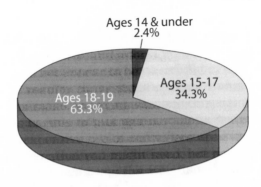

Figure 27.4. *Pregnancy among Females by Age Group, Ages 15–19, 1999*

Abortion Rates and Birth Rates Have Declined in the Past Decade

During the 1990s, birth and abortion rates fell among adolescents ages 15–19. Between 1991 and 2001, the adolescent birth rate (per 1,000) fell 26%, from 60.3 to 45.3 (Henshaw, 2003). Black non-Hispanic and White non-Hispanic adolescents experienced the steepest declines, while declines were smaller for Hispanic, American Indian/Alaskan Native, and Asian/Pacific Islander adolescents (Martin et al., 2003). With a 39% decrease, the adolescent abortion rate (per 1,000) fell even more steeply, going from 40.5 in 1990 to 24.7 in 1999. Abortion rates are higher for Black non-Hispanic (58.1) and Hispanic (32.1) adolescents than for White non-Hispanic (15.5) (Ventura et al., 2003). Because the decline in abortion rates is greater than the decline in birth rates, a greater proportion of adolescent pregnancies ended in birth than abortion (Henshaw, 2003).

Eighty Percent of Births among Adolescents Occur among Unmarried Females

Out-of-wedlock births account for four in five births (80%) to adolescents ages 15–19 a figure that varies significantly by race/ethnicity. Among children born to Black non-Hispanic adolescents, 95.9% were born out of wedlock, compared to 75.4% and 73.9% for White non-Hispanic and Hispanic adolescents, respectively. The racial/ethnic disparity for out-of-wedlock births is larger among older adolescents than younger adolescents (Martin et al., 2003).

About Four in Ten Black Male Students Have Had Sex with Four or More People during Their Lifetime

In 2001, nearly 40% of Black non-Hispanic male students reported having four or more sex partners during their lifetime, a decrease from 58.8% in 1993. Male students are 1.5 times more likely to report this behavior than their female peers (Grunbaum et al., 2002; Kann et al., 1995). Adolescents and young adults are more likely than other age groups to have multiple sex partners, to engage in unprotected sex, and, for young women, to choose sexual partners older than themselves, all of which are risk factors for sexually transmitted infections among adolescents (CDC, 2000).

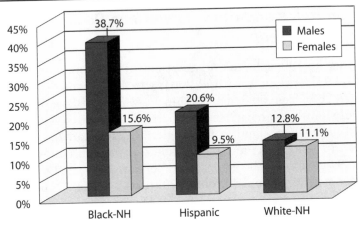

Figure 27.5. Four or More Sex Partners during Lifetime by Race/Ethnicity and Gender, High School Students, 2001

Prevalence of Chlamydia Is Over Six Times Higher for Female Adolescents Than Their Male Peers

The chlamydia rate (per 100,000) for females ages 15–19 is 6.4 times that of same-age males (2,626.4 vs. 411.7). Black non-Hispanic female adolescents have the highest rates of chlamydia: two to nine times that of same-age females in other racial/ethnic groups and five times that of same-age Black non-Hispanic males (CDC, 2003). Overall, chlamydia rates for adolescents have increased from 1080.8 in 1996 to 1488.3 in 2002 (CDC, 2001; CDC, 2003).

Note: Increased screening and testing for sexually transmitted infections (STI) may affect the trend of increased rates of STI among adolescents.

Black Female Adolescents Have the Highest Prevalence of Gonorrhea

Gonorrhea is less prevalent than chlamydia; the rate of gonorrhea is a third that of chlamydia. The gonorrhea rate (per 100,000) for Black non-Hispanic female adolescents ages 15–19 is 5 to 31 times that of same-age females in other racial/ethnic groups and twice that of same-age Black non-Hispanic males. Although the prevalence of gonorrhea among Black non-Hispanic adolescents declined from 2924.9 in 1996 to 2484.9 in 2002, this group accounted for more than three-quarters of all reported adolescent cases in 2002 (CDC, 2001; CDC, 2003).

218

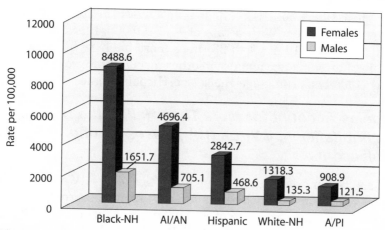

Figure 27.6. *Chlamydia Rates by Race/Ethnicity and Gender, Ages 15–19, 2002*

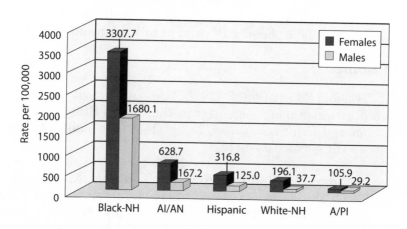

Figure 27.7. *Gonorrhea Rates by Race/Ethnicity and Gender, Ages 15–19, 2002*

Black Female Adolescents Have the Highest Rates of Syphilis, a Less Common Disease

Syphilis (primary and secondary) is relatively uncommon among adolescents: gonorrhea and chlamydia are 280 and 875 times more prevalent, respectively. Syphilis rates (per 100,000) decreased from 6.1 in 1996 to 1.7 in 2002 (CDC, 2001; CDC, 2003). As with chlamydia and gonorrhea, Black non-Hispanic female adolescents have higher rates of syphilis infection. With a rate of 11.3/100,000, Black non-Hispanic females ages 15–19 are 7 to 28 times more likely to be infected with syphilis than same-age females in other racial/ethnic groups, and about twice as likely as same-age Black non-Hispanic males (CDC, 2003).

Females Account for More Than Half of the Human Immunodeficiency Virus (HIV) Cases among Adolescents

Females comprise an increasing proportion of all HIV and AIDS cases among youth. Among adolescents ages 13–19, females comprise 57% of new HIV infections and 48% of new AIDS cases reported in 2001. Adolescents ages 13–19 account for 3.8% of all cumulative HIV cases and 0.5% of all AIDS cases. Among adolescents and young adults (ages 13–24), Black non-Hispanic account for over half (56%) of all HIV cases and 44% of all AIDS cases ever reported for this age group. While men account for 71% of AIDS cases among young adults ages 20–24, they only account for about 60% of new HIV cases in this age group (CDC, 2002).

Data Sources:

Abma, J. C., and Sonenstein, F. L. (2001). Sexual activity and contraceptive practices among teenagers in the United States, 1988 and 1995. *Vital and Health Statistics*, 23(21), 1–79. [Available at (12/03): http://www.cdc.gov/nchs/nsfg.html]

Brener, N., Lowry, R., Kann, L., Kolbe, L., Lehnherr, J., Janssen, R., et al. (2002). Trends in sexual risk behaviors among high school students-United States, 1991–2001. *Morbidity and Mortality Weekly Report*, 51(38), 856–859. [Available at (12/03): http://www.cdc.gov/mmwr/preview/mmwrhtml/mm5138a2.html]

Centers for Disease Control and Prevention [CDC]. (2000). *Tracking the hidden epidemics: Trends in STDs in the United States, 2000*. Atlanta, GA: Author, National Center for HIV, STD and TB Prevention, Division of Sexually Transmitted Diseases. [Available at (12/03): http://www.cdc.gov/nchstp/dstd/Stats_Trends/Trends2000.pdf]

Centers for Disease Control and Prevention [CDC]. (2001). *Sexually transmitted disease surveillance report, 2000*. Atlanta, GA: Author, National Center for HIV, STD and TB Prevention, Division of

Sexually Transmitted Diseases. [Available at (12/03): http://www.cdc .gov/nchstp/dstd/Stats_Trends/Stats_and_Trends.htm]

Centers for Disease Control and Prevention [CDC]. (2002). *HIV/AIDS surveillance report, 2001*. Atlanta, GA: Author, National Center for HIV, STD, and TB Prevention, Division of HIV/AIDS Prevention. [Available at (12/03): http://www.cdc.gov/hiv/stats/hasr1302.htm]

Centers for Disease Control and Prevention [CDC]. (2003). *Sexually transmitted disease surveillance report, 2002*. Atlanta, GA: Author, National Center for HIV, STD and TB Prevention, Division of Sexually Transmitted Diseases. [Available at (12/03): http://www.cdc.gov/ nchstp/dstd/Stats_Trends/Stats_and_Trends.htm]

Darroch, J. E., and Singh, S. (1999). *Why is teenage pregnancy declining? The roles of abstinence, sexual activity, and contraceptive use* (Occasional Report No. 1). New York: The Alan Guttmacher Institute. [Available at (12/03): http://www.agi-usa.org/pubs/or_teen_preg_decline.html]

Grunbaum, J. A., Kann, L., Kinchen, S. A., Williams, B., Ross, J. G., Lowry, R., et al. (2002). Youth Risk Behavior Surveillance-United States, 2001. *Morbidity and Mortality Weekly Report*, 51(No. SS-4), 1–62. [Available at (12/03): http://www.cdc.gov/mmwr/PDF/ss/ss5104.pdf]

Henshaw, S. K. (2003). *U.S. teenage pregnancy statistics*. New York: Alan Guttmacher Institute. [Available at (12/03): http://www .agi-usa.org/ pubs/teen_stats.pdf]

Kann, L., Warren, C. W., Harris, W. A., Collins, J. L., Douglas, K. A., Collins, M. E., et al. (1995). Youth Risk Behavior Surveillance-United States, 1993. *Morbidity and Mortality Weekly Report*, 44(No. SS-1), 1–55. [Available at (12/03): http://www.cdc.gov/nccdphp/dash/yrbs/ MMWR_summaries.htm]

Martin, J. A., Hamilton, B. E., Sutton, P. D., Ventura, S. J., Menacker, F., and Munson, M. L. (2003). Births: Final data for 2002. *National Vital Statistics Reports*, 52(10), 1–114. [Available at (12/03): http:// www.cdc.gov/nchs/data/nvsr/nvsr52/nvsr52_10.pdf]

Ventura, S. J., Abma, J. C., Mosher, W. D., and Henshaw, S. (2003). Revised pregnancy rates, 1990–1997, and new rates for 1998–99: United States. *National Vital Statistics Reports*, 52(7), 1–15. [Available at (12/ 03): http://www.cdc.gov/nchs/data/nvsr/nvsr52/nvsr52_07.pdf]

Table 27.1. Trends in the Prevalence of Sexual Behaviors, 1991–2003, U.S.

	1991	1993	1995	1997	1999	2001	2003	Changes from 1991–2003[1]	Change from 2001–2003[2]
Ever had sexual intercourse	54.1	53.0	53.1	48.4	49.9	45.6	46.7	Decreased, 1991–2003	No change
Had four or more sex partners during lifetime	8.7	18.7	17.8	16.0	16.2	14.2	14.4	Decreased, 1991–2003	No change
Currently sexually active (Had sexual intercourse during the three months preceding the survey.)	37.5	37.5	37.9	34.8	36.3	33.4	34.3	No change 1991–2003	No change
Condom use during last sexual intercourse (Among currently sexually active students.)	46.2	52.8	54.4	56.8	58.0	57.9	63.0	Increased 1991–2003	Increased
Birth control pill use before last sexual intercourse (Among currently sexually active students.)	20.8	18.4	17.4	16.6	16.2	18.2	17.0	Decreased, 1991–1999; No change, 1999–2003	No change
Alcohol or drug use before last sexual intercourse (Among currently sexually active students.)	21.6	21.3	24.8	24.7	24.8	25.6	25.4	Increased, 1991–2003	No change
Taught about AIDS or HIV infection in school	83.3	86.1	86.3	91.5	90.6	89.0	87.9	Increased, 1991–1997; Decreased, 1997–2003	No change

[1]Based on linear and quadratic trend analyses using a logistic regression model controlling for sex, race/ethnicity, and grade.
[2]Based on T-test analyses.

Youth Risk Behavior Surveillance System [YRBSS], Division of Adolescent and School Health, Centers for Disease Control and Prevention. (2003a). YRBS 2001, *Data and documentation files* [Private data run]. [Available at (12/03): http://www.cdc.gov/nccdphp/dash/yrbs/data/index.htm]

Youth Risk Behavior Surveillance System [YRBSS], Division of Adolescent and School Health, Centers for Disease Control and Prevention. (2003b). *Youth 2001 Online* [Online Database]. [Available at (12/03): http://www.cdc.gov/nccdphp/dash/yrbs/2001/youth01online.htm]

In all cases, the most recent available data were used. Some data are released one to three years after collection. For questions regarding data sources or availability, please contact the National Adolescent Health Information Center (NAHIC). For racial/ethnic data, the category names presented are those of the data sources used. Every attempt was made to standardize age ranges. When this was not possible, age ranges were those of the data sources used.

Trends in the Prevalence of Sexual Behaviors, National Youth Risk Behavior Survey: 1991–2003

What is the National Youth Risk Behavior Survey (YRBS)?

The national YRBS monitors priority health risk behaviors that contribute to the leading causes of death, disability, and social problems among youth and adults in the United States. The national YRBS is conducted every two years during the spring semester and provides data representative of 9th through 12th grade students in public and private schools throughout the United States.

Additional Information

National Adolescent Health Information Center
School of Medicine
University of California, San Francisco
UCSF Box 0503
San Francisco, CA 94143-0503
Phone: 415-502-4856
Fax: 415-502-4858
Website: http://nahic.ucsf.edu
E-mail: nahic@ucsf.edu

Healthy Youth

Centers for Disease Control and Prevention (CDC)
P.O. Box 8817
Silver Spring, MD 20907
Toll-Free: 888-231-6405
Toll-Free TTY: 888-232-6348
Website: http://www.cdc.gov/healthyYouth
E-mail: CDC-INFO@cdc.gov

Chapter 28

Sexually Transmitted Diseases (STDs)

Chapter Contents

Section 28.1

Commonly Asked Questions about STDs

U.S. Department of Health and Human Services: Office of Public Health and Science—Office of Population Affairs, March 2003.

What is an STD?

STD stands for sexually transmitted disease. These infections are passed from person to person during sexual activity (vaginal, oral, or anal intercourse). Some infections are curable, while others are not. It is estimated that more than 15 million new cases of STDs occur in the U.S. each year. Approximately one-quarter (3.75 million) of the new cases occur among teenagers.

Who can get an STD?

Anyone who engages in sexual activity.

How do I know if I have an STD?

Since many STDs do not have any obvious symptoms, the only sure way to know is by having a medical exam and lab tests.

Do latex condoms protect you from getting an STD?

For sexually active people, the most effective strategy for reducing the risk of STDs and preventing human immunodeficiency virus/acquired immune deficiency syndrome (HIV/AIDS) is correct and consistent use of latex condoms. However, research shows that condoms may not provide as much protection against some STDs such as human papillomavirus (HPV) also called genital warts. Abstinence—not having sex—is the only 100% sure way to avoid an STD.

Who can I talk to?

A parent, teacher, school nurse, family doctor, clergyman, or other responsible adult.

Health Consequences of STDs

Gonorrhea and Chlamydia: These STDs can cause serious health problems if not diagnosed and treated early. Specific health problems include:

- pelvic inflammatory disease (PID) which can damage fallopian tubes and make it difficult or impossible to have a baby (infertility);

- chronic pain in the lower abdomen;

- tubal pregnancy (also called ectopic pregnancy)—a condition where the pregnancy grows in the fallopian tube rather than the uterus. It is dangerous and requires immediate medical care.

HPV (genital warts): Infection with some types of HPV has been linked to cancer of the cervix.

Syphilis: This STD can cause blindness, heart disease, mental illness, joint damage, and death if not diagnosed and treated early.

HIV/AIDS: People who develop AIDS have severely weakened immune systems, which can lead to infections and death. STDs increase the risk of getting and transmitting HIV/AIDS. There is no cure for AIDS at this time.

Males who are infected with STDs can transmit the infection to their partners, who, if pregnant, can transmit the infection to their babies.

Common Myths

Myth: If I don't have symptoms, that means I don't have an STD.

Fact: You can be infected with an STD and not know it. The only sure way to know if you have an STD is by having a medical exam and lab tests.

Myth: HIV/AIDS is the only STD that can't be cured.

Fact: STDs caused by viruses—genital herpes, genital warts, and HIV/AIDS—cannot be cured, although some medications may reduce the severity and/or delay the appearance of symptoms.

STDs caused by bacteria (like chlamydia, gonorrhea, and syphilis) can usually be cured with antibiotics. If they are not treated early, serious long-term problems, like pain and infertility, can develop.

Symptoms of Common STDs

If you experience any of the following symptoms, go to a doctor or clinic as soon as possible.

- Chlamydia symptoms include:
  - no symptoms for three-quarters of infected women and half of infected men
  - discharge from the genital organs
  - burning with urination
  - in women, lower abdominal and/or back pain; pain during intercourse

- Gonorrhea symptoms include:
  - discharge from the genital organs
  - burning or itching during urination
  - pelvic pain
  - frequently no symptoms in females

- Syphilis causes painless sores on genitals (ten days to three months after infection) followed by a rash (3–6 weeks after sores appear).
- HIV/AIDS (human immunodeficiency virus/acquired immune deficiency syndrome) may have no symptoms appear for years until symptoms of AIDS occur.
- HPV (human papillomavirus) causes genital warts (sometimes warts are not visible).
- Genital herpes causes itching, burning, or pain in the genital area, and/or blisters or sores (sores always heal but can reappear throughout your life).

How can I prevent an STD?

Abstinence (not having vaginal, anal, or oral sex) is the best and only 100 percent effective way to prevent getting a sexually transmitted disease. Only having sex with one person who has been tested for STDs is the next best way to prevent getting HIV/AIDS and other STDs. Teens who choose to have multiple sexual partners should always use latex condoms. Latex condoms can help protect against STDs and HIV/AIDS, but they do not provide perfect protection against all STDs. To those teens involved in high-risk behaviors and relationships and to those who may have relations with high-risk populations, the message is: the latex condom is the only contraception method that may protect against some STDs, including HIV/AIDS.

If I am taking birth control pills, can I still get an STD?

Yes. Birth control pills only protect against pregnancy, not STDs. People who take birth control pills or use hormonal injections, implants, or patches to prevent pregnancy should also use latex condoms to reduce the risk for getting an STD, including HIV/AIDS.

What should I do if I think I have an STD?

If you think you have been exposed to an STD, you should go to a clinic or doctor as soon as possible to be tested and treated. Health departments, which diagnose and treat STDs, are located in almost every county and city. They provide confidential information and will help answer any questions you may have about STDs.

When should I have a checkup?

All sexually active teens should be seen by a health provider to be screened for STDs. Teens who have had sex with more than one person are at greater risk of getting an STD or HIV/AIDS.

Section 28.2

Human Immunodeficiency Virus/Acquired Immune Deficiency Syndrome (HIV/AIDS) among Youth

"HIV/AIDS among Youth: Fact Sheet," Centers for Disease Control and Prevention (CDC), May 2005.

Young people in the United States are at persistent risk for human immunodeficiency virus (HIV) infection. This risk is especially notable for youth of minority races and ethnicity. Continual prevention outreach and education efforts are required as new generations replace the generations that benefited from earlier prevention strategies. Unless otherwise noted, this section defines youth, or young people, as persons who are 13–24 years of age.

Statistics

Cumulative Effects of HIV Infection and Acquired Immune Deficiency Syndrome (AIDS) through 2003

- An estimated 38,490 young people in the United States received a diagnosis of AIDS. They accounted for about 4% of the 929,985 total estimated AIDS diagnoses.[1]

- An estimated 10,041 young people with AIDS died. They accounted for about 2% of the 524,060 total deaths of people with AIDS.[1]

- The proportion of young people with a diagnosis of AIDS increased. In 1999, 3.9% of all persons with a diagnosis of AIDS were aged 13–24. In 2003, 4.7% were aged 13–24.[1]

- According to data from the Centers for Disease Control and Prevention (CDC) reported through December 2001, African Americans were the largest group of young people affected by HIV. They accounted for 56% of all HIV infections ever reported among those aged 13–24.[2]

- Young men who have sex with men (MSM), especially those of minority races or ethnicity, were at high risk for HIV infection. In the seven cities that participated in CDC's Young Men's Survey during 1994–1998, 14% of African American MSM and 7% of Hispanic MSM aged 15–22 were infected with HIV.[3]

AIDS in 2003

- An estimated 2,050 young people received a diagnosis of AIDS (4.7% of the 43,171 estimated total with an AIDS diagnosis), and 237 young people with AIDS died.[1]

- An estimated 7,081 young people were living with AIDS, a 37% increase since 1999, when 5,159 young people were living with AIDS.[1]

- Young people who received a diagnosis of AIDS during 1995–2002 lived longer than persons with AIDS in any other age group except those who were younger than age 13. Nine years after receiving a diagnosis of AIDS, 72% of those aged 13–24 were alive, compared with 76% of those younger than age 13, 70% of those aged 25–34, 66% of those aged 35–44, 60% of those aged 45–54, and 50% of those aged 55 and older.[1]

HIV/AIDS in 2003

- An estimated 3,897 young people received a diagnosis of HIV/AIDS, representing about 12% of the persons given a diagnosis during that year.[1]

- In large proportions of young people who received a diagnosis of HIV infection—83% of those aged 15–24 and 78% of those aged 13–14—their infection did not progress to AIDS within 12 months. Of all persons given a diagnosis of HIV infection in the 33 areas with confidential name-based HIV reporting, 62% did not have AIDS within the first year after their HIV diagnosis.[1]

Risk Factors and Barriers to Prevention

Sexual Risk Factors

- **Heterosexual transmission.** Young women, especially those of minority races or ethnicity, are increasingly at risk for HIV infection through heterosexual contact. According to data from a CDC study of HIV prevalence among disadvantaged youth during the early to mid-1990s, the rate of HIV prevalence among young women aged 16–21 was 50% higher than the rate among young men in that age group.[4] African American women in this study were seven times as likely as white women and eight times as likely as Hispanic women to be HIV-positive. Young women are at risk for sexually transmitted HIV for several reasons, including biologic vulnerability, lack of recognition of their partners' risk factors, and having sex with older men who are more likely to be infected with HIV.

- **MSM.** Young MSM are at high risk for HIV infection, but their risk factors and the prevention barriers they face differ from those of persons who become infected through heterosexual contact. According to a CDC study of 5,589 MSM, 55% of young men (aged 15–22) did not let other people know they were sexually attracted to men.[5] MSM who do not disclose their sexual orientation are less likely to seek HIV testing, so if they become infected, they are less likely to know it. Because MSM who do not disclose their sexual orientation are likely to also have one or more female sex partners, MSM who become infected may transmit the virus to women as well as to men.

- **Sexually transmitted diseases (STDs).** The presence of an STD greatly increases a person's likelihood of acquiring or transmitting HIV.[6] Some of the highest STD rates in the country are those among young people, especially those of minority races and ethnicity.[7]

Substance Abuse

Young people in the United States use alcohol, tobacco, and other drugs at high rates.[8] Both casual and chronic substance users are more likely to engage in high-risk behaviors, such as unprotected sex, when they are under the influence of drugs or alcohol.[9] Runaways and other homeless young people are at high risk for HIV infection if they are exchanging sex for drugs or money.

Lack of Awareness

Research has shown that a large proportion of young people are not concerned about becoming infected with HIV.[10] Adolescents need accurate, age-appropriate information about HIV infection and AIDS, including the concept that abstinence is the only 100% effective way to avoid infection, how to talk with their parents or other trusted adults about HIV and AIDS, how to reduce and eliminate risk, how to talk with a potential partner about risk, where to get tested for HIV, and how to use a condom correctly.

Poverty and Out-of-School Youth

Nearly one in four African Americans and one in five Hispanics live in poverty.[11] Studies have found a direct relationship between higher AIDS incidence and lower income. In addition, studies have shown that the socioeconomic problems associated with poverty, including lack of access to high-quality health care, can directly or indirectly increase the risk for HIV infection.[12] Research has shown that young people who have dropped out of school are more likely to become sexually active at younger ages and to fail to use contraception.[13]

The Coming of Age of HIV-Positive Children

Many young people who contracted HIV through perinatal transmission are facing decisions about becoming sexually active. They will require ongoing counseling and prevention education to ensure that they do not transmit HIV.

Prevention

Following are some CDC prevention programs that state and local health departments and community-based organizations can provide for youth.

- Teens Linked to Care focuses on young people aged 13–29 who are living with HIV.

- Street Smart is an HIV/AIDS and STD prevention program for runaway and homeless youth.

- PROMISE (Peers Reaching Out and Modeling Intervention Strategies for HIV/AIDS Risk Reduction in their Community) is a community-level HIV prevention intervention that relies on role-model stories and peers from the community.

CDC research has shown that early, clear parent-child communication regarding values and expectations about sex is an important step in helping adolescents delay sexual initiation and make responsible decisions about sexual behaviors later in life. Parents have unique opportunities to engage their children in conversations about HIV, STDs, and teen pregnancy prevention because the discussions can be ongoing and timely.[14] Schools also can be important partners for reaching youth before high-risk behaviors are established.

References

1. CDC. *HIV/AIDS Surveillance Report, 2003*. Vol. 15. Atlanta: U.S. Department of Health and Human Services, CDC; 2004:1–40. Also available at http://www.cdc.gov/hiv/stats/2003surveillancereport.pdf. Accessed March 2, 2005.

2. CDC. *HIV Prevention in the Third Decade*. Atlanta: U.S. Department of Health and Human Services, CDC; 2003. Available at http://www.cdc.gov/hiv/HIV_3rdDecade/. Accessed August 16, 2004.

3. CDC. HIV incidence among young men who have sex with men—seven U.S. cities, 1994–2000. *MMWR* 2001; 50:440–444.

4. Valleroy LA, MacKellar DA, Karon JM, Janssen RS, Hayman DR. HIV infection in disadvantaged out-of-school youth: prevalence for U.S. Job Corps entrants, 1990 through 1996. *Journal of Acquired Immune Deficiency Syndromes* 1998; 19:67–73.

5. CDC. HIV/STD risks in young men who have sex with men who do not disclose their sexual orientation—six US cities, 1994–2000. *MMWR* 2003; 52:81–85.

6. Fleming DT, Wasserheit JN. From epidemiological synergy to public health policy and practice: the contribution of other sexually transmitted diseases to sexual transmission of HIV infection. *Sexually Transmitted Infections* 1999; 75:3–17.

7. CDC. *Sexually Transmitted Disease Surveillance*, 2003. Atlanta: U.S. Department of Health and Human Services, CDC; September 2004. Also available at http://www.cdc.gov/std/stats/toc2003.htm. Accessed March 3, 2005.

8. Substance Abuse and Mental Health Services Administration. *2003 National Survey on Drug Use & Health*. Available at http://www.oas.samhsa.gov/nhsda.htm. Accessed April 11, 2005.

9. Leigh B, Stall R. Substance use and risky sexual behavior for exposure to HIV: issues in methodology, interpretation, and prevention. *American Psychologist* 1993; 48:1035–1043.

10. The Kaiser Family Foundation. *National survey of teens on HIV/AIDS, 2000.* Available at http://www.kff.org/youthhivstds/loader.cfm?url=/commonspot/security/getfile.cfm&pageid=13570. Accessed March 3, 2005.

11. U.S. Census Bureau. *Poverty: 1999.* Census 2000 Brief. May 2003. Available at http://www.census.gov/prod/2003pubs/c2kbr-19.pdf. Accessed March 3, 2005.

12. Diaz T, Chu S, Buehler J, et al. Socioeconomic differences among people with AIDS: results from a multistate surveillance project. *American Journal of Preventive Medicine* 1994; 10:217–222.

13. Office of the Surgeon General. *The Surgeon General's call to action to promote sexual health and responsible sexual behavior, 2001.* Available at http://www.surgeongeneral.gov/library/sexualhealth/call.htm. Accessed March 3, 2005.

14. Dittus P, Miller KS, Kotchick BA, Forehand R. Why Parents Matter! The conceptual basis for a community-based HIV prevention program for the parents of African American youth. *Journal of Child and Family Studies* 2004; 13:5–20.

Additional Information

CDC National Prevention Information Network
P.O. Box 6003
Rockville, MD 20849-6003
Toll-Free: 800-458-5231
Toll-Free TTY: 800-243-7012
Fax/Fax-on-demand: 888-282-7681
Website: http://www.cdcnpin.org
E-mail: info@cdcnpin.org

Chapter 29

How to Avoid Teen Pregnancy

Chapter Contents

Section 29.1

Contraception

"What You Should Know about Contraception," U.S. Department of Health and Human Services (HHS), 2003; and excerpts from "Table 17," *Health, United States, 2005*, Centers for Disease Control and Prevention (CDC).

The Basics of Contraception

Contraception (also known as birth control) refers to the many different methods of preventing pregnancy. Abstinence from sexual activity until marriage is the only 100% sure contraception. Also, abstinent teens are not at risk for pregnancy or sexually transmitted disease (STD), including human immunodeficiency virus/acquired immune deficiency syndrome (HIV/AIDS). Teens who choose to be sexually active should remain faithful (not have sex with anyone else) to reduce the possibility of getting or giving someone an STD or HIV/AIDS. The latex condom is the only contraceptive method that may provide protection against some STD, including HIV/AIDS. Research shows that latex condoms may not be effective against some STD such as human papilloma virus (HPV—the virus that causes genital warts.)

Who needs contraception?

Anyone who has sex and does not want to get pregnant or get someone pregnant needs contraception. Any time you have sex, there is a risk of pregnancy. Not having sex—abstinence—is the only 100% sure way to avoid pregnancy.

Are some methods of contraception better than others at preventing pregnancy?

Yes. Abstinence is the only 100% sure way to not get pregnant. If you choose to have sex, know that some contraception methods are more effective than others, but no other method offers you total assurance. To be effective, whatever method you choose must be used correctly and consistently. Always read and follow the package instructions. It is a good idea to discuss this with your health provider.

Is the condom the only kind of contraception for males?

No. Vasectomy is a permanent method of contraception. But the condom is the most common method used by young males. Remember, the condom not only protects you from getting (or getting someone) pregnant, it may also provide protection against HIV/AIDS and some other STD.

How do I decide which method of contraception to use?

Your health care provider can help you decide which method is best for you. Remember, even if you are using a method like the pill, the latex condom is the only method that may provide some protection against HIV/AIDS and some STD.

Do I need a prescription to get contraception?

Latex condoms can be purchased without a prescription, but other methods require one. Even if you use a nonprescription method, it is a good idea to see a health care provider on a regular basis.

Hormonal Methods

Hormonal methods prevent pregnancy by interrupting the normal process for becoming pregnant. Hormonal methods do not protect against STD.

Emergency Contraception—Hormonal pills that are taken within 72 hours of unprotected sex or method failure (for example, the condom broke or you forgot to take your pill). Emergency contraception is the only method that can be used after having sex to prevent pregnancy.

Hormonal Implant—Small capsules inserted under the skin of a woman's upper arm that release small amounts of a hormone.

Hormonal Injection—A hormone injection (shot) that is injected into a woman's arm or buttock on a regular basis (every one to three months, depending on the hormones).

Hormonal Patch—A thin beige patch containing hormones that a woman applies to her skin once a week for three weeks. Hormones that prevent pregnancy are released during the time the patch is on.

The woman removes it for one week, during which time she has her period.

The Pill—A pill for women that must be taken at the same time every day.

Vaginal Ring—A ring containing hormones that a woman puts into her vagina and leaves there for three weeks. Hormones that prevent pregnancy are released for that time. The woman removes it for one week, during which time she has her period.

Barrier Methods

Barrier methods prevent sperm from reaching the egg.

Condom/Rubber—A cover for the penis or vagina. Latex condoms may provide protection against some STD, including HIV/AIDS.

Diaphragm/Cervical Cap—A shallow latex cup which the woman puts into her vagina, covering the cervix, before having sex. The diaphragm is generally used with a spermicidal jelly or cream that stops or kills sperm.

Other Contraceptive Methods

Abstinence—Not having vaginal, oral, or anal intercourse. Abstinence is the only 100% effective way to prevent pregnancy and STD, including HIV/AIDS.

Intra-Uterine Device (IUD)—An IUD is a small plastic device that is inserted into a woman's uterus by a trained clinician. Those used in the U.S. contain copper or hormones. This method is not generally recommended for teens, but is excellent for faithful married couples.

Natural Family Planning—Not having sex during the five or six days of the month when it is possible for the woman to get pregnant. Specialized training is essential for using this method.

Spermicide—A cream, foam, jelly, or insert which kills sperm. Spermicides do not protect against STD or HIV/AIDS. Nonoxynol-9, the most common spermicide, may increase the risk of HIV/AIDS in individuals who are at risk for an STD or HIV/AIDS.

Sterilization—A permanent, surgical form of contraception that blocks the fallopian tubes in women (tubal ligation) and the vas deferens in men (vasectomy).

Withdrawal—Removing the penis from the vagina before ejaculation. It may not prevent pregnancy, because some semen may leak before ejaculation.

Table 29.1. Contraceptive use and method of contraception among women 15–19 years of age by race, United States, 1982, 1988, 1995, 2002 (Data are based on household interviews of samples of women in the childbearing ages.)

Race, Hispanic origin, and year
Percent of women 15–19 years of age using contraception

	1982	1988	1995	2002
All women	24.2	32.1	29.8	31.5
White (Not Hispanic or Latino)	23.6	34.0	30.5	35.0
Black or African-American	29.8	35.7	36.1	23.9
Hispanic or Latino	*	*18.3	26.1	20.4

Method of contraception and year
Percent of women 15–19 years of age using this type of contraception

	1982	1988	1995	2002
Injectable[1]	N/A	N/A	9.7	13.9
Birth control pill	63.9	58.8	43.8	53.8
Condom	20.8	32.8	45.8	44.6
Withdrawal	2.9	3.0	13.2	15.0

*Estimates are considered unreliable. Data preceded by an asterisk have a relative standard error of 20–30 percent.

[1]Data collected starting the 1995 survey.

Source: Centers for Disease Control and Prevention, National Center for Health Statistics, National Survey of Family Growth.

Section 29.2

Facts about Sexual Abstinence

Information for Teens

- **Not everybody is doing it.** The percentage of high school males who have ever had sex declined from 57% in 1991 to 48% in 2003. The proportion of high school girls who reported having sex decreased from 51% in 1991 to 45% in 2001.[1]

- **Teens do not think it is embarrassing to say they are virgins.** The vast majority of teens (73%) surveyed recently do not think it is embarrassing for teens to say they are virgins.[2]

- **Most teens who have had sex wish they had waited.** Sixty-seven percent of teens surveyed who have had sexual intercourse wish they had waited longer. Of those who have had sex, more than one-half of teen boys (60%) and the great majority of teen girls (77%) said they wish they had waited longer to have sex.[3]

- **Teens say sex is not acceptable for high school-age teens.** Close to six in ten teens (58%) surveyed said sexual activity for high school-age teens is not acceptable, even if precautions are taken against pregnancy and sexually transmitted diseases.[4]

- **Teens say they should be given a strong abstinence message.** Ninety-four percent of teens say that it is important for teens to be given a strong message from society that they should abstain from sex until they are at least out of high school.[5]

- **Teens decide to delay becoming sexually active for many different reasons.** In one survey of teen girls, "values and morals" was the most common reason given. Others included wanting to avoid pregnancy and sexually transmitted diseases, or because they were waiting for the right partner.[6]

- **Teen males' approval of premarital sex is declining.** The proportion of adolescent males aged 17–19 who approve of premarital sex when a couple does not plan to marry decreased from 80% in 1988 to 71% in 1995.[7]

- **College freshmen are less likely to approve of casual sex.** A record low 40% of college freshmen (down from a record high of 52% in 1987) agree that "if two people really like each other, it's all right for them to have sex even if they've known each other for a very short time."[8]

References

1. Brener, N., Lowry, R., Kann, L., Kolbe, L., Lehnherr, J., Janssen, R., and Jaffe, H. (2002). Trends in sexual risk behaviors among high school students—United States, 1991-2001. *MMWR*, 51(38), 856-859. Centers for Disease Control and Prevention. (2004). Youth Risk Behavior Surveillance—United States, 2003. MMWR, 53(SS-2).

2. National Campaign to Prevent Teen Pregnancy. (2003). *With one voice: America's adults and teens sound off about teen pregnancy*. Washington, DC: Author.

3. National Campaign to Prevent Teen Pregnancy. (2003). *With one voice: America's adults and teens sound off about teen pregnancy*. Washington, DC: Author.

4. National Campaign to Prevent Teen Pregnancy. (2000). *The cautious generation? Teens tell us about sex, virginity, and "the talk."* Washington, DC: Author.

5. National Campaign to Prevent Teen Pregnancy. (2003). *With one voice: America's adults and teens sound off about teen pregnancy*. Washington, DC: Author.

6. Anderson Moore, K., Driscoll, A., and Duberstein Lindberg, L. (1998). *A statistical portrait of adolescent sex, contraception, and childbearing*. Washington, DC: The National Campaign to Prevent Teen Pregnancy.

7. Ku, L., et al (1998). Understanding changes in sexual activity among young metropolitan men: 1979–1995. *Family Planning Perspectives*, 30(6), 256–262.

8. UCLA. 27 Jan. 1999. College Freshmen: Acceptance of abortion, casual sex at all-time low. *Kaiser Daily Reproductive Health*

Report online. http://report.kff.org/archive/repro/1999/01/
kr990127.6.html.

Section 29.3

Advice from Teens

"Useful Tips–Thinking about the Right-Now," © 2002 The National
Campaign to Prevent Teen Pregnancy. Reprinted with permission. For
additional information, visit http://www.teenpregnancy.org.

When it comes to teen pregnancy—why it happens and how to prevent it—teens get loads of advice from adults, but they are not often asked to offer their own. Along with *Teen People* magazine, the National Campaign to Prevent Teen Pregnancy set out to change this by asking teens directly what they would say to other teens about preventing pregnancy.

The advice in this section is based on suggestions offered by readers of *Teen People*. The Campaign's own Youth Leadership team and teen visitors to the Campaign's website also played a key role in making these tips what they are.

As so many teens have made clear, the teen years should not be about pregnancy, parenting, midnight feedings, and diapers. We hope that you find these ideas useful—and perhaps see your own views and opinions reflected in them.

1. Thinking "it won't happen to me" is stupid; if you don't protect yourself, it probably will. Sex is serious. Make a plan.

2. Just because you think "everyone is doing it," doesn't mean they are. Some are, some aren't—and some are lying.

3. There are a lot of good reasons to say "no, not yet." Protecting your feelings is one of them.

4. You are in charge of your own life. Don't let anyone pressure you into having sex.

5. You can always say no—even if you've said yes before.

6. Carrying a condom is just being smart—it does not mean you are pushy or easy.

7. If you think birth control ruins the mood, consider what a pregnancy test will do to it.

8. If you are drunk or high, you cannot make good decisions about sex. Don't do something you might not remember or might really regret.

9. Sex will not make him yours, and a baby will not make him stay.

10. Not ready to be someone's father? It's simple: Use protection every time or do not have sex.

Section 29.4

Myths about Sex and Contraception

"You Can't Get Pregnant if You Do It Standing Up and Other Myths," © 2002 The National Campaign to Prevent Teen Pregnancy. Reprinted with permission. For additional information, visit http://www.teenpregnancy.org.

Myths about Getting Pregnant

You cannot get pregnant if:

- It's your first time.
- If you are both virgins.
- When the girl is having her period.
- If the guy pulls out before he ejaculates or if he doesn't go all the way in.
- If you have sex in a pool or hot tub.
- If the girl douches after sex.
- If both partners do not orgasm at the same time.
- If the girl jumps up and down after sex (to get all the sperm out).

- If the girl pushes really hard on her belly button after sex.
- If the girl takes a shower or bath right away.
- If the girl is on top during sex.
- If the guy drinks a two-liter Mountain Dew before sex (to kill the sperm).
- If the girl makes herself sneeze for fifteen minutes after sex.

Myths about Contraception

- Having contraception readily available makes you a slut (girls) or makes it look like you are expecting sex (boys).
- If you use birth control pills now, you will have trouble having kids later.
- It is okay to use your friend or sister's birth control pills.
- You can use plastic wrap if you do not have a condom.
- You only take birth control pills when you are going to have sex.
- Girls can get cancer if they are on the pill.
- After a certain point in the relationship you do not have to use condoms anymore.

Myths about Health and Sex

- Sex equals love and commitment.
- People cannot get sexually transmitted disease (STD) from having oral sex.
- If you use a tampon before you have sex, you are not a virgin anymore.
- A guy/girl will know if you are a virgin.
- If you stop having sex with a guy once he is aroused, he will be in serious pain.
- If you only have sex with healthy people, you do not need a condom.

Section 29.5

Tips to Help Your Teen Avoid Pregnancy

"Ten Tips for Parents to Help Their Children Avoid Teen Pregnancy," © 2002 The National Campaign to Prevent Teen Pregnancy; and excerpts from "Where and When Teens First Have Sex," © 2003 The National Campaign to Prevent Teen Pregnancy. Reprinted with permission. For additional information, visit http://www.teenpregnancy.org.

Tips for Parents

The National Campaign to Prevent Teen Pregnancy has reviewed recent research about parental influences on children's sexual behavior and talked to many experts in the field, as well as to teens and parents themselves. From these sources, it is clear that there is much parents and adults can do to reduce the risk of kids becoming pregnant before they have grown up.

Presented here as tips, many of these lessons will seem familiar because they articulate what parents already know from experience—like the importance of maintaining strong, close relationships with children and teens, setting clear expectations for them, and communicating honestly and often with them about important matters. Research supports these common sense lessons: not only are they good ideas generally, but they can also help teens delay becoming sexually active, as well as encourage those who are having sex to use contraception carefully.

Finally, although these tips are for parents, they can be used by adults more generally in their relationships with teenagers. Parents—especially those who are single or working long hours—often turn to other adults for help in raising their children and teens. If all these caring adults are on the same wavelength about the issues covered here, young people are given more consistent messages.

Be Clear about Your Own Sexual Values and Attitudes

Communicating with your children about sex, love, and relationships is often more successful when you are certain in your own mind about these issues. To help clarify your attitudes and values, think about the following kinds of questions:

247

- What do you really think about school-aged teenagers being sexually active—perhaps even becoming parents?

- Who is responsible for setting sexual limits in a relationship and how is that done, realistically?

- Were you sexually active as a teenager and how do you feel about that now? Were you sexually active before you were married? What do such reflections lead you to say to your own children about these issues?

- What do you think about encouraging teenagers to abstain from sex?

- What do you think about teenagers using contraception?

Talk with Your Children Early and Often about Sex, and Be Specific

Kids have lots of questions about sex, and they often say that the source they would most like to go to for answers is their parents. Start the conversation, and make sure that it is honest, open, and respectful. If you cannot think of how to start the discussion, consider using situations shown on television or in movies as conversation starters. Tell them candidly and confidently what you think and why you take these positions; if you are not sure about some issues, tell them that, too. Be sure to have a two-way conversation, not a one-way lecture. Ask them what they think and what they know so you can correct misconceptions. Ask what, if anything, worries them.

Age-appropriate conversations about relationships and intimacy should begin early in a child's life and continue through adolescence. Resist the idea that there should be just one conversation about all this—you know, the talk. The truth is that parents and kids should be talking about sex and love all along. This applies to both sons and daughters and to both mothers and fathers. All kids need a lot of communication, guidance, and information about these issues, even if they sometimes do not appear to be interested in what you have to say. And if you have regular conversations, you will not worry so much about making a mistake or saying something not quite right, because you will always be able to talk again.

Many inexpensive books and videos are available to help with any detailed information you might need, but do not let your lack of technical information make you shy. Kids need as much help in understanding the meaning of sex as they do in understanding how all the body parts work. Tell them about love and sex, and what the difference is.

And remember to talk about the reasons that kids find sex interesting and enticing; discussing only the downside of unplanned pregnancy and disease misses many of the issues on teenagers' minds.

Here are the kinds of questions kids say they want to discuss:

- How do I know if I am in love? Will sex bring me closer to my girlfriend/boyfriend?

- How will I know when I am ready to have sex? Should I wait until marriage?

- Will having sex make me popular? Will it make me more grown-up and open up more adult activities to me?

- How do I tell my boyfriend that I do not want to have sex without losing him or hurting his feelings?

- How do I manage pressure from my girlfriend to have sex?

- How does contraception work? Are some methods better than others? Are they safe?

- Can you get pregnant the first time?

In addition to being an approachable parent, be a parent with a point of view. Tell your children what you think. Do not be reluctant to say, for example:

- I think kids in high school are too young to have sex, especially given today's risks.

- Whenever you do have sex, always use protection against pregnancy and sexually transmitted disease until you are ready to have a child.

- Our family's religion says that sex should be an expression of love within marriage.

- Finding yourself in a sexually charged situation is not unusual; you need to think about how you will handle it in advance. Have a plan. Will you say no? Will you use contraception? How will you negotiate all this?

- It is okay to think about sex and to feel sexual desire. Everybody does! But it is not okay to get pregnant or get somebody pregnant as a teenager.

- One of the many reasons I am concerned about teens drinking is that it often leads to unprotected sex.

- (For boys) Having a baby does not make you a man. Being able to wait and acting responsibly does.

- (For girls) You do not have to have sex to keep a boyfriend. If sex is the price of a close relationship, find someone else.

Research clearly shows that talking with your children about sex does not encourage them to become sexually active. Also, remember that your own behavior should match your words. The "do as I say, not as I do" approach is bound to lose with children and teenagers, who are careful and constant observers of the adults in their lives.

Supervise and Monitor Your Children and Adolescents

Establish rules, curfews, and standards of expected behavior, preferably through an open process of family discussion and respectful communication. If your children get out of school at 3 p.m. and you do not get home from work until 6 p.m., who is responsible for making certain that your children are not only safe during those hours, but also are engaged in useful activities? Where are they when they go out with friends? Are there adults around who are in charge? Supervising and monitoring your kids' whereabouts does not make you a nag; it makes you a parent.

Know Your Children's Friends and Their Families

Friends have a strong influence on each other, so help your children and teenagers become friends with kids whose families share your values. Some parents of teens even arrange to meet with the parents of their children's friends to establish common rules and expectations. It is easier to enforce a curfew that all your child's friends share rather than one that makes him or her different—but even if your views do not match those of other parents, hold fast to your convictions. Welcome your children's friends into your home and talk to them openly.

Discourage Early, Frequent, and Steady Dating

Group activities among young people are fine and often fun, but allowing teens to begin steady, one-on-one dating much before age 16 can lead to trouble. Let your child know about your strong feelings about this throughout childhood—do not wait until your young teen proposes a plan that differs from your preferences in this area; otherwise, he or she will think you just do not like the particular person or invitation.

Discourage Significant Age Differences

Take a strong stand against your daughter dating a boy significantly older than she is. And do not allow your son to develop an intense relationship with a girl much younger than he is. Older guys can seem glamorous to a young girl—sometimes they even have money and a car to boot. But the risk of matters getting out of hand increases when the guy is much older than the girl. Try setting a limit of no more than a two- (or at most three-) year age difference. The power differences between younger girls and older boys or men can lead girls into risky situations, including unwanted sex and sex with no protection.

Encourage Future Options That Are More Attractive Than Early Parenthood

Help your teenagers to have options for the future that are more attractive than early pregnancy and parenthood. The chances that your children will delay sex, pregnancy, and parenthood are significantly increased if their future appears bright. This means helping them set meaningful goals for the future, talking to them about what it takes to make future plans come true, and helping them reach their goals. Tell them, for example, that if they want to be a teacher, they will need to stay in school in order to earn various degrees and pass certain exams. It also means teaching them to use free time in a constructive way, such as setting aside certain times to complete homework assignments. Explain how becoming pregnant—or causing pregnancy—can derail the best of plans; for example, child care expenses can make it almost impossible to afford college. Community service, in particular, not only teaches job skills, but can also put teens in touch with a wide variety of committed and caring adults.

Let Your Kids Know That You Value Education Highly

Encourage your children to take school seriously and set high expectations about their school performance. School failure is often the first sign of trouble that can end in teenage parenthood. Be very attentive to your children's progress in school and intervene early if things are not going well. Keep track of your children's grades and discuss them together. Meet with teachers and principals, guidance counselors, and coaches. Limit the number of hours your teenager gives to part-time jobs (20 hours per week should be the maximum) so that there is enough time and energy left to focus on school. Know about homework assignments and support your child in getting them done. Volunteer at the school, if possible. Schools want more parental involvement and will often try to accommodate your work schedule, if asked.

Know What Your Kids Are Watching, Reading, and Hearing

The media (television, radio, movies, music videos, magazines, the Internet) are chock full of material sending the wrong messages. Sex rarely has meaning, unplanned pregnancy seldom happens, and few people having sex ever seem to be married or even especially committed to anyone. Is this consistent with your expectations and values? If not, it is important to talk with your children about what the media portray and what you think about it. If certain programs or movies offend you, say so, and explain why. Be media literate—think about what you and your family are watching and reading. Encourage your kids to think critically: ask them what they think about the programs they watch and the music they hear. You can always turn the television off, cancel subscriptions, and place certain movies off limits. You will probably not be able to fully control what your children see and hear, but you can certainly make your views known and control your own home environment.

Build Strong Relationships

These tips for helping your children avoid teen pregnancy work best when they occur as part of strong, close relationships with your children that are built from an early age. Strive for a relationship that is warm in tone, firm in discipline, and rich in communication, and one that emphasizes mutual trust and respect. There is no single way to create such relationships, but the following habits of the heart can help:

- Express love and affection clearly and often. Hug your children, and tell them how much they mean to you. Praise specific accomplishments, but remember that expressions of affection should be offered freely, not just for a particular achievement.

- Listen carefully to what your children say and pay thoughtful attention to what they do.

- Spend time with your children engaged in activities that suit their ages and interests, not just yours. Shared experiences build a "bank account" of affection and trust that forms the basis for future communication with them about specific topics, including sexual behavior.

- Be supportive and be interested in what interests them. Attend their sports events; learn about their hobbies; be enthusiastic about their achievements, even the little ones; ask them questions that show you care and want to know what is going on in their lives.

- Be courteous and respectful to your children and avoid hurtful teasing or ridicule. Do not compare your teenager with other family members (for example: Why can't you be like your older sister?). Show that you expect courtesy and respect from them in return.

- Help them to build self-esteem by mastering skills; remember, self-esteem is earned, not given, and one of the best ways to earn it is by doing something well.

- Try to have meals together as a family as often as possible, and use the time for conversation, not confrontation.

It is never too late to improve a relationship with a child or teenager. Do not underestimate the great need that children feel—at all ages—for a close relationship with their parents and for their parents' guidance, approval, and support.

Where and When Teens First Have Sex

Almost half (46%) of high school-aged teens in the United States have had sexual intercourse. Because of continued concern about teenage sexual activity and support for messages that encourage young people to delay sexual debut, where and when teens first have sex is a matter of interest to those who run programs for teens, to policy makers, and to parents.

Location of First Sex

Two-thirds (68%) of 16 to 18-year-olds who reported a first sexual experience in 2000 report they first had sexual intercourse in their family home, their partner's family home, or a friend's house.

Gender and Location of First Sexual Experience

- One-quarter of sexually experienced teen males first have sex at home, compared to 18% of sexually experienced teen females. Almost four in ten teen females (39%) first have sex in their partner's home compared to 29% of teen males.

253

- Teen males were also more likely than teen females to have first sex in a friend's house (15% versus 8%).

- More than twice as many teen females as teen males had sex in their own or in a partner's own home, apartment, or dorm (17% versus 8%). This difference is mostly due to first sexual experience in a partner's own home, which may reflect older partners, on average, among females.

Table 29.2 Where 16–18 Year Olds First Have Sex

Location	Percent
Family's Home	22%
Partner's Family Home	34%
Friend's House	12%
Partner or Own Apt/Dorm/Home	12%
Car/Truck/Park	4%
Hotel/Motel	3%
Someplace Else	10%

Data: National Longitudinal Survey of Youth 1997 (NLSY97), Waves 1–4.

Timing of First Sex

Among teens who have had sex, more than two-thirds (70%) report they first had sexual intercourse in the evening or night.

Table 29.3. When 16–18 Year Olds First Have Sex

Time	Percent
7 a.m.–Noon	4%
Noon–3 p.m.	10%
3 p.m.–6 p.m.	15%
6 p.m.–10 p.m.	28%
10 p.m.–7 a.m.	42%

Data: National Longitudinal Survey of Youth 1997 (NLSY97), Waves 1–4.

Time of Day of First Sex Varies by Race/Ethnicity

- Among sexually experienced teens, African-Americans were more likely to first have sex during the late afternoon or after school hours of 3 p.m. to 6 p.m. (24%) than Hispanic (16%) and White teens (13%).

- Hispanic teens (23%) were more likely than African-American (12%) or White (14%) teens to report that their first sexual experience occurred during typical school-day hours (before 3 p.m.).

- More than two out of five White and African-American teens and about one-third of Hispanic teens first had sex between 10 p.m. and 7 a.m.

What Else Is Known About When Teens First Have Sex?

- When examining which month teens first have sex, there does not appear to be much difference between school year months (September–April) and summer months (June–August). For example, 28% of the sample reported first having sex during the summer months of June–August (or about one-third of the sample during one-third of the calendar year). However, June is the month of the year with the highest proportion of teens reporting that they first had sex (13.7%).

- Moreover, there are no significant differences in the time of day that teens report first having sex (for example, early morning, afternoon/school hours, evening, or night) among those who first had sex during the school year compared with those who first had sex during the summer months.

- While the study used in this brief uses a data set that did not include questions on day of the week first sex occurred, several small area data sets (not nationally representative) have looked at this issue. A recent study conducted in an urban, African-American school district found that 82.6% of sexually experienced youth reported that their most recent episode of sexual intercourse occurred at a time other than weekdays between 3 and 6 p.m.[1] An earlier study asked teen girls who had been diagnosed with a sexually transmitted disease (STD) to keep a diary of sexual activity, and found that over an average period of ten weeks, sex was most likely to occur on Friday or Saturday, and least likely to occur on Sunday.[2]

What It All Means

This research has several possible implications for those working with young people, policy makers, and parents and other caring adults (teachers, coaches, faith leaders).

- Parents and other caring adults need to be aware that adolescents' first sexual experience may very well occur when parents are in the home. Consequently, the primary message to parents is: Whether young people are at home, their partner's home, or the home of a friend, parents should be more aware of their activities. Parents should not be shy about making their presence known around the house. Parents should make sure that a responsible adult is present and paying attention when their children are at the home of a boyfriend/girlfriend or friend. Other research shows that the likelihood of first sexual experience increases with the number of hours teens spend unsupervised (Cohen et al., 2002). If parents or other responsible adults are not with teenagers, they should take advantage of adult-supervised activities that constructively engage teens.

- While parents clearly cannot determine their children's decisions about sex, the quality of their relationships with their children can make a real difference. Overall closeness between parents and their children, shared activities, parental presence in the home, and parental caring and concern are all associated with a reduced risk of early sex and teen pregnancy. (Blum and Rinhart 1998).

- Many program leaders have come to believe that teenage sexual activity primarily occurs in the unsupervised hours many teens have immediately after school. These data show that the after-school hours are not the time when most teens first initiate sexual activity. (Information is not available on where and when teens had their most recent sexual experience.) After-school programs may delay sexual activity by keeping teens engaged in programs during times when they may not otherwise be monitored. After-school and pregnancy prevention programs also have a role in helping teens make responsible decisions during non-program hours. In addition, there appears to be a need for supervised activities that occur after 6 p.m. Programs that offer game nights, dances, or sports activities provide teens with a supervised evening activity that may help delay early sexual debut.

References

1. Cohen, D.A., Farley, T.A., Taylor, S.N., Martin, D.H., and Schuster, M.A. (2002). When and where do youths have sex? The potential role of adult supervision. *Pediatrics*, 110(6). Online at http://www.pediatrics.org/cgi/content/full/110/ 6/e66.

2. Fortenberry, J.D., Orr, D.P., Zimet, G.D., and Blythe, M.J. (1997).Weekly and seasonal variation in sexual behaviors among adolescent women with sexually transmitted diseases. *Journal of Adolescent Health*, 20(6), 420–25.

Chapter 30

Teen Pregnancy

Chapter Contents

Section 30.1

Information for Teens Who Are Having a Baby

This information was provided by Teens Health, one of the largest resources online for medically reviewed health information written for parents, kids, and teens. For more articles like this one, visit www.teens Health.org, or www.KidsHealth.org. © 2004 The Nemours Center for Children's Health Media, a division of The Nemours Foundation.

Having a Healthy Pregnancy

If you're a pregnant teen, you're not alone. About half a million adolescents give birth each year. Most teens who have babies didn't plan on becoming pregnant. You may have been surprised when you found out or even hoped it wasn't true. You may have been terrified to tell your parents. You may have worried how this might affect your relationships with your family, friends, and the baby's father. Sharing the news of your pregnancy can be one of the most difficult conversations to have.

Whether you feel confused, worried, scared, or excited, you'll want to know how your life will change, what you can do to have a healthy baby, and what it takes to become a good parent. The most important thing you can do is to take good care of yourself so that you and your baby will be healthy. Girls who get the proper care and make the right choices have a very good chance of having healthy babies.

Prenatal Care

If you are pregnant, you need to see a doctor as soon as possible to begin getting prenatal care (medical care during pregnancy). The sooner you start to get medical care, the better your chances that you and your baby will be healthy.

If you can't afford to go to a doctor or clinic for prenatal care, there are social service organizations that can help you. Ask your parent, school counselor, or another trusted adult to help you locate resources in your community.

During your first visit, your doctor will ask you lots of questions including the date of your last period. This is so he or she can estimate how long you have been pregnant and your due date. Doctors measure pregnancies in weeks. It's important to remember that your due date is only an estimate: Most babies are born between 38 and 42 weeks after the first day of a woman's last menstrual period, or 36 to 38 weeks after conception (when the sperm fertilizes the egg). Only a small percentage of women actually deliver exactly on their due dates.

A pregnancy is divided into three phases, or trimesters. The first trimester is from conception to the end of week 13. The second trimester is from week 14 to the end of week 26. The third trimester is from week 27 to the end of the pregnancy.

The doctor will examine you and perform a pelvic exam. He or she will also perform blood tests, a urine test, and tests for sexually transmitted diseases (STDs), including a test for human immunodeficiency virus (HIV), which is on the rise in teens. (Some STDs can cause serious medical problems in newborns, so it's important to get treatment to protect the baby.)

The doctor will explain the types of physical and emotional changes you can expect during pregnancy. He or she will also teach you to how to recognize the signs of possible problems during pregnancy (called complications). This is especially important because teens are more at risk for certain complications such as anemia, high blood pressure, miscarriage, and delivering a baby earlier than usual (called premature delivery).

Your doctor will want you to start taking prenatal vitamins that contain the minerals folic acid, calcium, and iron as soon as possible. The vitamins may be prescribed by the doctor, or he or she may recommend a brand that you can buy over the counter. These vitamins and minerals help ensure the baby's and mother's health as well as prevent some types of birth defects.

Ideally, you should see your doctor once each month for the first 28 to 30 weeks of your pregnancy, then every two to three weeks until 36 weeks, then once a week until you deliver the baby. If you have a medical condition such as diabetes that needs careful monitoring during your pregnancy, your doctor will probably want to see you more often.

During visits, your doctor will check your weight, blood pressure, and urine, and will measure your abdomen to keep track of the baby's growth. Once the baby's heartbeat can be heard with a special device, the doctor will listen for it at each visit. Your doctor will probably also send you for some other tests during the pregnancy, such as an ultrasound, to make sure that everything is okay with your baby.

One part of prenatal care is attending classes where expectant mothers can learn about having a healthy pregnancy and delivery and the basics of caring for a new baby. These classes may be offered at hospitals, medical centers, schools, and colleges in your area.

It can be difficult for adults to talk to their doctors about their bodies and even more difficult for teens to do so. Your doctor is there to help you stay healthy during pregnancy and have a healthy baby— and there's probably not much he or she hasn't heard from expectant mothers. So don't be afraid to ask questions. Think of your doctor both as a resource and a friend who you can confide in about what's happening to you. And always be honest when your doctor asks questions about issues that could affect your baby's health.

Changes to Expect in Your Body

Pregnancy causes lots of physical changes in the body. Here are some common ones.

Breast Growth

An increase in breast size is one of the first signs of pregnancy, and the breasts may continue to grow throughout the pregnancy. You may go up several bra sizes during the course of your pregnancy.

Skin Changes

Don't be surprised if people tell you your skin is glowing when you are pregnant—pregnancy causes an increase in blood volume, which can make your cheeks a little pinker than usual. And hormonal changes increase oil gland secretion, which can give your skin a shinier appearance. Acne is also common during pregnancy for the same reason.

Other skin changes caused by pregnancy hormones may include brownish or yellowish patches on the face called chloasma and a dark line on the midline of the lower abdomen, known as the linea nigra. Also, moles or freckles that you had prior to pregnancy may become bigger and darker. Even the areola, the area around the nipples, becomes darker. Stretch marks are thin pink or purplish lines that can appear on your abdomen, breasts, or thighs. Except for the darkening of the areola, which is usually permanent, these skin changes will usually disappear after you give birth.

Mood Swings

It's very common to have mood swings during pregnancy. Some girls may also experience depression during pregnancy or after delivery. If you have symptoms of depression such as sadness, changes in sleep patterns, or bad feelings about yourself or your life for more than two weeks, tell your doctor so he or she can help you to get treatment.

Pregnancy Discomforts

Pregnancy can cause some uncomfortable side effects. These include nausea and vomiting, especially early in the pregnancy; leg swelling; varicose veins in the legs and the area around the vaginal opening; hemorrhoids; heartburn and constipation; backache; fatigue; and sleep loss. If you experience one or more of these side effects, keep in mind that you're not alone. Ask your doctor for advice on how to deal with these common problems.

Things to Avoid

Smoking, drinking, and taking drugs when you are pregnant put you and your baby at risk for a number of serious problems.

Alcohol

Doctors now feel that it's not safe to drink any amount of alcohol when you are pregnant. Drinking can harm a developing fetus, putting a baby at risk for birth defects and mental problems.

Smoking

The risks of smoking during pregnancy include stillbirths (when a baby dies while inside the mother), low birth weight (which increases a baby's risk for health problems), prematurity (when babies are born earlier than 37 weeks), and sudden infant death syndrome (SIDS). SIDS is the sudden, unexplained death of an infant who is younger than one year old.

Drugs

Using illegal drugs such as cocaine or marijuana during pregnancy can cause miscarriage, prematurity, and other medical problems. Babies can also be born addicted to certain drugs. Ask your doctor for help if you are having trouble quitting smoking, drinking, or drugs. Check with your doctor before taking any medication while you are pregnant, including over-the-counter medications, herbal remedies and supplements, and vitamins.

Table 30.1. Teenage childbearing, according to race and Hispanic origin of mother: United States, selected years 1980–2003.

Maternal age, race, and Hispanic origin of mother	1980	1990	2000	2003
Age of mother under 18 years	Percent of live births			
All races	5.8	4.7	4.1	3.4
White	4.5	3.6	3.5	3.0
Black or African American	12.5	10.1	7.8	6.6
American Indiana or Alaska Native	9.4	7.2	7.3	6.6
Asian or Pacific Islander	1.5	2.1	1.5	1.1
Chinese	0.3	0.4	0.2	*
Japanese	1.0	0.8	0.6	*
Filipino	1.6	2.0	1.6	*
Hawaiian	6.6	6.5	5.7	*
Other Asian or Pacific Islander	1.2	2.4	1.7	*
Hispanic or Latino	7.4	6.6	6.3	5.4
Mexican	7.7	6.9	6.6	5.8
Puerto Rican	10.0	9.1	7.8	6.9
Cuban	3.8	2.7	3.1	2.4
Central and South American	2.4	3.2	3.3	2.8
Other and unknown Hispanic or Latino	6.5	8.0	7.6	6.3
Age of mother 18–29 years	Percent of live births			
All races	9.8	8.1	7.7	6.9
White	9.0	7.3	7.1	6.4
Black or African American	14.5	13.0	11.9	10.7
American Indiana or Alaska Native	14.6	12.3	12.4	11.6
Asian or Pacific Islander	3.9	3.7	3.0	2.4
Chinese	1.0	0.8	0.7	*
Japanese	2.3	2.0	1.4	*
Filipino	4.0	4.1	3.7	*
Hawaiian	13.3	11.9	11.7	*
Other Asian or Pacific Islander	3.8	3.9	3.2	*
Hispanic or Latino	11.6	10.2	9.9	8.9
Mexican	12.0	10.7	10.4	9.5
Puerto Rican	13.3	12.6	12.2	11.0
Cuban	9.2	5.0	4.4	5.5
Central and South American6.0	5.9	6.5	5.6	
Other and unknown Hispanic or Latino	10.8	11.1	11.3	9.6

*Data not available.

Source: Excerpted from "Table 9" from *Health, United States 2005*, Centers for Disease Control and Prevention (CDC).

Unsafe Sex

Talk to your doctor about sex during pregnancy. If you are sexually active while you are pregnant, you must use a condom to help prevent getting an STD. Some STDs can cause blindness, pneumonia, or meningitis in newborns, so it's important to protect yourself and your baby.

Taking Care of Yourself during Pregnancy

Eating

Many girls worry about how their bodies look and are afraid to gain weight during pregnancy. But now that you are eating for two, this is not a good time to cut calories or go on a diet. Don't try to hide your pregnancy by dieting—both you and your baby need certain nutrients to grow properly. Eating a variety of healthy foods, drinking plenty of water, and cutting back on high-fat junk foods will help you and your developing baby to be healthy.

Doctors generally recommend adding about 250 calories a day to your diet to provide adequate nourishment for the developing fetus. Depending on your prepregnancy weight, you should gain about 25 to 35 pounds during pregnancy, most of this during the last six months. Your doctor will advise you about this based on your individual situation.

Eating additional fiber—20 to 30 grams a day—and drinking plenty of water can help to prevent common problems such as constipation. Good sources of fiber are fresh fruits and vegetables and whole-grain breads, cereals, or muffins.

Exercise

Exercising during pregnancy is good for you as long as you choose appropriate activities. Doctors generally recommend low-impact activities such as walking, swimming, and yoga. Contact sports and high-impact aerobic activities that pose a greater risk of injury should generally be avoided. Also, working at a job that involves heavy lifting is not recommended for women during the last trimester of pregnancy. Talk to your doctor if you have questions about whether particular types of exercise are safe for you and your baby.

Sleep

It's important to get plenty of rest while you are pregnant. Early in your pregnancy, try to get into the habit of sleeping on your side.

Lying on your side with your knees bent is likely to be the most comfortable position as your pregnancy progresses. Also, it makes your heart's job easier because it keeps the baby's weight from applying pressure to the large vein that carries blood back to the heart from your feet and legs.

Some doctors specifically recommend that girls who are pregnant sleep on the left side. Because your liver is on the right side of your abdomen, lying on your left side helps keep the uterus off that large organ. Ask what your doctor recommends—in most cases, lying on either side should do the trick and help take some pressure off your back.

Stress can interfere with sleep. Maybe you're worried about your baby's health, about delivery, or about what your new role as a parent will be like. All of these feelings are normal, but they may keep you up at night. Talk to your doctor if you are having problems sleeping during your pregnancy.

Emotional Health

It's common for pregnant teens to feel a range of emotions, such as fear, anger, guilt, and sadness. It may take a while to adjust to the fact that you're going to have a baby. It's a huge change, and it's natural for pregnant teens to wonder whether they're ready to handle the responsibilities that come with being a parent.

How a girl feels often depends on how much support she has from the baby's father, from her family (and the baby's father's family), and from friends. Each girl's situation is different. Depending on your situation, you may need to seek more support from people outside your family. It's important to talk to the people who can support and guide you and help you share and sort through your feelings. Your school counselor or nurse can refer you to resources in your community that can help.

School and the Future

Some girls plan to raise their babies themselves. Sometimes grandparents or other family members help. Some girls decide to give their babies up for adoption. It takes a great deal of courage and concern for the baby to make these difficult decisions.

Girls who complete high school are more likely to have good jobs and enjoy more success in their lives. If possible, finish high school now rather than trying to return later. Ask your school counselor or an adult you trust for information about programs and classes in your community for pregnant teens.

Some communities have support groups especially for teen parents. Some high schools have child-care centers on campus. Perhaps a family member or friend can care for your baby while you're in school.

Life takes unexpected turns. These changes often bring opportunities to learn and grow and develop new strengths. You can stay informed by reading books, attending classes, or checking out reputable websites on child-raising. Keep communications open in your own family and talk to your parents about this new phase in your life. Your baby's doctor, your parents, family members, or other adults can all help guide you while you are pregnant and when you become a parent.

Section 30.2

Adoption Options

"Are You Pregnant and Thinking of Adoption?" National Adoption Information Clearinghouse, 2000. Despite the date of this document, the guidelines described are still deemed pertinent.

If you are pregnant and not sure that you want to keep the baby, you might be thinking about adoption. Pregnancy causes many changes, both physical and emotional. It can be a very confusing time for a woman, even in the best of circumstances. Talking to a counselor about your options might help. But how do you start? This section gives you, the birth mother, information about counseling and adoption. It addresses many questions you might have:

Who can I talk to about my options?

If you want to talk to a professional about your options, there are different places you can go. Counseling at the places listed will be free or cost very little.

- Crisis pregnancy center—This is a place where they talk only to pregnant women. It might even have a maternity center attached where you could live until the baby is born.

- Family planning clinic—This is a place where women get birth control information or pregnancy tests.

- Adoption agency—This choice is good if you are already leaning strongly in the direction of adoption.

- Health Department or Social Services—A food stamps or welfare worker can tell you which clinic or department is the right one.

- Mental health center or family service agency—Counselors at these places help all kinds of people in all kinds of situations.

No matter where you go for counseling, a counselor should always treat you with respect. A counselor may have strong feelings about adoption, abortion, and parenting a child. Nevertheless, those feelings should not influence their professional advice nor the treatment provided to you. In order to make up your own mind, it is important for you to get clear answers from your counselor to these three questions:

- If I feel I cannot carry my pregnancy to term, how will you help me?

- If I decide to take care of my baby myself, how will you help me do that?

- If I want to place my baby for adoption, will you help me find an adoption agency or attorney who will listen to what I think is right for us?

If you are not happy with the answers you get, you may wish to find a counselor at another place. The National Adoption Information Clearinghouse can tell you about crisis pregnancy centers and adoption agencies in each State, and can also help you find other counseling agencies in your area.

Should I place my child for adoption?

The decision to place a child for adoption is a difficult one. It is an act of great courage and much love. Remember, adoption is permanent. The adoptive parents will raise your child and have legal authority for his or her welfare. You need to think about these questions as you make your decision.

Have I explored all possibilities?

Pregnancy can affect your feelings and emotions. Are you only thinking about adoption because you have money problems, or because your living situation is difficult? These problems might be temporary. Have you called Social Services to see what they can do, or asked friends and family if they can help? If you have done these things and still want adoption, you will feel more content with your decision.

Will the adoptive parents take good care of my child?

Prospective adoptive parents are carefully screened and give a great deal of information about themselves. They are visited in their home several times by a social worker and must provide personal references. They are taught about the special nature of adoptive parenting before an adoption takes place. By the time an agency has approved adoptive parents for placement, they have gotten to know them very well, and feel confident they would make good parents. This does not promise that they will be perfect parents, but usually decent people who really want to care for children.

Will my child wonder why I placed him (or her) for adoption?

Probably. Most adopted adults realize that their birth parents placed them for adoption out of love, and because it was the best they knew how to do. Hopefully, your child will come to realize that a lot of his or her wonderful traits come from you. And if you have an open adoption, it is likely that you will be able to explain to the child why you chose adoption.

Why am I placing my child for adoption?

If your answer is because it is what you, or you and your partner, think is best, then it is a good decision. Now it is time to move forward, and not feel guilty.

Different Types of Adoption

There are two types of adoptions, confidential and open.

Confidential: The birth parents and the adoptive parents never know each other. Adoptive parents are given background information about you and the birth father that they would need to help them take care of the child, such as medical information.

Open: The birth parents and the adoptive parents know something about each other. There are different levels of openness.

- Least open—You will read about several possible adoptive families and pick the one that sounds best for your baby. You will not know each other's names.

- More open—You and the possible adoptive family will speak on the telephone and exchange first names.

- Even more open—You can meet the possible adoptive family. Your social worker or attorney will arrange the meeting at the adoption agency or attorney's office.

- Most open—You and the adoptive parents share your full names, addresses, and telephone numbers. You stay in contact with the family and your child over the years, by visiting, calling, or writing each other. Fifteen States have enacted laws that recognize post-adoption contact between adoptive and birth families if the parties have voluntarily agreed to this plan.

Talk to your counselor about the type of adoption that is best for you. Do you want to help decide who adopts your child? Would you mind if a single person adopted your child, or a couple of a different race than you? Would you like to be able to share medical information with your child's family that may only become known in the future?

If you have strong feelings about these things, work with an agency or attorney who you feel will listen to what you want. If you do not have strong feelings about these things, the adoption agency or attorney will decide who adopts your child based on who they think can best care for the child.

Arranging an Adoption through an Agency

In all States, you can work with a licensed child placing (adoption) agency. In all but four States, you can also work directly with an adopting couple or their attorney without using an agency.

Private adoption agencies arrange most infant adoptions. There are several types of private adoption agencies. Some are for profit and some are nonprofit. Some work with prospective adoptive parents of a particular religious group, though they work with birth parents of all religions.

When you contact adoption agencies, ask the social workers as many questions as you need to ask so that you understand the agencies' rules. Some questions you will want to ask are:

- Will I get counseling all through my pregnancy, after I sign the papers allowing my child to be adopted, and after my baby is gone?

- Can my baby's father and other people who are important to me join me in counseling if they want to?

- What kind of financial help can I get? What kind of medical and legal help will I have? Can I get help with medical and legal expenses?

- What will I get to know about the people who adopt my baby? May I tell you what I think are important traits for parents to have? How do you know the adoptive parents are good people? May I meet them if I want, or know their names? Will I ever be able to have contact with them or my child? Will I ever know how my child turns out?

- What information will you provide to the adoptive parents about me and my family?

The agency social worker will ask you questions to find out some information about you and the baby's father, such as your medical histories, age, race, physical characteristics, whether you have been to see a doctor since you became pregnant, whether you have been pregnant or given birth before, and whether you smoked cigarettes, took any drugs, or drank any alcohol since you became pregnant. The social worker asks these questions so that the baby can be placed with parents who will be fully able to care for and love the baby, not so that she can turn you down.

Arranging a Private Adoption

An adoption arranged without an adoption agency is called an independent or private adoption. It is legal in all States except Connecticut, Delaware, Massachusetts, and Minnesota. With a private adoption, you need to find an attorney to represent you. Look for an attorney who will not charge you a fee if you decide not to place your baby for adoption. You also need to find adoptive parents. Here's how you find both of these.

Finding an Attorney

Legal Aid—This is a service available in most communities for people who cannot afford a private attorney. Sometimes it is located at a university law school. Note: Some States allow the adopting parents to pay your legal fees, so going to Legal Aid may not be necessary.

State Attorney Association or the American Academy of Adoption Attorneys—These groups can refer you to an attorney who handles adoptions in your area.

Finding Adoptive Parents

Personal Ads—Some newspapers carry personal ads from people seeking to adopt. You call the number in the ad and get to know each other over the telephone. If you think you want to work with the couple, have your attorney call their attorney. The attorneys will work out all the arrangements according to what you and the adoptive parents want and the laws of your State.

Your Doctor—He or she may know about couples who are seeking a child, and be able to help arrange the adoption.

Adoptive Parent Support Groups—Parents who have already adopted may know other people seeking to adopt.

National Matching Services—These services help birth parents and adoptive parents find one another.

Personal referrals—Ask friends and family if they know any adoption attorneys or possible adoptive parents.

Arranging for Possible Future Contact

If you decide on a confidential adoption, you may still wish to make sure that your child can contact you in the future. There are things you can do now to make that happen.

Many people who are adopted as children later want to meet their birth parents. With the exception of Alabama, Alaska, Delaware,

Kansas, Oregon, and Tennessee, State laws do not permit them to see their original birth certificate. Because of these problems, many States, and some private national organizations, have set up adoption registries to help people find one another.

A registry works like this: You leave the information about the birth of the child and your address and telephone number. You must keep your address and telephone number current. You can register at any time, even years after the child is born.

When your child is an adult, he or she can call or write this registry. If what the child knows about his or her birth matches what the registry has, the registry will release your current address and telephone number to the child, and you could be contacted.

There is another way to ensure that your child can contact you if he or she wishes. Some adoption agencies and attorneys who arrange private adoptions will hold a letter in their file in which you say why you chose adoption and how to get in touch with you if the child ever wants to. If the agency or attorney that you are working with will not agree to do this, you may wish to work with somebody else.

There are several national organizations that offer ongoing advice and support to birth parents, information about contact and reunion with their children, and many other things. People in these organizations have already gone through what you are going through. They will be very helpful and understanding if you need someone to talk to.

Additional Information

American Academy of Adoption Attorneys
P.O. Box 33053
Washington, DC 20033-0053
Phone: 202-832-2222
Website: http://www.adoptionattorneys.org
E-mail: info@adoptionattorneys.org

National Adoption Information Clearinghouse
Children's Bureau/ACYF
1250 Maryland Ave. SW, 8th Floor
Washington, DC 20024
Toll-Free: 888-251-0075
Phone: 703-352-3488
Fax: 703-385-3206
Website: http://naic.acf.hhs.gov
E-mail: NAIC@caliber.com

Concerned United Birthparents

P.O. Box 503475
San Diego, CA 92150-3475
Toll-Free: 800-822-2777
Toll-Free Fax: 866-589-9624
Fax: 858-712-3317
Website: http://www.cubirthparents.org

American Adoption Congress

P.O. Box 42730
Washington, DC 20015
Phone: 202-483-3399
Website: http://www.americanadoptioncongress.org

International Soundex Reunion Registry

P.O. Box 2312
Carson City, NV 89702
Phone: 775-882-7755
Website: http://www.isrr.net

Section 30.3

Terminating a Pregnancy

Reproduced with permission from "Ending Your Pregnancy," July 2005, http://familydoctor.org/846.xml. Copyright © 2005 American Academy of Family Physicians. All Rights Reserved.

What is abortion?

Abortion means ending a pregnancy. Most abortions are done in the first trimester (the first three months of the pregnancy). They are done by a doctor and other health care professionals in a hospital, doctor's office, or health center. There are two types of abortion: medical and surgical.

What is medical abortion?

It is an abortion caused by medicine. It can only be done in the first nine weeks of pregnancy. The medicine used for medical abortions is called mifepristone (brand name: Mifeprex). This is a pill that blocks progesterone, a hormone needed for pregnancy. It causes the lining of the womb (uterus) to thin.

After taking mifepristone, the woman goes home. She comes back to the doctor a few days later to take another medicine called misoprostol (brand name: Cytotec). This medicine makes the uterus contract and empty. Many women have bleeding for about 13 days after taking it. Light bleeding or discharge (called spotting) can continue for several weeks.

What does medical abortion feel like?

For most women, it feels like a bad menstrual period with strong cramps, diarrhea, and upset stomach. Acetaminophen (one brand name: Tylenol) or ibuprofen (one brand name: Motrin) can help the cramps. These symptoms are normal. However, the doctor will want to know if any of these occur:

- bleeding through more than two sanitary pads in an hour

- fever above 100 degrees for more than four hours

- pain even after taking acetaminophen or ibuprofen

How effective is medical abortion?

Mifepristone is about 97% effective. In rare cases when medical abortion does not work, surgical abortion may be tried.

What is surgical abortion?

It is a procedure done by a doctor to remove the lining of the womb. There are two common types: manual vacuum aspiration (MVA) and dilatation and suction curettage (D and C). They both use suction to empty the womb. MVA uses a handheld tool. D and C is done with a suction machine and tools.

MVA can be done in the first ten weeks of pregnancy. D and C can be done after the first month of pregnancy but before the end of the 13th week.

- For both types, medicine can be given to help the woman feel calm. Then the doctor injects the opening to the womb (cervix) with a medicine to make it numb. The cervix is stretched open with a tool called a dilator and the doctor inserts a tube. The uterus is emptied through this tube.

Table 30.2. Legal abortions by age, United States, 1980, 1990, 2000, and 2001

Data are based on reporting by State health departments and hospitals and other medical facilities.

	Abortions per 100 live births			
Age	1980	1990	2000	2001
Under 15 years	139.7	81.8	70.8	74.4
15–19 years	71.4	51.1	36.1	36.6
20–24 years	39.5	37.8	30.0	30.4
25–29 years	23.7	21.8	19.8	20.0
30–34 years	23.7	19.0	14.5	14.7
35–39 years	41.0	27.3	18.1	18.0
40 years and over	80.7	50.6	30.1	30.4

Source: Excerpted from Table 16, *United States Health, 2005*, Centers for Disease Control and Prevention.

What does surgical abortion feel like?

- For most women, it feels like strong menstrual cramps. Women are usually given medicine to help with the pain and told to rest when they get home. Acetaminophen or ibuprofen can also help. Bleeding may continue off and on for a few weeks.

How effective is surgical abortion?

It is nearly 100% effective.

Are abortions safe?

When done by health care professionals, both medical and surgical abortions are generally very safe. Serious complications are rare. Abortion generally does not reduce a woman's ability to get pregnant in the future.

Section 30.4

The Need to Prevent Teen Pregnancy

"Teen Pregnancy–So What?" © 2004 National Campaign to Prevent Teen Pregnancy. Reprinted with permission. For additional information, visit http://www.teenpregnancy.org.

The National Campaign to Prevent Teen Pregnancy, organized in 1996, is based on the concept that reducing the nation's rate of teen pregnancy is one of the most strategic and direct means available to improve overall child well-being and to reduce persistent child poverty. Teen pregnancy has serious consequences for the teen mother, the child, and to society in general.

Despite the recently declining teen pregnancy rates, 34% of teenage girls get pregnant at least once before they reach age 20, resulting in more than 820,000 teen pregnancies a year.[1, 2] At this level, the United States has the highest rate of teen pregnancy in the fully industrialized world.[3]

Teen Pregnancy Is Bad for the Mother

Decline of Future Prospects

Future prospects for teenagers decline significantly if they have a baby. Teen mothers are less likely to complete school and more likely to be single parents. Less than one-third of teens who begin their families before age 18 ever earn a high school diploma. Only 1.5% earn a college degree by the age of 30.[4]

Health Risks

There are serious health risks for adolescents who have babies. Common medical problems among adolescent mothers include poor weight gain, pregnancy-induced hypertension, anemia, sexually transmitted disease (STD), and cephalopelvic disproportion. Later in life, adolescent mothers tend to be at greater risk for obesity and hypertension than women who were not teenagers when they had their first child.[5]

A sixteen year-old mother relates: "I absolutely hate hearing everyone talk about that great party on the weekend or how they are going out of town over spring break. It seems that I am missing out on my childhood years. Where my daughter grows up and asks me what I did when I was a teen, all I will be able to say is 'I changed your diapers and prepared you formula.' I really wish I could go back and do things differently. I am sick of the constant worrying about how we are ever going to live once we move out of my mother's house."

Social and Economic Effects of Teen Pregnancy

Teen pregnancy is closely linked to poverty and single parenthood. A 1990 study showed that almost one-half of all teenage mothers and over three-quarters of unmarried teen mothers began receiving welfare within five years of the birth of their first child.[6] The growth in single-parent families remains the single most important reason for increased poverty among children over the last twenty years, as documented in the *1998 Economic Report of the President.*

Out-of-wedlock childbearing (as opposed to divorce) is currently the driving force behind the growth in the number of single parents, and half of first out-of-wedlock births are to teens.[7] Therefore, reducing teen pregnancy and child-bearing is an obvious place to anchor serious efforts to reduce poverty in future generations.

Teen Pregnancy Is Bad for the Child

Low Birth Weight and Related Health Problems

Children born to teen mothers suffer from higher rates of low birth weight and related health problems. The proportion of babies with low birth weights born to teens is 21 percent higher than the proportion for mothers age 20–24.[8] Low birth weight raises the probabilities of infant death, blindness, deafness, chronic respiratory problems, mental retardation, mental illness, and cerebral palsy. In addition, low birth weight doubles the chances that a child will later be diagnosed as having dyslexia, hyperactivity, or another disability.[4]

Insufficient Health Care

Children of teens often have insufficient health care. One mother relates: "I got pregnant a month before my 17th birthday. I live in an emergency shelter for teen moms. I raise my son alone. In his whole life, his father has only taken care of him by himself one time. He does not pay me child support. My son was born two months early and with a hole in his heart. He requires constant care, so I have little time for myself. I love my son more than anything in the world, but it would have been a lot better if this had happened when I was like 27 instead of 17."

Despite having more health problems than the children of older mothers, the children of teen mothers receive less medical care and treatment. In his or her first 14 years, the average child of a teen mother visits a physician and other medical providers an average of 3.8 times per year, compared with 4.3 times for a child of older childbearers.[4] And when they do visit medical providers, more of the expenses they incur are paid by others in society. One recent study suggested that the medical expenses paid by society would be reduced dramatically if teenage mothers were to wait until they were older to have their first child.[4]

Inadequate Parenting

Children born to teen mothers are at higher risk of poor parenting because their mothers—and often their fathers as well—are typically too young to master the demanding job of being a parent. Still growing and developing themselves, teen mothers are often unable to provide the kind of environment that infants and very young children require for optimal development. Recent research, for example, has

279

clarified the critical importance of sensitive parenting and early cognitive stimulation for adequate brain development.[4] Given the importance of careful nuturing and stimulation in the first three years of life, the burden borne by babies with parents who are too young to be in this role is especially great.

Abuse and Neglect Rates Are Higher

Children with adolescent parents often fall victim to abuse and neglect. A recent analysis found that there are 110 reported incidents of abuse and neglect per 1,000 families headed by a young teen mother. By contrast, in families where the mothers delay childbearing until their early twenties, the rate is less than half this level—or 51 incidents per 1,000 families.[4] Similarly, rates of foster care placement are significantly higher for children whose mothers are under 18. In fact, over half of foster care placements of children with these young mothers could be averted by delaying child-bearing, thereby saving taxpayers nearly $1 billion annually in foster care costs alone.[4]

School Difficulties

Children of teenagers often suffer from poor school performance. Children of teens are 50 percent more likely to repeat a grade; they perform much worse on standardized tests; and ultimately they are less likely to complete high school than if their mothers had delayed childbearing.[6]

Teen Pregnancy Is Bad for Everyone

The U.S. still leads the fully industrialized world in teen pregnancy and birth rates—by a wide margin. In fact, the U.S. rates are nearly double Great Britain's, at least four times those of France and Germany, and more than ten times that of Japan.[3]

Teen pregnancy costs society billions of dollars a year. There are nearly half a million children born to teen mothers each year. Most of these mothers are unmarried, and many will end up poor and on welfare. Each year the federal government alone spends about $40 billion to help families that began with a teenage birth.[10]

Teen pregnancy hurts the business community's bottom line. Too many children start school unprepared to learn, and teachers are overwhelmed trying to deal with problems that start in the home. Forty-five percent of first births in the United States are to women who are either unmarried, teenagers, or lacking a high school degree, which means that too many children—tomorrow's workers—are born into families that are not prepared to help them succeed.[6] In addition, teen mothers often do not finish high school themselves. It's not easy for a teen to learn work skills and be a dependable employee while caring for children.

A new crop of kids becomes teenagers each year. This means that prevention efforts must be constantly renewed and reinvented. And between 1995 and 2010, the number of girls aged 15–19 is projected to increase by 2.2 million.[6]

References

1. National Campaign to Prevent Teen Pregnancy. (2004). *Fact sheet: How is the 34% statistic calculated?* Washington, DC: Author.

2. Henshaw, S.K. (2004). *U.S. Teenage Pregnancy Statistics with Comparative Statistics for Women Aged 20–24.* New York: The Alan Guttmacher Institute.

3. Singh, S., and Darroch, J.E. (2000). Adolescent pregnancy and childbearing: Levels and trends in developed countries. *Family Planning Perspectives, 32*(1), 14–23.

4. Maynard, R.A. (Ed.). (1996). *Kids Having Kids: A Robin Hood Foundation Special Report on the Costs of Adolescent Childbearing.* New York: The Robin Hood Foundation.

5. Brown, S., and Eisenberg, L. (Eds.) (1995). *The Best Intentions: Unintended Pregnancy and the Well-Being of Children and Families.* Committee on Unintended Pregnancy. Washington, DC: Author.

6. National Campaign to Prevent Teen Pregnancy. (1997). *Whatever Happened to Childhood? The Problem of Teen Pregnancy in the United States.* Washington, DC: Author.

7. Sawhill, I.V. (1998). Teen pregnancy prevention: Welfare reform's missing component. *Brookings Policy Brief, 38,* 1–8.

8. Martin, J.A., Hamilton, B.E., Ventura, S.J., Menacker, F., Park, M.M., and Sutton, P.D. (2002). Births: Final data for 2001. *National Vital Statistics Reports, 51* (2).

9. Carnegie Task Force on Meeting the Needs of Children. (1994). *Starting Points: Meeting the Needs of Our Youngest Children.* New York: Author.

10. Flinn, S.K., and Hauser, D. (1998). *Teenage Pregnancy: The Case for Prevention. An Analysis of Recent Trends and Federal Expenditures Associated with Teenage Pregnancy.* Washington, DC: Advocates for Youth.

Additional Information

National Campaign to Prevent Teen Pregnancy
1776 Massachusetts Ave. NW, Suite 200
Washington, DC 20036
Phone: 202-478-8500
Fax: 202-478-8588
Website: http://www.teenpregnancy.org
E-mail: campaign@teenpregnancy.org

Part Five

Adolescent Injury

Chapter 31

Sports Injuries

In recent years, increasing numbers of people of all ages have been heeding their health professionals' advice to get active for all of the health benefits exercise has to offer. But for some people—particularly those who overdo or who do not properly train or warm up—these benefits can come at a price: sports injuries.

Fortunately, most sports injuries can be treated effectively, and most people who suffer injuries can return to a satisfying level of physical activity after an injury. Even better, many sports injuries can be prevented if people take the proper precautions.

What Are Sports Injuries?

The term sports injury, in the broadest sense, refers to the kinds of injuries that most commonly occur during sports or exercise. Some sports injuries result from accidents; others are due to poor training practices, improper equipment, lack of conditioning, or insufficient warm up and stretching. Although virtually any part of your body can be injured during sports or exercise, the term is usually reserved for injuries that involve the musculoskeletal system, which includes the muscles, bones, and associated tissues like cartilage. Following are some of the most common sports injuries.

Excerpted from "Handout on Health: Sports Injuries," National Institute of Arthritis and Musculoskeletal and Skin Diseases (NIAMS), NIH Publication No. 04–5278, April 2004.

Sprains and Strains

A sprain is a stretch or tear of a ligament, the band of connective tissues that joins the end of one bone with another. Sprains are caused by trauma such as a fall or blow to the body that knocks a joint out of position and, in the worst case, ruptures the supporting ligaments. Sprains can range from first degree (minimally stretched ligament) to third degree (a complete tear). Areas of the body most vulnerable to sprains are ankles, knees, and wrists. Signs of a sprain include varying degrees of tenderness or pain; bruising; inflammation; swelling; inability to move a limb or joint; or joint looseness, laxity, or instability.

A strain is a twist, pull, or tear of a muscle or tendon, a cord of tissue connecting muscle to bone. It is an acute, noncontact injury that results from overstretching or excessive contraction. Symptoms of a strain include pain, muscle spasm, and loss of strength. While it's hard to tell the difference between mild and moderate strains, severe strains not treated professionally can cause damage and loss of function.

Knee Injuries

Because of its complex structure and weight-bearing capacity, the knee is the most commonly injured joint. Each year, more than 5.5 million people visit orthopaedic surgeons for knee problems.

Knee injuries can range from mild to severe. Some of the less severe, yet still painful and functionally limiting knee problems are runner's knee (pain or tenderness close to or under the knee cap at the front or side of the knee), iliotibial band syndrome (pain on the outer side of the knee), and tendonitis, also called tendinosis (marked by degeneration within a tendon, usually where it joins the bone). More severe injuries include bone bruises or damage to the cartilage or ligaments.

Knee injuries can result from a blow to or twist of the knee; from improper landing after a jump; or from running too hard, too much, or without proper warmup.

Compartment Syndrome

In many parts of the body, muscles (along with the nerves and blood vessels that run alongside and through them) are enclosed in a compartment formed of a tough membrane called fascia. When muscles become swollen, they can fill the compartment to capacity, causing interference with nerves and blood vessels as well as damage to the muscles themselves. The resulting painful condition is referred to as compartment syndrome.

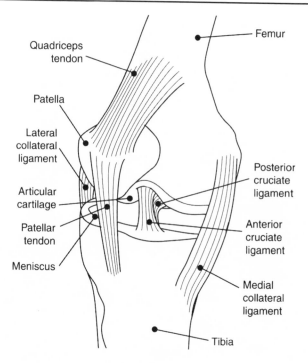

Figure 31.1. Lateral View of the Knee

Compartment syndrome may be caused by a one-time traumatic injury (acute compartment syndrome), such as a fractured bone or a hard blow to the thigh, by repeated hard blows (depending upon the sport), or by ongoing overuse (chronic exertional compartment syndrome), which may occur, for example, in long-distance running.

Shin Splints

While the term shin splints has been widely used to describe any sort of leg pain associated with exercise, the term actually refers to pain along the tibia or shin bone, the large bone in the front of the lower leg. This pain can occur at the front outside part of the lower leg, including the foot and ankle (anterior shin splints) or at the inner edge of the bone where it meets the calf muscles (medial shin splints).

Shin splints are primarily seen in runners, particularly those just starting a running program. Risk factors for shin splints include overuse or incorrect use of the lower leg; improper stretching, warmup, or exercise technique; overtraining; running or jumping on hard surfaces; and running in shoes that do not have enough support. These injuries are often associated with flat (over-pronated) feet.

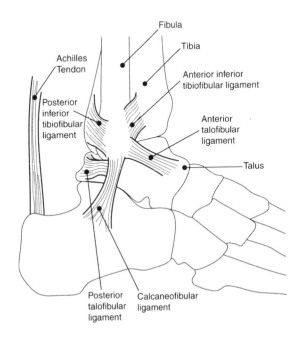

Figure 31.2. *Lateral View of the Ankle*

Achilles Tendon Injuries

A stretch, tear, or irritation to the tendon connecting the calf muscle to the back of the heel, Achilles tendon injuries can be so sudden and agonizing that they have been known to bring down charging professional football players in shocking fashion. Achilles tendon injuries are common in athletes who may not exercise regularly or take time to stretch properly before an activity.

Fractures

A fracture is a break in the bone that can occur from either a quick, one-time injury to the bone (acute fracture) or from repeated stress to the bone over time (stress fracture).

Acute fractures: Acute fractures can be simple (a clean break with little damage to the surrounding tissue) or compound (a break in which the bone pierces the skin with little damage to the surrounding tissue). Most acute fractures are emergencies. One that breaks the skin is especially dangerous because there is a high risk of infection.

Stress fractures: Stress fractures occur largely in the feet and legs and are common in sports that require repetitive impact, primarily running/jumping sports such as gymnastics or track and field. Running creates forces two to three times a person's body weight on the lower limbs.

The most common symptom of a stress fracture is pain at the site that worsens with weight-bearing activity. Tenderness and swelling often accompany the pain.

Dislocations

When the two bones that come together to form a joint become separated, the joint is described as being dislocated. Contact sports such as football and basketball, as well as high-impact sports and sports that can result in excessive stretching or falling cause the majority of dislocations. A dislocated joint is an emergency situation that requires medical treatment.

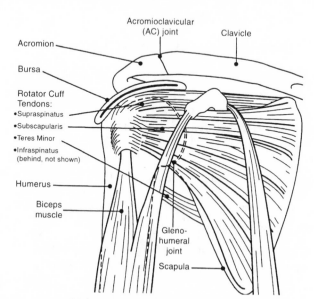

Figure 31.3. *The Shoulder Joint*

The joints most likely to be dislocated are some of the hand joints. Aside from these joints, the joint most frequently dislocated is the shoulder. Dislocations of the knees, hips, and elbows are uncommon.

What Is the Difference between Acute and Chronic Injuries?

Acute injuries, such as a sprained ankle, strained back, or fractured hand, occur suddenly during activity. Signs of an acute injury include:

- sudden, severe pain
- swelling
- inability to place weight on a lower limb
- extreme tenderness in an upper limb
- inability to move a joint through its full range of motion
- extreme limb weakness
- visible dislocation or break of a bone

Chronic injuries usually result from overusing one area of the body while playing a sport or exercising over a long period. Signs of a chronic injury include pain when performing an activity, a dull ache when at rest, and/or swelling.

What Should I Do If I Suffer an Injury?

Whether an injury is acute or chronic, there is never a good reason to try to work through the pain of an injury. When you have pain from a particular movement or activity—stop! Continuing the activity only causes further harm. Some injuries require prompt medical attention, while others can be self-treated.

You should call a health professional if:

- the injury causes severe pain, swelling, or numbness;
- you cannot tolerate any weight on the area;
- the pain or dull ache of an old injury is accompanied by increased swelling or joint abnormality or instability.

If you do not have any of the above symptoms, it is probably safe to treat the injury at home—at least at first. If pain or other symptoms worsen, it is best to check with your health care provider. Use the RICE (rest, ice, compression, elevation) method to relieve pain and inflammation and speed healing. Follow these four steps immediately after injury and continue for at least 48 hours:

- *Rest.* Reduce regular exercise or activities of daily living as needed. If you cannot put weight on an ankle or knee, crutches may help. If you use a cane or one crutch for an ankle injury, use it on the uninjured side to help you lean away and relieve weight on the injured ankle.

- *Ice.* Apply an ice pack to the injured area for 20 minutes at a time, four to eight times a day. A cold pack, ice bag, or plastic bag filled with crushed ice and wrapped in a towel can be used. To avoid cold injury and frostbite, do not apply the ice for more than 20 minutes. (Note: Do not use heat immediately after an injury. This tends to increase internal bleeding or swelling. Heat can be used later on to relieve muscle tension and promote relaxation.)

- *Compression.* Compression of the injured area may help reduce swelling. Compression can be achieved with elastic wraps, special boots, air casts, and splints. Ask your health care provider for advice on which one to use.

- *Elevation.* If possible, keep the injured ankle, knee, elbow, or wrist elevated on a pillow, above the level of the heart, to help decrease swelling.

Who Is at Greatest Risk for Sports Injuries?

Anyone who plays sports can be injured. Three groups—children and adolescents, middle-aged athletes, and women—are particularly vulnerable.

Children and Adolescents

While playing sports can improve children's fitness, self-esteem, coordination, and self-discipline, it can also put them at risk for sports injuries: some minor, some serious, and still others that may result in lifelong medical problems.

Young athletes are not small adults. Their bones, muscles, tendons, and ligaments are still growing and that makes them more prone to injury. Growth plates—the areas of developing cartilage where bone growth occurs in growing children—are weaker than the nearby ligaments and tendons. As a result, what is often a bruise or sprain in an adult can be a potentially serious growth-plate injury in a child. Also, a trauma that would tear a muscle or ligament in an adult would be far more likely to break a child's bone. Because young athletes of the same age can differ greatly in size and physical maturity, some may try to perform at levels beyond their ability in order to keep up with their peers.

Women

More women of all ages are participating in sports than ever before. In women's sports, the action is now faster and more aggressive and powerful than in the past. As a result, women are sustaining many more injuries, and the injuries tend to be sport specific.

Female athletes have higher injury rates than men in many sports, particularly basketball, soccer, alpine skiing, volleyball, and gymnastics. Female college basketball players are about six times more likely to suffer a tear of the knee's anterior cruciate ligament (ACL) than men are, according to a study of 11,780 high school and college players.

While poor conditioning has not been related to an increased incidence of ACL injuries specifically, it has been associated with an increase in injuries in general. For most American women, the basic level of conditioning is much lower than that of men. Studies at the U.S. Naval Academy revealed that overuse injuries were more frequent in women; however, as women became used to the rigors of training, the injury rates for men and women became similar.

Aside from conditioning level, other possible factors in women's sports injuries include structural difference of the knee and thigh muscles, fluctuating estrogen levels caused by menstruation, the fit of athletic shoes, and the way players jump, land, and twist. Also, the female triad, a combination of disordered eating, curtailed menstruation (amenorrhea), and loss of bone mass (osteoporosis), is increasingly more common in female athletes in some sports. Its true prevalence is unknown, but it appears to be greater in athletes, adolescents, and young adults, especially in people who are perfectionists and overachievers.

Preventing Sports Injuries

Anyone who exercises is potentially at risk for a sports injury and should follow the injury prevention tips. But additional measures can be taken by groups at higher risk of injury.

Children and Adolescents

Preventing injuries in children and adolescents is a team effort, requiring the support of parents, coaches, and the kids themselves. Here's what each should do to reduce injury risk.

What Parents and Coaches Can Do

- Try to group youth according to skill level and size, not by chronological age, particularly during contact sports. If this is not practical, modify the sport to accommodate the needs of children with varying skill levels.

- Match the child to the sport, and do not push the child too hard into an activity that she or he may not like or be physically capable of doing.

- Try to find sports programs where certified athletic trainers are present. These people, in addition to health care professionals, are trained to prevent, recognize, and give immediate care to sports injuries.

- See that all children get a preseason physical exam.

- Do not let (or insist that) a child play when injured. No child (or adult) should ever be allowed to work through the pain.

- Get the child medical attention if needed. A child who develops any symptom that persists or that affects athletic performance should be examined by a health care professional. Other clues that a child needs to see a health professional include inability to play following a sudden injury, visible abnormality of the arms and legs, and severe pain that prevents the use of an arm or leg.

- Provide a safe environment for sports. A poor playing field, unsafe gym sets, unsecured soccer goals, etc., can cause serious injury to children.

What Children and Adolescents Can Do

- Be in proper condition to play the sport.
- Get a preseason physical exam.
- Follow the rules of the game.
- Wear appropriate protective gear.
- Know how to use athletic equipment.

- Avoid playing when very tired or in pain.

- Make warm ups and cool downs part of your routine. Warmup exercises, such as stretching or light jogging, can help minimize the chances of muscle strain or other soft tissue injury. They also make the body's tissues warmer and more flexible. Cool down exercises loosen the muscles that have tightened during exercise.

Tips for Preventing Injury

Whether you have never had a sports injury and you are trying to keep it that way or you have had an injury and do not want another, the following tips can help.

- Avoid bending knees past 90 degrees when doing half knee bends.

- Avoid twisting knees by keeping feet as flat as possible during stretches.

- When jumping, land with your knees bent.

- Do warmup exercises not just before vigorous activities like running, but also before less vigorous ones such as golf.

- Do not overdo.

- Do warmup stretches before activity. Stretch the Achilles tendon, hamstring, and quadriceps areas and hold the positions. Do not bounce.

- Cool down following vigorous sports. For example, after a race, walk or walk/jog for five minutes so your pulse comes down gradually.

- Wear properly fitting shoes that provide shock absorption and stability.

- Use the softest exercise surface available, and avoid running on hard surfaces like asphalt and concrete. Run on flat surfaces. Running uphill may increase the stress on the Achilles tendon and the leg itself.

Women

Increased emphasis on muscle strength and conditioning should be a priority for all women. Women should also be encouraged to maintain a normal body weight and avoid excessive exercise that affects the menstrual cycle. In addition, women should follow precautions listed for other groups.

Additional Information

American College of Sports Medicine
P.O. Box 1440
Indianapolis, IN 46206-1440
Phone: 317-637-9200
Fax: 317-634-7817
Website: http://www.acsm.org

National Athletic Trainers Association
2952 Stemmons Freeway
Dallas, TX 75247-6916
Toll-Free: 800-TRY-NATA (800-879-6282)
Phone: 214-637-6282
Fax: 214-637-2206
Website: http://www.nata.org

National Institute of Arthritis and Musculoskeletal and Skin Diseases (NIAMS) Information Clearinghouse
1 AMS Circle
Bethesda, MD 20892-3675
Toll-Free: 877-22-NIAMS (64267)
Phone: 301-495-4484
TTY: 301-565-2966
Fax: 301-718-6366
Website: http:www.niams.nih.gov
E-mail: niamsinfo@mail.nih.gov

Chapter 32

Growth Plate Injuries

Growth plates are located on the long bones of children and young people. These plates are areas of growing tissue near the end of the bones. Each long bone has at least two growth plates—one at each end. This is where the long bones grow. When young people finish growing, the growth plates close and are replaced by solid bone. Growth plate injuries occur mainly at the wrist, bones of the legs, or in the ankle, foot, or hip bones.

Who gets growth plate injuries?

Growth plate injuries happen to children and young people. The growth plate is the weakest part of the growing skeleton. Injuries to the plates are called fractures. Growth plate fractures happen twice as often in boys as in girls. And, fractures are most likely in 14- to 16-year-old boys and 11- to 13-year-old girls.

What causes growth plate injuries?

Growth plate injuries happen for many reasons. Most occur after a sudden accident, such as falling or being hit hard on the leg. People who sometimes get injuries from overuse include:

- gymnasts who practices for hours on the uneven bars
- long-distance runners
- baseball pitchers perfecting their curve balls

"Fast Facts about Growth Plate Injuries," National Institute of Arthritis and Musculoskeletal and Skin Diseases (NIAMS), March 2005.

The top reasons for growth plate injuries are:

- falling down
- competitive sports (like football)
- recreational activities
- car, motorcycle, and all-terrain-vehicle accidents (only in a small number of cases)

Other reasons for growth plate injuries are:

- child abuse
- injury from extreme cold (for example, frostbite)
- radiation (used to treat certain cancers)
- neurological disorders that cause people to lose their balance and fall
- some inherited disorders
- bone infections

When to See a Doctor

A child or adolescent should never have to work through the pain. Parents should take their child to see a doctor for the following situations:

- The child has to stop playing because of pain after a sudden injury.
- The child is less able to play because of an old injury.
- The child's arm or leg bends the wrong way.
- The child cannot move an arm or leg because of pain.
- The pain continues after overuse or injury.[1]

[1]Source: Adapted from *Play It Safe, a Guide to Safety for Young Athletes*, with permission of the American Academy of Orthopaedic Surgeons.

How are growth plate fractures diagnosed?

First, the doctor will find out how the injury happened. Second, the doctor will examine the child and use x-rays to find out what kind of fracture it is. Third, a treatment plan is chosen. Sometimes other tests are used to look at the fracture, including computed tomography (CT) scan (a special x-ray), and ultrasound (uses sound waves to look inside the body).

What kind of doctor treats growth plate injuries?

An orthopaedic surgeon (a doctor who treats bone and joint problems) treats most growth plate injuries. At other times, the child will see a pediatric orthopaedic surgeon (a doctor who treats bone and joint problems in children).

How are growth plate injuries treated?

The treatment depends on the type of fracture. However, with all fractures, treatment should start as soon as possible. Treatment usually involves a mix of the following:

- immobilization (a cast or splint)
- manipulation or surgery (depending on where and how serious the injury is, and the patient's age)
- exercises (only after the fracture heals)
- long-term followup (including x-rays)

How well do children grow after a growth plate injury?

Most growth plate fractures get better and do not cause any lasting problems. Occasionally, the bone stops growing and ends up shorter than the other limb. For example, a fractured leg might end up shorter than the other leg. Or, if only part of the growth plate is injured, the limb can become crooked when only part of the bone keeps growing. Lasting problems are most common with injuries to the knee.

Additional Information

National Institute of Arthritis and Musculoskeletal and Skin Diseases (NIAMS) Information Clearinghouse
1 AMS Circle
Bethesda, MD 20892-3675
Toll-Free: 877-22-NIAMS (64267)
Phone: 301-495-4484
TTY: 301-565-2966
Fax: 301-718-6366
Website: http:www.niams.nih.gov
E-mail: niamsinfo@mail.nih.gov

Chapter 33

Teen Drivers:
Injury and Mortality Facts

Facts about Teen Drivers

Two out of five deaths among U.S. teens are the result of a motor vehicle crash (CDC 2004).

Occurrence and Consequences

- In 2002, more than 5,000 teens ages 16 to 19 died of injuries caused by motor vehicle crashes (CDC 2004).

- The risk of motor vehicle crashes is higher among 16- to 19-year-olds than among any other age group. In fact, per mile driven, teen drivers ages 16 to 19 are four times more likely than older drivers to crash (IIHS 2005).

- In 2003, teenagers accounted for 10 percent of the U.S. population and 13 percent of motor vehicle crash deaths (IIHS 2005).

- The presence of teen passengers increases the crash risk of unsupervised teen drivers; the risk increases with the number of teen passengers (Chen 2000).

This chapter includes: "Teen Drivers: Fact Sheet," Centers for Disease Control and Prevention (CDC), October 7, 2005; and excerpts from "Safety Belts and Teens 2003 Report," U.S. Department of Transportation, DOT HS 809 578, March 2003.

Cost

In 2002, the estimated economic cost of police-reported crashes (both fatal and nonfatal) involving drivers ages 15 to 20 was $40.8 billion (NHTSA 2003).

Groups at Risk

- In 2002, the motor vehicle death rate for male occupants age 16 to 19 was nearly twice that of their female counterparts (23 per 100,000 compared with 12 per 100,000) (CDC 2004a).

- Crash risk is particularly high during the first year that teenagers are eligible to drive (IIHS 2005).

Risk Factors

- Teens are more likely than older drivers to underestimate hazardous situations or dangerous situations or not be able to recognize hazardous situations (Jonah 1987).

- Teens are more likely than older drivers to speed, run red lights, make illegal turns, ride with an intoxicated driver, and drive after using alcohol or drugs (Jonah 1987).

- Among male drivers between 15–20 years of age who were involved in fatal crashes in 2003, 39% were speeding at the time of the crash (NHTSA 2004a).

- Compared with other age groups, teens have the lowest rate of seat belt use. In 2003, 18% of high school students reported they rarely or never wear seat belts when riding with someone else (CDC 2004b).

  - Male high school students (22%) were more likely than female students (15%) to rarely or never wear seat belts (CDC 2004b).

  - African-American students (21%) and Hispanic students (20%) were more likely than white students (17%) to rarely or never wear seat belts (CDC 2004b).

- At all levels of blood alcohol concentration (BAC), the risk of involvement in a motor vehicle crash is greater for teens than for older drivers (IIHS 2004).

- In 2003, 25% of drivers ages 15 to 20 who died in motor vehicle crashes had a BAC of 0.08 g/dl or higher (NHTSA 2004).

- In a national survey conducted in 2003, 30% of teens reported that within the previous month, they had ridden with a driver who had been drinking alcohol. One in eight reported having driven after drinking alcohol within the same one-month period (CDC 2004b).

- In 2003, among teen drivers who were killed in motor vehicle crashes after drinking and driving, 74% were unrestrained (NHTSA 2004b).

- In 2003, 54% of teen deaths from motor vehicle crashes occurred on Friday, Saturday, or Sunday; 42% occurred between 9 p.m. and 6 a.m. (IIHS 2005).

References

Centers for Disease Control and Prevention. Web-based Injury Statistics Query and Reporting System (WISQARS) [Online]. (2004a). National Center for Injury Prevention and Control, Centers for Disease Control and Prevention (producer). Available from: URL: www.cdc.gov/ncipc/wisqars. [Cited 2004 Dec 13].

Centers for Disease Control and Prevention. *Youth Risk Behavior Surveillance—United States, 2003* [Online]. (2004b). National Center for Chronic Disease Prevention and Health Promotion (producer). Available from: URL: http://apps.nccd.cdc.gov/yrbss/CategoryQuestions .asp?cat=1&desc=Unintentional%20Injuries%20and%20Violence. [Cited 2005 Jan 14].

Chen L, Baker SP, Braver ER, Li G. Carrying passengers as a risk factor for crashes fatal to 16- and 17-year old drivers. *JAMA* 2000; 283(12):1578–82.

Insurance Institute for Highway Safety (IIHS). *Fatality facts: teenagers 2003*. Arlington (VA): The Institute; 2005 [cited 2005 June 19]. Available from: URL: www.hwysafety.org/research/fatality_facts/pdf/teenagers.pdf

Insurance Institute for Highway Safety (IHHS). *Q&A teenagers: underage drinking*. Arlington (VA): The Institute; 2004 [cited 2005 June 19]. Available from: URL: www.hwysafety.org/research/qanda/underage.html.

Jonah BA, Dawson NE. Youth and risk: age differences in risky driving, risk perception, and risk utility. *Alcohol, Drugs and Driving* 1987; 3:13–29.

National Highway Traffic Safety Administration (NHTSA), Dept. of Transportation (US). *Traffic safety facts 2003: overview.* Washington (DC): NHTSA; 2004a [cited 2005 June 19]. Available from: URL: www-nrd.nhtsa.dot.gov/pdf/nrd-30/NCSA/TSF2003/809767.pdf.

National Highway Traffic Safety Administration (NHTSA), Dept. of Transportation (US). *Traffic safety facts 2003: young drivers.* Washington (DC): NHTSA; 2004b [cited 2005 June 19]. Available from: URL: www-nrd.nhtsa.dot.gov/pdf/nrd-30/NCSA/TSF2003/809774.pdf.

National Highway Traffic Safety Administration (NHTSA), Department of Transportation (US). *Traffic safety facts 2002: young drivers.* Washington (DC): NHTSA; 2003 [cited 2003 Sept 15]. Available from: URL: www-nrd.nhtsa.dot.gov/pdf/nrd-30/NCSA/TSF2002/2002ydrfacts.pdf.

Safety Belts and Teens 2003 Report

Teens, young people ages 16–20, have the highest fatality rate in motor vehicle crashes than any other age group.[1] There are many reasons; for instance, while teens are learning the new skills needed for driving, many frequently engage in high-risk behaviors, such as speeding and/or driving after using alcohol or drugs. Studies also have shown that teens may be easily distracted while driving.[2] One key reason for high traffic fatalities among this age group is that they have lower safety belt use rates than adults.[3] Because teens have an increased exposure to potentially fatal traffic crashes, it is imperative that efforts to increase safety belt use among this age group be given the highest priority. In addition, the youth population has increased by more than 12 percent since 1993, and is expected to increase by another seven percent by 2005.[4] As this age group increases as a percentage of the population, the personal and societal costs associated with deaths and injuries from motor vehicle crashes also will rise.

Safety Belts Save Lives and Dollars

- In 2001, the estimated economic cost of police-reported crashes involving drivers between 15 and 20 years old was $42.3 billion.[5]

- Safety belts saved more than 12,000 American lives in 2001. Yet, during that same year, nearly two-thirds (60 percent) of passenger vehicle occupants killed in traffic crashes were unrestrained.[6]

- Research has shown that lap/shoulder belts, when used properly, reduce the risk of fatal injury to front-seat passenger car occupants by 45 percent and the risk of moderate to critical injury by 50 percent. For light truck occupants, safety belts reduce the risk of fatal injury by 60 percent and moderate-to-critical injury by 65 percent.[7]

- Safety belts should always be worn, even when riding in vehicles equipped with air bags. Air bags are designed to work with safety belts, not alone. Air bags, when not used with safety belts, have a fatality-reducing effectiveness rate of only 12 percent.[8]

- Safety belt usage saves society an estimated $50 billion annually in medical care, lost productivity, and other injury-related costs.[9]

- Conversely, safety belt nonuse results in significant economic costs to society. The needless deaths and injuries from safety belt nonuse account for an estimated $26 billion in economic costs to society annually.[10] The cost goes beyond the lost lives of unbuckled drivers and passengers: We all pay—in higher taxes and higher health care and insurance costs.

Strong Safety Belt Laws Can Make a Difference

- There are two types of safety belt laws: primary and secondary. A primary safety belt law allows law enforcement officers to stop a vehicle and issue a citation when the officer simply observes an unbelted driver or passenger. A secondary safety belt law means that a citation for not wearing a safety belt can only be written after the officer stops the vehicle or cites the offender for another infraction.

- In June 2002, the average safety belt use rate in States with primary enforcement laws was 11 percentage points higher than in States without primary enforcement laws.[11] (Safety belt use was 80 percent in primary law States versus 69 percent in States without primary enforcement.)

- Many teens support primary enforcement safety belt laws. Of more than 500 youth age 16–20 years of age surveyed in a 2000 nationwide survey, 60 percent voiced their support for primary enforcement laws.[12]

- Young drivers are more likely to use safety belts in States with a primary safety belt law versus States with a secondary law. California, Maryland, Michigan, North Carolina, and Oregon have primary safety belt laws that are among the strongest in the nation and have the highest teenage safety belt use.[13]

References

1. *Traffic Safety Facts 2001* (Book), National Highway Traffic Safety Administration, DOT HS 809 484, pg. 21.

2. Williams, Alan F. 2001. *Teenage Passengers in Motor Vehicle Crashes: A Summary of Current Research.* Insurance Institute for Highway Safety.

3. NHTSA Research Notes, August 2001. DOT HS 809 318.

4. U.S. Census Bureau

5. *Traffic Safety Facts 2001.* Younger Driver, National Highway Traffic Safety Administration, DOT HS 809 483.

6. *Traffic Safety Facts 2001*, Overview, National Highway Traffic Safety Administration, DOT HS 809 476, p. 10.

7. Motor Vehicle Traffic Crash Fatality and Injury Estimates for 2000, National Highway Traffic Safety Administration, November 2001.

8. *Traffic Safety Facts, 2000*, Occupant Protection, National Highway Traffic Safety Administration, DOT HS 809 327.

9. *The Economic Impact of Motor Vehicle Crashes, 2000.* National Highway Traffic Safety Administration, DOT HS 809 446, p. 55.

10. *Ibid.*

11. *Safety Belt and Helmet Use in 2002—Overall Results.* National Highway Traffic Safety Administration. DOT HS 809 500. September 2002.

12. *Motor Vehicle Occupant Safety Survey, 2000, Volume Two*, p. 147. National Highway Traffic Safety Administration, DOT HS 809 389.

13. McCartt A.T., and Shabanova, V.I. (2002). *Teenage Seat Belt Use*: White Paper. The National Safety Council's Air Bag and Seat Belt Safety Campaign.

Additional Information

CDC-INFO Contact Center
Toll-Free: 800-CDC-INFO (232-4636)
Toll-Free TTY: 888-232-6348
Website: http://www.cdc.gov
E-mail: cdcinfo@cdc.gov

National Highway Traffic Safety Administration (NHTSA)
400 Seventh St. SW
Washington, DC 20590
Toll-Free: 888-327-4236
Toll-Free TTY: 800-424-9153
Website: http://www.nhtsa.dot.gov

Chapter 34

Testicular Trauma

Because the testicles are located within the scrotum, which hangs outside of the body, they do not have the protection of muscles and bones. This makes it easier for the testicles to be struck, hit, kicked, or crushed. The following information should help explain why timely evaluation and proper management are critical for the best outcomes.

What happens under normal conditions?

As the producers of sperm and testosterone, the testicles are paired organs essential for every reproductive and sexual function enjoyed by men. But they are also prone to injuries that can leave damage to either the entire gland or essential parts of it.

Suspended in the scrotum, a skin pouch below the penis, each testicle is surrounded by the tunica albuginea, a tough, fibrous covering that often takes the hit of trauma to the gland. Like the shell of an egg, it can be easily fractured or shattered when confronted by a blunt or violent force.

But while this covering is injury-prone, other parts of the scrotal sac, most notably the adjacent epididymis, are also vulnerable. Lying along the backside of the testicle, this rubbery gland contains a single coiled tube formed by the merger of thousands of sperm-producing ducts, seminiferous tubules, originating inside the testicle.

Sperm stop briefly in the epididymis to mature before exiting in semen through the vas deferens, a tube that connects with the urethra. Unlike the vas, which is covered by a thick muscle wall, the epididymis has a coating that is both thin and fragile. As such, it puts the gland at higher risk for inflammation or injury.

What are the causes of testicular injury?

While testicular injuries fall into three categories, they all have the potential of inflicting similar injuries: partial or complete ripping of the testicle as well as loss of the entire gland. An injury can be sustained as the result of a penetrating object such as a knife or bullet that punctures the scrotal sac, causing a minor scrape to the skin or major impediment of the blood flow to the testicle itself. An injury might be caused by a moving object—such as a kick or baseball to the groin—hitting the scrotal sac with a force so strong the energy causes injury. Or an injury can result from the scrotum striking a solid object, such as in a fall or car accident.

What are the symptoms of testicular injury?

While trauma to the testicle or scrotal sac usually produces severe pain as a first symptom, it can also result in actual physical injury to any of its contents. When the testicle's hard covering is shattered or ripped blood flows from the injury, stretching the normally elastic scrotal sac until it is tense. While that collection of blood can trigger infection, there also may be additional fertility problems due to the ultimate loss of a testicle or immune system problems that affect the remaining testicle. In very severe cases of testicular injury, the entire testicle is ripped with either part of the testicle that cannot be saved or the entire testicle injured beyond repair.

Considerable pain not caused by a defect in the testicle's covering, may be due to epididymitis. Because the epididymis, the lengthy coil alongside the testicle, is a very thin-walled gland it easily becomes red and swollen either by infection or injury. If left untreated, the condition can lead to a loss of the testicle due to blockage of the blood supply to the testicle.

The symptoms mentioned above may indicate a very treatable, benign problem but they may also indicate testicular cancer. A substantial number of malignancies are discovered after minor injuries.

But many men are not aware of the painless, solid lump, bulging from the smooth testicular covering, until they're injured in the groin and are examining themselves.

Do not make the mistake of many men who postpone medical care, thinking they are dealing with a simple bruise. This is a medical emergency. While testicular cancer caught early is generally curable, malignancies discovered late often require prolonged treatment involving surgery, radiation, and chemotherapy.

Men who suffer anything more than a minor injury to the scrotum should seek an evaluation by a urologist. Reasons to seek medical care include:

- swelling of the scrotal sac

- any penetrating injury to the scrotal sac

- prolonged pain in the scrotal sac

- bruising and swelling of the scrotal sac

- fevers after testicular injury

- any other symptom that develops after injury to the scrotal sac

How are testicular injuries treated?

A urologist (particularly an expert in scrotal injury) can probably determine the extent of any injury to the testicle with a simple physical examination. After the urologist asks questions about how the injury occurred as well as other medical history questions, he will examine the contents of the scrotal sac. In doing so, the hard covering overlying the testicle can generally be easily felt as well as the narrow, soft epididymis. The structures that run into the testicle including the artery, vein, and vas would then be felt to ensure that they are normal.

If everything appears normal, with no injury present, the urologist will probably prescribe pain medication such as acetaminophen or ibuprofen. A patient will also be advised to wear a jock strap, which provides good support for the scrotum.

If it is not clear that an injury has occurred, the urologist may request a scrotal ultrasound scan. Based on the same sonar sound waves that guide submarines, this device can safely and effectively image parts of the sac, including the testicle, epididymis, and spermatic cord. More specialized versions can also track blood flow.

Although no imaging test is 100 percent perfect, ultrasound is an attractive alternative because it is easy to perform, uses no x-rays, and clearly shows the physical structure of the scrotum. On rare occasions, the urologists may request a magnetic resonance image (MRI), a more sophisticated imaging technique, if the ultrasound leaves more questions than answers.

If any imaging study reveals evidence of or suggests testicular injury, the usual course of action is an operation in which the urologists opens the scrotal sac and visually inspects as well as repairs any injury. Under anesthesia, an incision is made in the sac and the entire contents are examined. If a rip of the testicle has occurred and the testicle can be repaired (if it has good blood supply and the remaining testicle has sufficient covering available), the urologist will usually repair the defect with stitches and then close the scrotal sac skin. Usually, the patient will leave surgery with a catheter, to drain blood and other fluids. While it is removed in a few days, the patient can expect to wear a protective jock strap for several weeks.

On occasion, the injury is so severe that the testicle cannot be repaired. If this occurs, the urologist will remove the testicle. However, that does not mean the patient cannot father a child. If the patient's other testicle is normal, he should be able to impregnate his partner. Also, the patient's hormone levels should remain steady since only one testicle is required for either function

If the patient's physical examination and ultrasound suggest that the injury has caused epididymitis, he will probably be treated conservatively, placed on an anti-inflammatory medication (such as ibuprofen) and encouraged again to wear a jock strap. If necessary, the urologist may also prescribe an antibiotic. It generally takes six to eight weeks for the swelling to subside. The patient may have to have several follow-up visits with the urologist to chart his progress. Further, if conservative measures (medications and jock strap) do not work, surgery may be required and the testicle may have to be removed.

Frequently Asked Questions

I have noticed pain in my scrotum and testicle, but I do not remember any injury. What should I do?

There are many possible causes of scrotal or testicle pain including epididymitis, inflammation of the testicle, and problems with other parts of the scrotum. Whatever the source, you should be examined by a urologist, a specialist trained in such problems.

I was hit by a knee during a basketball game and have since noticed a new lump in my scrotal sac. It does not hurt, but should I do anything about it?

Like many young men, you are probably examining yourself for the first time now that you have had a sporting injury. There is a good chance that the lump or new mass you have just felt is your epididymis. But it could be an injury or even testicular cancer. Any new lump should be checked immediately by the trained eyes of a urologist. With his/her expertise, a urologist will ease your mind and point you to swift and accurate treatment.

I'm 55 years old and noticed a lump in my scrotum after being hit in the groin during pick-up game of baseball. Could this be testicular cancer or am I too old for that?

Testicular cancer can occur at any age, even though the most cases are between 15 and 35. Anyone with a new lump in the scrotum should call a urologist immediately. Often you will not need any further tests because the urologist can make a diagnosis with a physical examination. However, the urologist may also request an ultrasound. While some masses are benign, 99 percent or more are malignant. The good news, however, is that testicular cancer can be treated effectively (with initial surgical removal of the gland) if caught early. So do not be afraid to contact a urologist.

I noticed blood in my urine after being hit with a baseball. I do not feel any lumps. Should I still report this to my doctor?

Absolutely. Blood in the urine that is visible to the naked eye is almost always due to a urologic problem. You need to see a urologist immediately for evaluation to sort out the possibilities.

What can I do to prevent injury to my testicles?

There are many common-sense steps you can take to reduce your risk of testicular trauma. Wear a seat belt when driving a car. Make sure your clothes are tucked in and you are not exposing loose belts or other items to machinery that has exposed chains or belts. Wear a jock strap when playing sports. If the activity could produce severe contact (as in baseball, football, or hockey), use a hard cup to reduce the risk. Finally, avoid any circumstances in which a moving object could hit your groin, particularly the scrotum.

Chapter 35

Fireworks-Related Injuries

How extensive is the problem?

- In 2003, four persons died and an estimated 9,300 were treated in emergency departments for fireworks-related injuries in the United States (Greene 2004).

- An estimated 5% of fireworks-related injuries treated in emergency departments required hospitalization (Greene 2004).

Who is most likely to be injured?

- About 45% of persons injured from fireworks are children ages 14 years and younger (Greene 2004).

- Males represent 72% of all injuries (Greene 2004).

- Children ages 5 to 9 years have the highest injury rate for fireworks-related injuries (Greene 2004).

- Persons who are actively participating in fireworks-related activities are more frequently injured, and sustain more severe injuries, than bystanders (Smith 1996).

When and where do these injuries happen?

- Injuries occur on and around holidays associated with fireworks celebrations, especially July 4th and New Year's Eve.

Centers for Disease Control and Prevention (CDC), August 5, 2004.

315

- Most of these injuries occur in homes. Other common locations include recreational settings, streets or highways, and parking lots or occupational settings (U.S. CPSC 1993).

What kinds of injuries occur?

- Fireworks-related injuries most frequently involve hands and fingers (26%), eyes (21%), and the head and face (18%). More than half of the injuries are burns (63%); contusions and lacerations were the second most frequent injuries (18%) (Greene 2002).

- Fireworks also can also cause life-threatening residential fires (NFPA 2002).

What types of fireworks are associated with the most injuries?

- Illegal large firecrackers represent 2% of all firecracker injuries (Greene 2002).

- Firecrackers (24%), rockets (18%), and sparklers (11%) accounted for most of the injuries seen in emergency departments during 2003 (Greene 2004).

- Sparklers were associated with the most injuries for children under five (Greene 2004).

- For children ages 5 to 14 years and people ages 15 to 24 years, firecrackers, rockets, and other devices (including sparklers) were the source of most injuries (Greene 2004).

How and why do these injuries occur?

Availability: In spite of federal regulations and varying state prohibitions, class C and class B fireworks are often accessible by the public. It is not uncommon to find fireworks distributors near state borders, where residents of states with strict fireworks regulations can take advantage of more lenient state laws.

Fireworks type: Among class C fireworks, which are sold legally in some states, bottle rockets can fly into one's face and cause eye injuries; sparklers can ignite one's clothing (sparklers burn at more than 1,000 degrees Fahrenheit); and firecrackers can injure one's hands or face if they explode at close range (U.S. CPSC 1996).

Being too close: Injuries may result from being too close to fireworks when they explode; for example, when someone bends over to look more closely at a firework that has been ignited, or when a misguided bottle rocket hits a nearby person (U.S. CPSC 1996).

Unsupervised use: One study estimates that children are 11 times more likely to be injured by fireworks if they are unsupervised (U.S. CPSC 1996).

Lack of physical coordination: Younger children often lack the physical coordination to handle fireworks safely.

Curiosity: Children are often excited and curious around fireworks, which can increase their chances of being injured for example, when they re-examine a firecracker dud that initially fails to ignite (U.S. CPSC 1996).

Experimentation: Homemade fireworks, such as those made of the powder from several firecrackers, can lead to dangerous explosions (U.S. CPSC 1996).

How much do these injuries cost each year?

In addition to medical costs directly and indirectly attributable to fireworks injuries, U.S. fire departments reported approximately 24,200 fireworks-related fires in 1999 that were estimated to have cost $17.2 million in direct property damage (NFPA 2002).

What effect do laws have on fireworks injuries?

Studies suggest that state laws regulating the sale and use of fireworks affect the number of injuries incurred. For example, in one state, the number of injuries seen in emergency departments more than doubled following the legalization of fireworks (McFarland 1984). Under the Federal Hazardous Substances Act, the federal government prohibits the sale of the most dangerous types of fireworks to consumers. These banned fireworks include large reloadable shells, cherry bombs, aerial bombs, M-80 salutes, and larger firecrackers that contain more than two grains of powder. Under this same Act, mail-order kits to build these fireworks are also prohibited (Banned Hazardous Substances 2001).

What is the safest way to prevent fireworks injuries?

The safest way to prevent fireworks-related injuries is to leave fireworks displays to trained professionals. See safety tips from the U.S. Consumer Product Safety Commission.

References

U.S. Consumer Product Safety Commission. Federal Hazardous Substances Act. [cited 25 June 2003]. Bethesda (MD): The Commission. Available at URL: http://www.cpsc.gov/businfo/fhsa.html

Greene MA, Race PM. *2003 Fireworks Annual Report: Fireworks-Related Deaths, Emergency Department Treated Injuries, and Enforcement Activities During 2003*. Washington (DC): U.S. Consumer Product Safety Commission; 2004 [cited 1 July 2004]. Available at URL: http://www.cpsc.gov/LIBRARY/2001fwreport.pdf

McFarland LV, Harris JR, Kobayashi JM, Dicker RC. Risk factors for fireworks-related injury in Washington State. *JAMA* 1984;251:3251–3254.

National Fire Protection Association. *Fireworks-related injuries, deaths, and fires.* Quincy (MA): NFPA; 2004.

Smith GA, Knapp JF, Barnett, TM, Shields BJ. The rockets' red glare, the bombs bursting in air: fireworks-related injuries to children. *Pediatrics* 1996; 98(1):1–9.

U.S. Consumer Product Safety Commission. *CPSC stops hazardous products at the docks: Preventing fireworks injuries and deaths.* [cited 5 May 1996] Arlington (VA): 1996. Available at URL: www.cpsc.gov/cpscpub/pubs/success/firework.html

U.S. Consumer Product Safety Commission. Safety commission holds seventh annual fireworks safety news conference. [cited 28 June 1993]. Arlington (VA): The Commission; 1993.

Additional Information

CDC-INFO Contact Center
Toll-Free: 800-CDC-INFO (232-4636)
Toll-Free TTY: 888-232-6348
Website: http://www.cdc.gov
E-mail: cdcinfo@cdc.gov

Chapter 36

Teen Injury
in the Workplace

Preventing Deaths, Injuries, and Illnesses of Young Workers

Many young workers die or are hospitalized each year from injuries at work. Many also suffer adverse health effects from hazardous exposures in the workplace. An average of 67 workers under age 18 died from work-related injuries each year during 1992–2000. In 1998, an estimated 77,000 required treatment in hospital emergency rooms.

Research surveys of students and parents suggest that 70% to 80% of teens have worked for pay at some time during their high school years. Between 1996 and 1998, a monthly average of 2.9 million workers aged 15 to 17 worked during school months, and 4.0 million worked during summer months. Workers aged 15 to 17 spend the most work hours in food preparation and service jobs, stock handler or laborer jobs, administrative support jobs, and farming, forestry, or fishing jobs.

Developmental factors in young workers and the nature of their employment may increase their risk of injury or illness on the job.

- Young workers commonly perform tasks outside their usual work assignments for which they may not have received training.

This chapter includes: Excerpts from "Preventing Deaths, Injuries, and Illnesses of Young Workers," Centers for Disease Control and Prevention (CDC), NIOSH Publication No. 2003-128, July 2003; and "Do You Have a Working Teen," Occupational Safety and Health Administration (OSHA).

- Young workers may lack the experience and physical and emotional maturity needed for certain tasks.

- Young workers may be unfamiliar with work requirements and safe operating procedures for certain tasks.

- Young workers may not know their legal rights and may not know which work tasks are prohibited by child labor laws.

- Young workers are experiencing rapid growth of organ and musculoskeletal systems, which may make them more likely to be harmed by exposure to hazardous substances or to develop cumulative trauma disorders.

- Young workers may be exposed to suspected asthma-causing agents and substances that disrupt the function or maturation of the endocrine and central nervous systems.

Fatalities

According to data from the U.S. Bureau of Labor Statistics (BLS), 603 workers under age 18 suffered fatal occupational injuries between 1992 and 2000, an average of 67 per year. Of these, 362 were aged 16 or 17, 119 were aged 14 or 15, and 122 were under age 14. More than 30% of all fatal injuries to young workers occurred in family businesses.

Table 36.1. Percentage of Work-Related Deaths by Industry: Workers Under Age 18 Compared with All Workers, United States, 1992–2000.*

Industry	Workers under 18	All workers
Agriculture, forestry, and fishing	42%	14%
Retail trade (e.g., restaurants, retail stores)	18%	11%
Construction	14%	18%
Services (e.g., nursing homes, amusement parks, swimming pools)	11%	14%
Manufacturing	6%	12%
All other	9%	32%

*Data do not include work-related deaths in New York City.
Source: Census of Fatal Occupational Injuries Special Research Files, BLS, analysis by NIOSH [2003].

Table 36.2. Percentage of Work-Related Deaths by Event: Workers Under Age 18 Compared with All Workers, United States, 1992–2000.*

Event	Workers under 18	All workers
Transportation incidents	45%	42%
Contact with objects and equipment	19%	16%
Assaults and violent acts	17%	18%
Exposure to harmful substances and environments	10%	9%
Falls	7%	11%
All other	2%	4%

*Data do not include work-related deaths in New York City.
Source: Census of Fatal Occupational Injuries Special Research Files, BLS, analysis by NIOSH [2003].

Nonfatal Injuries

Information from national surveys indicates that only one-third of work-related injuries are seen in emergency departments; therefore, it is likely that nearly 230,000 teens suffered work-related injuries that year. According to emergency department data, workers aged 15 to 17 had a substantially higher rate of work-related injuries or illnesses in 1998 than did all workers aged 15 or older: 4.9 per 100 versus 2.9 per 100 full-time equivalent (FTE) workers.

Compared with adult workers, injuries to young workers result in slightly fewer days away from work. However, injury severity for young workers may be underestimated because days away from work are counted only if the injured worker was scheduled to work on those days.

Special Risks for Young Workers in Agricultural Work

Agriculture is the most dangerous industry for young workers, accounting for 42% of all work-related fatalities of young workers between 1992 and 2000. Unlike other industries, half the young victims in agriculture were under age 15. For young agricultural workers aged 15–17, the risk of fatal injury is four times the risk for young workers in other workplaces. Young workers employed in agriculture may be directly hired workers, employees of labor contractors, or farm residents working in the family business. Agricultural work exposes young workers to safety hazards such as machinery, confined spaces, work at elevations, and work around livestock. Young workers may also be exposed to agricultural chemicals (for example, pesticides or fertilizers), noise, respiratory irritants, and toxic gases.

Workers may legally perform any agricultural task after they reach age 16, whereas they are prohibited from some jobs in other industries until they reach age 18. Furthermore, child labor laws do not cover workers under age 16 who work on their parents' or guardians' farms. Between 1992 and 2000, 76% of the fatal injuries to agricultural workers under age 16 involved work in a family business.

Special Risks for Young Workers in Retail Trades

The second highest number of workplace fatalities among workers younger than age 18 occurred in the retail trades (for example, restaurants and retail stores). Between 1992 and 2000, 63% of these deaths were due to assaults and violent acts, most of which were homicides. Homicide associated with robbery is the probable cause for one-fourth to one-half of all young worker fatalities in retail trades. Handling cash, working alone or in small numbers, and working in the late evening and early morning hours may contribute to workplace homicides.

In 1998, more than half of all work-related nonfatal injuries to young workers occurred in retail trades, more than 60% of which were eating and drinking establishments. Cuts in retail trades were the most common type of injury treated in emergency departments, followed by burns in eating and drinking establishments, and bruises, scrapes, and scratches in other retail settings. Common hazards in restaurants include using knives to prepare food, handling hot grease from fryers, working near hot surfaces, and slipping on wet or greasy floors.

Transportation: Motor Vehicles and Mobile Machinery

Persons aged 16 to 20 in the general population have higher fatality and injury rates due to motor vehicle crashes than any other age group. In the workplace, 45% of all fatal injuries to workers under age 18 between 1992 and 2000 resulted from transportation incidents. Transportation incidents include incidents occurring on or off the highway involving motor vehicles as well as industrial vehicles (such as tractors and forklifts) in which at least one vehicle was in operation. Child labor laws prohibit workers under age 18 from operating many types of motor vehicles or mobile machinery. Operating a motor vehicle at work is prohibited for workers aged 16 and allowed only under limited circumstances for those aged 17. Despite current restrictions, transportation-related fatalities and injuries among young workers continue to occur. Ensuring safe operation of vehicles on the job by young workers poses special challenges for employers. In addition to being new to the workplace, young employees are new to driving, which compounds the risk of injury.

Construction

The complex and ever-changing construction work environment presents multiple safety hazards. Overall, more U.S. workers are killed working in construction than in any other industry. Construction workers risk injury from a wide range of events, including falls, electrocution, collapsing structures, machinery-related incidents, falling objects, and motor vehicle crashes. Child labor laws prohibit workers aged 14 and 15 from working in construction, except when performing office work away from the construction site. Other laws that apply to all workers under age 18 prohibit several tasks associated with construction, yet they do not address all hazards on the job site.

Safety Regulations that Protect Young Workers

The Occupational Safety and Health Administration (OSHA) within the U.S. Department of Labor (DOL) is the Federal agency with primary responsibility for setting and enforcing standards to promote safe and healthful working conditions for all workers. Employers are responsible for becoming familiar with standards applicable to their establishments and for ensuring a safe working environment.

A workplace may be fully compliant with OSHA regulations and yet may place young workers at risk of injury or illness if applicable Federal and State child labor laws are not followed. One study estimated that more than three-fourths of employers of young workers were unfamiliar with child labor laws. Lack of awareness of occupational safety and health laws by young workers, adults, and employers has been identified as a major obstacle to preventing injury and illness in young workers.

The primary Federal law governing the employment of workers under age 18 is the Fair Labor Standards Act (FLSA) of 1938, which is enforced by the Wage and Hour Division of the Employment Standards Administration within DOL. The FLSA does not cover all young workers. The FLSA applies to an entire business enterprise if the enterprise has annual gross revenues of $500,000 or more. Some States extend coverage of child labor laws to all businesses, regardless of revenues. Even if an entire enterprise is not covered, the FLSA applies to individual workers engaged in producing, transporting, loading, or receiving goods for interstate commerce. Interstate commerce also includes workers who handle documents related to interstate commerce, such as credit card transactions.

Child Labor Regulation No. 3 restricts hours and specifies allowable employment activities for workers aged 14 and 15. Two other groups of regulations define work prohibited for young workers in terms of Hazardous Orders—occupations declared hazardous for young workers by the Secretary of Labor. The first of these defines hazardous farm work prohibited for workers under age 16. However, no Federal child labor laws cover children working on their parents' or guardians' farms. Another group of regulations applicable to nonagricultural businesses, including family businesses, defines jobs prohibited for adolescents under age 18. DOL reviews Federal child labor laws on an ongoing basis to ensure that they provide adequate protection to young workers.

States may also have their own child labor laws that are stricter than Federal laws. For example, Maine and Massachusetts prohibit all workplace driving by workers under age 18, whereas Federal law allows occasional and incidental driving by workers aged 17, although in limited circumstances. If a State child labor law is less protective than Federal law, or if no applicable State law exists, Federal child labor laws apply (if the business meets the requirements for coverage under Federal laws).

Conclusions

Employment of young workers can have many benefits for businesses and for young workers. However, the potential for serious injury and death must be recognized and addressed by everyone involved. Employers, educators, parents, and young workers may not be aware of safety and health laws designed to protect young workers on the job. Safety and health regulations alone cannot control or eliminate all the factors that may contribute to risk of injury for young workers. One or more of the following circumstances are commonly present when young workers are injured or killed at work:

- Young workers may not be trained to perform assigned tasks safely.

- Young workers may be assigned to perform incidental tasks for which they have no training or experience, or they may take it upon themselves to perform these tasks.

- Young workers may not be adequately supervised.

- Young workers lack the experience and maturity needed to recognize and deal with injury hazards. More specifically, they may not yet have a sufficient understanding of work processes to recognize hazardous situations.

- Young workers may not have the training or experience to handle emergencies or injuries.

- Young workers, their employers, and parents may disregard or be unaware of child labor laws that specify the jobs and the hours that young workers may not work.

Recommendations for Young Workers and Their Employers

Young workers should take the following steps to protect themselves:

- Know about and follow safe work practices:

  - Recognize the potential for injury at work.
  - Follow safe work practices.
  - Seek information about safe work practices from employers, school counselors, parents, State labor departments, and the Department of Labor (DOL).

- Ask about training: Participate in training programs offered by your employer, or request training if none is offered.

- Ask about hazards: Don't be afraid to ask questions if you are not sure about the task you are asked to do. Discuss your concerns with your supervisor or employer first.

- Know your rights: Be aware that you have the right to work in a safe and healthful work environment free of recognized hazards.

  - You have the right to refuse unsafe work tasks and conditions.

  - You have the right to file complaints with DOL when you feel your rights have been violated or your safety has been jeopardized.

  - You are entitled to workers' compensation for a work-related injury or illness.

- Know the laws: Before you start work, learn what jobs young workers are prohibited from doing. State child labor laws may be more restrictive than Federal laws, and they vary considerably from State to State.

Employers should take the following steps to protect young workers:

- Recognize the hazards:

  - Reduce the potential for injury or illness in young workers by assessing and eliminating hazards in the workplace.

  - Make sure equipment used by young workers is safe and legal.

- Supervise young workers:

  - Make sure that young workers are appropriately supervised.

  - Make sure that supervisors and adult coworkers are aware of tasks young workers may or may not perform.

  - Label equipment that young workers cannot use, or color-code uniforms of young workers so that others will know they cannot perform certain jobs.

- Provide training:

  - Provide training in hazard recognition and safe work practices.

  - Have young workers demonstrate that they can perform assigned tasks safely and correctly.

  - Ask young workers for feedback about the training.

- Know and comply with child labor laws and occupational safety and health regulations that apply to your business. State laws may be more restrictive than Federal laws, and they vary considerably from State to State. Post these regulations for workers to read.

- Involve supervisors and experienced workers in developing a comprehensive safety program that includes an injury and illness prevention program and a process for identifying and solving safety and health problems. OSHA consultation programs are available in every State to help employers identify hazards and improve their safety and health management programs.

Do You Have a Working Teen?

It is important to realize that teens and all workers are entitled to a safe and healthful work environment. Do not assume your teen-agers are aware of their rights or that employers are aware of child labor laws for teenagers.

Take an active role in the employment decisions of your children. Some work sites are safer than others. Know where your teens are working and what they are doing. Frequently ask teens what they did at work and discuss any problems or concerns.

Discuss with your teen the types of work they are involved with and the training and supervision provided by the employer.

Watch for signs that the job is taking too much of a physical or mental toll on your teen. How is your child's performance at school? If there is loss of interest in or energy for school, the job may be too demanding. Other signs of concern could include increased stress levels, anxiety, fatigue, depression, and use of alcohol or other drugs.

Support your teen in reporting hazards to managers or, if necessary, to OSHA or your state department of labor, if the work environment seems to be unsafe.

Know Federal and State Child Labor Laws

Know the Federal child labor laws and the State child labor laws for the area in which you live, so you can recognize if employers are following the law. For example, are employers working your teen longer hours than allowed or in unsafe conditions?

Federal law limits the number and hours that 14- and 15-year-olds can work in non-agricultural work sites. They are not permitted to work during school hours, or before 7 a.m. or after 7 p.m. between Labor Day and June 1. During the summer, they can work only between 7 a.m. and 9 p.m. (Again, state laws may be more stringent.) When school is in session, teens are not allowed to work more than 18 hours each week, more than three hours on a school day, or more than eight hours on a weekend day or holiday. When school is not in session, they are prohibited from working more than 40 hours each week or eight hours per day.

Examples of jobs and work-related activities that the federal government prohibits—some states have even stricter regulations—for non-agricultural workers under age 18 include:

- driving a motor vehicle as a regular part of the job or operating a forklift
- operating many types of power equipment such as meat slicers, power saws, and bakery machinery
- wrecking, demolition, excavation, or roofing
- logging, mining, or working in sawmills
- meat packing or slaughtering
- any job involving exposure to radiation
- any job where explosives are manufactured or stored

Anyone age 14 or 15 is also banned from the following jobs or work-related activities:

- baking or cooking
- operating power-driven machines such as lawnmowers and electric hedge clippers. (Low-risk machines like photocopiers and computers are all right.)
- climbing ladders or scaffolding
- working in warehouses
- manufacturing, building, or working in construction
- loading or unloading trucks, railroad cars, or conveyors

Youth of any age may be employed at any time, in any occupation in agriculture on a farm owned or operated by their parent or guardian.

Additional Information

U.S. Department of Labor (DOL)
Information Referral Service
Frances Perkins Building
200 Constitution Ave. NW
Washington DC 20210
Toll-Free: 866-487-2365
Toll-Free TTY: 877-889-5627
Website: http://www.dol.gov

Chapter 37

Trends in
Adolescent Injuries

Unintentional Injuries Are the Leading Cause of Death for Adolescents and Young Adults

Unintentional injuries account for the greatest number of adolescent and young adult deaths. Among young people ages 10–24 in 2001, 15,964 died as a result of unintentional injuries, representing 44.1% of all deaths in this age group.[1] Over seven out of ten unintentional injury deaths involved motor vehicle accidents. The unintentional injury mortality rate for this age group has decreased during the past two decades, from 43.2/100,000 in 1981 to 26.1/100,000 in 2001.[2]

Unintentional Injury Mortality Is Highest for Older Adolescent and Young Adult Males

Among adolescents and young adults, males ages 18–19 had the highest mortality rates in 2001, followed by males ages 20–24. After young adulthood, mortality due to unintentional injury decreases throughout the lifespan. Males have a higher unintentional injury mortality rate than females, and this gender disparity increases with age: males ages 10–14 were 1.8 times as likely to die as same-age females, while males ages 20–24 were 3.5 times as likely to die as their female peers.[2]

Reprinted with permission of the National Adolescent Health Information Center. 2004. Fact Sheet on Unintentional Injury: Adolescents and Young Adults, San Francisco, CA. University of California, San Francisco.

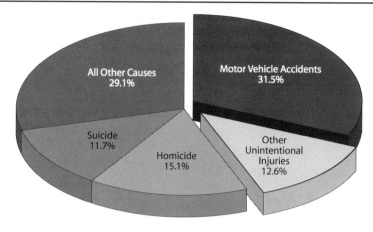

Figure 37.1. Leading Causes of Death, Ages 10–24, 2001[2]

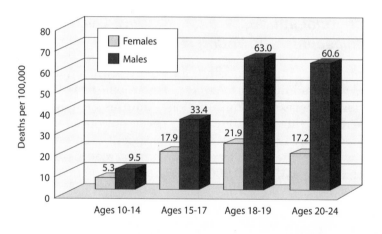

Figure 37.2. Unintentional Injury Mortality by Age and Gender, Ages 10–24, 2001[2]

Motor Vehicle Accidents Account for 71% of Unintentional Injury Deaths among Adolescents/Young Adults

In 2001, motor vehicle accidents (MVA) accounted for almost three-fourths of all unintentional injury mortality and one-third of all mortality for adolescents and young adults.[2] Alcohol use and lack of seat belt use contribute to MVA mortality at all ages. Lack of driving experience is also a contributing factor for adolescents.[3] Other unintentional injuries included poisoning, drowning, fires/burns, suffocation and falls. Non Hispanic American Indian/Alaskan Native youth were 1.8 to 3.6 times more likely to die from unintentional injury than their peers in other racial/ethnic groups.[2]

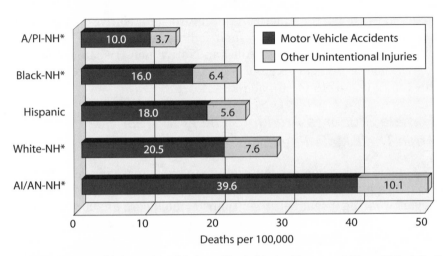

Figure 37.3. *Unintentional Injury Mortality by Type and Race/Ethnicity,* Ages 10–24, 2001*[2]

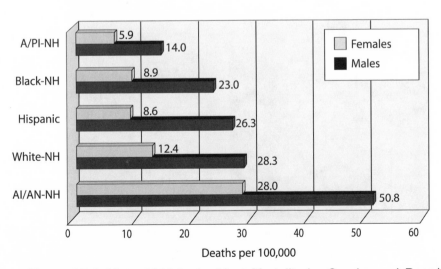

Figure 37.4. *Motor Vehicle Accident Mortality by Gender and Race/ Ethnicity,* Ages 10–24, 2001*[2]

Motor Vehicle Accident Mortality Is Highest for Young American Indian/Alaskan Native Males

Among males ages 10–24, the motor vehicle accident mortality rate is two times higher for non Hispanic American Indians/Alaskan Natives than same-age males in other racial/ethnic groups. Among females ages 10–24, the American Indian/Alaskan Native-non Hispanic rate is 2.6 times greater than their female peers in other racial/ethnic groups. American Indian/Alaskan Native-non Hispanics have the highest motor vehicle accident mortality rates (per 100,000) at ages 10–14 (12.0), 15–19 (49.6), and 20–24 (61.8).[2]

Female Students Are More Likely to Wear Seat Belts Than Their Male Peers.

Female high school students are more likely to wear seat belts than same-age males. Male students were more likely to report "rarely or never" wearing a seat belt than their female peers in 2003 (21.5% vs. 14.6%, respectively). These figures varied little by race/ethnicity. Seat belt use among high school students increased over the last decade, with 18.2% reporting "rarely or never" wearing a seat belt in 2003, compared to 25.9% in 1991.[4] Motor vehicle accidents are less likely to end in fatality when seat belts are used.[5]

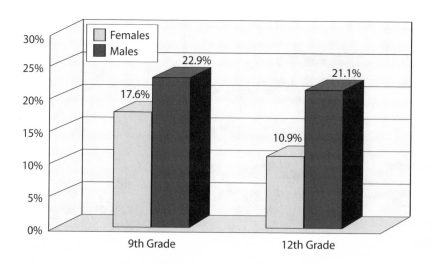

Figure 37.5. *"Rarely/Never Wore" Seat Belts by Gender and Grade Level, High School Students, 2003[4]*

Male Students Are almost Twice as Likely to Drink and Drive as Their Female Peers

Male high school students are much more likely to drink and drive than female students. In 2003, 12.1% of high school students reported driving after drinking, a decrease from 16.7% in 1991. Both genders are almost equally likely to ride with a driver who has been drinking. Hispanic students (36.4%) were more likely than Black-non Hispanic (30.9%) and White-non Hispanic (28.5%) students to report riding with a driver who had been drinking. In 2003, 30.2% of high school students reported this behavior—a large decrease from 40% in 1991.[4] In 2002, 30% of fatal motor vehicle accidents among adolescents and young adults ages 16–24 involved a driver who had been drinking.[5]

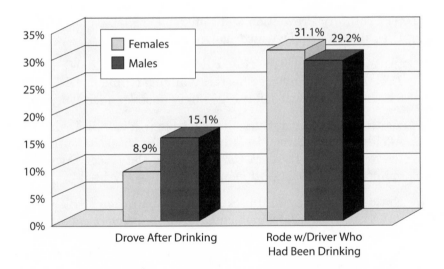

Figure 37.6. *Driving and Drinking Behavior by Gender, High School Students, 2003[4]*

Unintentional Injury Mortality Has Decreased in the Past Two Decades for Adolescents and Young Adults

Mortality rates for unintentional injury among older adolescents and young adults have decreased by one-third in the past two decades. The decrease in MVA mortality plays a large role in the overall decline.[2]

A contributing factor may be the decrease in alcohol-related MVA mortality (deaths per 100,000), which fell from 16.3 in 1990 to 9.0 in 2001 among adolescents ages 16–20.[2, 5]

*NH(s)=non Hispanic(s); AI/AN=American Indian/Alaskan Native; A/PI=Asian/Pacific Islander.

Data and Figure Sources

1. Anderson, R.N., and Smith, B.L. (2003). *Deaths: Leading causes for 2001.* National Vital Statistics Reports, 52(9), 1-86. [Available online at URL (9/04): http://www.cdc.gov/nchs/products/pubs/pubd/nvsr/nvsr52/nvsr52_09.pdf]

2. National Center for Injury Prevention and Control [NCIPC]. (2004). *Mortality reports database* [Online Database]. Atlanta, GA: Centers for Disease Control and Prevention, National Center for Injury Prevention and Control. [Available online at URL (9/04): http://www.cdc.gov/ncipc/wisqars/]

3. Insurance Institute for Highway Safety [IIHS]. (2004). *Q&A: Teenagers* [Online Fact Sheet]. [Available online at URL (9/04): http://www.hwysafety.org/ safety_facts/qanda/teens.htm]

4. Youth Risk Behavior Surveillance System [YRBSS], Division of Adolescent and School Health, Centers for Disease Control and Prevention. (2004). *Youth Online* [Online Database]. [Available online at URL (9/04): http://apps.nccd.cdc.gov/yrbss/]

5. National Highway Traffic Safety Administration [NHTSA]. (2004). *Traffic safety facts 2002: A compilation of motor vehicle crash data from the fatality analysis reporting system and the general estimates system.* Washington, DC: National Highway Traffic Safety Administration, National Center for Statistics and Analysis, U.S. Department of Transportation. [Available online at URL (9/04): http://www.nrd.nhtsa.dot.gov/pdf/nrd30/NCSA/TSFAnn/TSF2002Final.pdf]

In all cases, the most recent available data were used. Some data are released 1–3 years after collection. In some cases, trend data with demographic breakdowns (e.g., racial/ethnic) are relatively limited. For racial/ethnic data, the category names presented are those of the data sources used. Every attempt was made to standardize age ranges; when this was not possible, age ranges are those of the data sources used.

Additional Information

National Adolescent Health Information Center
School of Medicine
University of California, San Francisco
UCSF Box 0503
San Francisco, CA 94143-0503
Phone: 415-502-4856
Fax: 415-502-4858
Website: http://nahic.ucsf.edu
E-mail: nahic@ucsf.edu

Chapter 38

Injury Prevention Tips for Teens

Car Crashes

Since car crashes are the most common cause of injury among teens, let's start with them. How are you going to keep yourself and others safe on the road? How many of you wear a safety belt every time you are in a car? One of the most important choices you can make is to wear a safety belt and make everyone in your car wear one too. Your safety belt is going to keep you behind the wheel, so you have a better chance of keeping control of the car, or securely in the passenger seat. Air bags save a lot of lives, but you have to stay 10–12 inches behind the airbag so it won't hurt or kill you. The air bag and the safety belt are designed to work together to reduce injuries. Options include:

- **No Airbag, no belt:** Without an air bag or safety belt, the person has no protection and is thrown into the steering column, windshield, or even out of the car, causing serious injury or death. If you think an air bag would hurt, how do you think it would feel to have the metal steering column go into your chest?

- **Airbag, no belt:** When the person doesn't buckle up and there is an air bag, the person is thrown closer than that 10–12 inch distance and the air bag explodes at speeds of up to 200 mph,

Excerpted from "Think First for Teens: Safety," Copyright © ThinkFirst National Injury Prevention Foundation, reprinted with permission. For more information visit www.thinkfirst.org.

causing severe injuries or death. You have to have the safety belt on to keep you back from that impact.

- **Airbag and belt:** With the safety belt on, the person is held back and the air bag protects him. This person will have the least amount of injury, or maybe no injury at all. Do not be afraid of the air bag: it inflates and deflates in less than a second, so with the safety belt, it will keep you from going into the steering column or through the windshield. What if you are in the back seat? Do you think you will be thrown any less of a distance than if you are in the front? No. So you need to be buckled no matter where you are in the car.

Bicycles and Motorcycles

Motorcycles, motocross, and all terrain vehicles do not have airbags, seat belts, and that protective frame a car offers you—so there's basically nothing between you and the pavement if you crash on a motorcycle. If you do choose to ride a motorcycle, we hope you also choose to wear a helmet and protective clothing, like leather, so if you hit that asphalt, you have something between your head, your skin, and that pavement. Unfortunately, there are not many good outcomes with these crashes. Consider that there is the speed of the bike, how far you are thrown, and how far you have to come down to land—the impact is usually too much to survive.

Bicycles are like motorcycles in one way; there is nothing between you and the pavement. Again helmets are about 85% effective in reducing brain injuries due to bike crashes, so if you have not started wearing a helmet yet, find one you like and get in the habit of using it.

Diving

Important things to remember when swimming and diving include:

- Never swim alone. Always swim with a buddy.
- Try to swim in supervised areas only.
- Know your swimming limits and stay within them.
- Know how to prevent, recognize, and respond to emergencies.
- Never drink alcohol and swim.
- Obey "No Diving" signs, which always indicate the area is unsafe for head first entries. A general rule is to enter the water

feet first rather than head first if you do not know the depth. The water should be eight feet deep or deeper.

- Watch out for the "dangerous too's"—too tired, too cold, too far from safety, too much sun, too much strenuous activity.

- Stay out of the water when overheated.

- Use common sense about swimming after eating. In general, you do not have to wait an hour after eating before you can swim. However, if you have eaten a large meal, it is best to digest before swimming.

- Know local weather conditions and prepare for electrical storms. It is best to get out of the water when you hear thunder. Do not wait for lightning to strike.

Team Sports

If you are involved in team sports such as football or hockey, make sure you are using the right equipment and the right technique. Be sure to condition well; remember your muscles protect other parts of your body. Try not to use unnecessary force. Keep in mind, a helmet is going to protect your head, but it is not going to do anything for your spinal cord.

Violence

Violence is another unnecessary cause of injury and death. This is not the way you want to be noticed or remembered; there are so many other great things to be filling your life with. We all need to make an effort to be thoughtful and forgiving of others and solve problems in non-violent ways. Do not get involved in gangs or use handguns.

Conflict Resolution

So much violence could be prevented if only we would stop and think about how to handle problems. How could we be smarter and better at resolving problems? It is easy to act tough; it takes a lot more to stay cool. Stop and think about the situation. Weigh your choices and the consequences of each choice. Focus on the problem, do not make it personal, and then, use some strategies. What are some possible strategies?

- **Avoidance:** Avoid the situation or remove yourself from a situation until you or the other person have regained control and calmed down.

- **Diffusion:** One example of diffusion is humor; use humor to laugh at or lighten the situation. Another type of diffusion is to agree with the person. If they say something rude or ridiculous, agree and walk away, diffusing the situation.

- **Confrontation:** Talk with them about the problem. Pick the right time to speak to the person and tell them in a controlled voice that what they said or did hurt, angered, or offended you, and ask them for an explanation.

- **Negotiation:** Talk about it and compromise. Tell them you are sorry that they are upset and agree to talk about it later, alone or with others involved. Agree that there was a misunderstanding. Apologize when appropriate and accept their apology if given.

Additional Information

ThinkFirst National Injury Prevention Foundation
26 S. La Grange Rd., Suite 103
La Grange, IL 60525
Toll-Free: 800-844-6556
Phone: 708-588-2000
Fax: 708-588-2002
Website: http://www.thinkfirst.org
E-mail: thinkfirst@thinkfirst.org

Part Six

Physical Disorders and Illnesses That May Affect Adolescents

Chapter 39

Asthma Management

Childhood Asthma

Asthma is the most common chronic disease of childhood, and yet many parents know little about it. In the United States, it is estimated that nearly five million youngsters under age 18 have this disease. In 1993 alone, asthma was the reason for almost 200,000 hospital stays and about 340 deaths among persons under age 25.

The number of young people and children with asthma is rising. In children ages 5–14 years, the rate of death from asthma almost doubled between 1980 and 1993. The disease is more common in blacks and in city-dwellers than in whites and those who reside in suburban and rural areas. A government survey of young people with asthma (those aged 15–24 years) showed that more blacks than whites died of the disease from 1980 to 1993. Among children aged 0–4 years in 1993, blacks were six times more likely to die from asthma than whites. Among children aged 5–14, blacks were four times more likely than whites to die of the illness.

Although asthma can occur in people of any age, even in infants, most children with the illness developed it by about age five.

This chapter includes: "Childhood Asthma," reprinted with permission from the Asthma and Allergy Foundation of America, © 2005. All rights reserved. For additional information about asthma and related topics visit the AAFA website at http://www.aafa.org. Also, excerpts from "Asthma Prevalence, Health Care Use, and Mortality, 2002," Centers for Disease Control and Prevention (CDC), August 23, 2005.

Asthma seems to be more common in boys than in girls in early childhood. The survey mentioned above showed that in 1993, boys aged 0–4 were 1.4 times more likely than girls the same age to die from asthma. This increased risk remained in boys aged 5–14, who were 1.3 times more likely to die from asthma than girls in that age group. By the teen years, the risk seems to even out between girls and boys.

These numbers can be cause for alarm, but the best defense against childhood asthma begins with knowledge of the disease. This is the best way to ensure that if your child does develop asthma you and your doctor can work together to control the illness.

What is asthma?

Asthma is a chronic (long-term) illness in which the airways become blocked or narrowed. This is usually temporary, but it causes shortness of breath, trouble breathing, and other symptoms. If asthma becomes severe, the person may need emergency treatment to restore normal breathing.

When you breathe in, air travels through your nose and/or mouth through a tube called the trachea (sometimes referred to as the windpipe). From there, it enters a series of smaller tubes that branch off from the trachea. These branched tubes are the bronchi, and they divide further into smaller tubes called the bronchioles. It is in the bronchi and bronchioles that asthma has its main effects.

The symptoms of asthma are triggered by things in the environment. These vary from person to person, but common triggers include cold air; exercise; allergens (things that cause allergies) such as dust mites, mold, pollen, animal dander, or cockroach debris; and some types of viral infections.

Here is how the process occurs. When the airways come into contact with one of these triggers, the tissue inside the bronchi and bronchioles becomes inflamed (inflammation). At the same time, the muscles on the outside of the airways tighten up (constriction), causing them to narrow. Then the fluid (mucus) is released into the bronchioles, which also become swollen. The breathing passages are narrowed still more, and breathing becomes very difficult.

This process can be normal, up to a point. Everyone's airways constrict somewhat in response to irritating substances. But in a person with asthma, the airways are hyperreactive. This means that their airways overreact to things that would just be minor irritants in people without asthma.

To describe the effects of asthma, some doctors use the term twitchy airways. This is a good description of how the airways of people with asthma are different from those without the disease. (Not all patients with hyperreactive airways have symptoms of asthma, though).

In mild cases of asthma, the symptoms usually subside on their own. Most people with asthma, though, need medication to control or prevent the episodes. The need for medication is based on how often asthma attacks occur and how severe they are. With the treatments available today, most children with asthma can do almost everything that children without the disease can do.

Who gets asthma and what triggers it?

Some traits make it more likely that a child will develop asthma. These risk factors can alert you to watch for signs of the disease so that your child can be treated promptly.

Heredity. To some extent, asthma seems to run in families. Children whose brothers, sisters, or parents have asthma are more likely to develop the illness themselves. If both parents have asthma, the risk is greater than if only one parent has it. For some reason, the risk appears to be greater if the mother has asthma than if the father does.

Atopy. Certain types of allergies can increase a child's risk of developing asthma. A person is said to have atopy (or to be atopic) when he or she is prone to have allergies. This tendency is passed on from the person's parents. It is not the same as inheriting a specific type of allergy. Rather, it is merely the tendency to develop allergies. In other words, both the child and the parent might be allergic to something, but not necessarily to the same thing.

Substances in the environment that cause allergies—things like dust mites, mold, or pollen—are known as allergens. Atopy causes the body to respond to allergens by producing *immunoglobulin E* (IgE) antibodies. Antibodies are proteins that form in response to foreign substances in the body. One way to test a person for allergies is to perform skin tests with extracts of the allergens or do blood tests for IgE antibodies to these allergens.

What are some asthma triggers?

It is important to be aware of the things in your environment that tend to make asthma worse. These factors vary from person to person. Some of the more common factors or triggers are described here.

Allergens. Some allergens (substances that cause allergies) are more likely to trigger an asthma attack. For instance, babies in particular may have food allergies that can bring on asthma symptoms. Some of the foods to which American children are commonly allergic are eggs, cow's milk, wheat, soybean products, tree nuts, and peanuts.

A baby with a food allergy may have diarrhea and vomiting. He or she is also likely to have a runny nose, a wet cough, and itchy, flaky skin. In toddlers, common allergens that trigger asthma include house dust mites, molds, and animal hair. In older children, pollen may be a trigger, but indoor allergens and molds are more likely to be a cause of asthma.

Viral infections. Some types of viral infections can also trigger asthma. Two of the most likely culprits are respiratory syncytial virus (RSV) and parainfluenza virus. The latter affects the respiratory tract in children, sometimes causing bronchitis (inflammation of the bronchi) or pneumonia (inflammation of the lining inside the lungs). RSV can cause diseases of the bronchial system known as bronchopneumonia and bronchiolitis. A young child who has wheezing with bronchiolitis is likely to develop asthma later in life.

Tobacco smoke. Today most people are aware that smoking can lead to cancer and heart disease. What you may not be aware of, though, is that smoking is also a risk factor for asthma in children and a common trigger of asthma for all ages.

It may seem obvious that people with asthma should not smoke, but they should also avoid the smoke from others' cigarettes. This secondhand smoke, or passive smoking, can trigger asthma symptoms in people with the disease. Studies have shown a clear link between secondhand smoke and asthma in young people. Passive smoking worsens asthma in children and teens and may cause up to 26,000 new cases of asthma each year.

Other irritants in the environment can also bring on an asthma attack. These irritants may include paint fumes, smog, aerosol sprays, and even perfume.

Exercise. Exercise—especially in cold air—is a frequent asthma trigger. A form of asthma called exercise-induced asthma is triggered by physical activity. Symptoms of this kind of asthma may not appear until several minutes of sustained exercise. (When symptoms appear sooner than this, it usually means that the person needs to adjust his or her treatment). The kind of physical activities that can bring on asthma symptoms include not only exercise, but also laughing, crying, holding one's breath, and hyperventilating (rapid, shallow breathing).

The symptoms of exercise-induced asthma usually go away within a few hours. With proper treatment, a child with exercise-induced asthma does not need to limit his or her overall physical activity.

Other triggers. Cold air, wind, rain, and sudden changes in the weather can sometimes bring on an asthma attack.

The ways in which children react to asthma triggers vary. Some children react to only a few triggers, others to many. Some children get asthma symptoms only when more than one trigger occurs at the same time. Others have more severe attacks in response to multiple triggers.

In addition, asthma attacks do not always occur right after exposure to a trigger. Depending on the type of trigger and how sensitive this child is to it, asthma attacks may be delayed.

Each case of asthma is unique to that particular child. It is important to keep track of the factors or triggers that you know provoke asthma attacks in your child. Because the symptoms do not always occur right after exposure, this may take a bit of detective work.

What are the symptoms of asthma?

Common symptoms of asthma include:

- **Wheezing** is a high-pitched, whistling sound that your child may make during an asthma attack. If you hear this sound as your child breathes, be sure to let your doctor know. Not all people who wheeze have asthma, and not all those who have asthma wheeze. In fact, if asthma is really severe, there may not be enough movement of air through a person's airways to produce this sound.

- **Chronic cough,** especially at night and after exercise or exposure to cold air, can be a symptom of asthma.

- **Shortness of breath,** especially during exercise, is another possible sign. All children get out of breath when they're running and jumping, but most resume normal breathing very quickly afterward. If your child doesn't, a visit to your doctor is in order.

- **Tightness in the chest** is a symptom that you may have to ask your child about. If you notice any of the signs just described, it's a good idea to ask your child whether he or she feels a tight, uncomfortable feeling in the chest.

Treatment for Asthma

Because each case of asthma is different, treatment needs to be tailored for each child. One general rule that does apply, though, is removing those things in the child's environment that you know act as triggers for asthma symptoms. When possible, keeping down levels of dust mites, mold, animal dander, and cockroach debris in the house—especially in the child's bedroom—can be helpful. When these measures are not enough, it may be time to try one of the many medications that are available to control symptoms.

New guidelines from the National Institutes of Health advise treating asthma with a stepwise approach. This means using the lowest dose of medication that is effective, then stepping up the dose and the frequency with which it is taken if the asthma gets worse. When the asthma gets under control, the medicines are then stepped down.

Asthma medications may be either inhaled or in pill form. These medications are divided into two types—quick-relief and long-term control. The first group (quick relief) is used to relieve the immediate symptoms of an asthma attack. The second group (long-term control) does not provide relief right away, but over time these medications help to lessen the frequency and severity of attacks.

Like any medication, asthma treatments often have side effects. Be sure to ask your doctor about the side effects of the medications your child is prescribed and what warning signs should prompt you to contact your doctor.

Quick-relief medications. Medications that provide immediate relief of asthma symptoms relax the muscles around the airways, making breathing easier. They begin to work within minutes after they are used, and their effects may last for up to six hours.

Most of the quick-relief medications are inhaled through a pocket-sized device that your child can easily learn to use when he or she feels symptoms coming on. These medications can also be used before exercise to help ward off asthma symptoms. Commonly used quick-relief treatments for asthma include albuterol, bitolterol, metaproterenol, pirbuterol, and terbutaline. In addition, ipratropium is an inhaled asthma medication that works more slowly than the above medications. It is not effective for exercise-induced asthma, but it is helpful in people, such as older adults, who cannot tolerate the side effects of the medications listed.

Other quick-relief medications are methylprednisolone, prednisolone, and prednisone. These oral corticosteroids are taken by mouth in short bursts to establish initial control or to control symptoms during a period of gradual deterioration.

Long-term control medications. The list of long-term control medications for asthma include both oral and inhaled medications. Unlike the quick-relief medications, long-term medicines do not provide quick relief in the midst of an asthma episode. Rather, they work over the long term to reduce the frequency and severity of attacks. Most of these medications take several weeks of regular use to achieve their full effect, and all work only when they are taken consistently.

The long-term control medications can be divided into four broad categories:

- inhaled anti-inflammatory agents
- oral corticosteroids
- long-acting bronchodilators
- oral leukotriene modifiers

Anti-inflammatory agents prevent and reduce airway inflammation. They also make airways less sensitive to asthma triggers.

Corticosteroids are the most potent and consistently effective long-term control medications. Children with moderate to severe persistent asthma take inhaled corticosteroids daily, while those with mild persistent asthma may take an inhaled corticosteroids or inhaled non-steroids such as cromolyn sodium or nedocromil.

Inhaled anti-inflammatory medications are taken through a metered-dose inhaler (MDI). This is a device that delivers a measured amount of medication each time it is used. Most can also be inhaled through a nebulizer. With this device, medication is turned into a vapor that is inhaled deeply into the lungs.

The non-steroids have very few mild side effects. Potential side effects of inhaled steroids are cough, hoarseness, oral thrush, and perhaps a slowing of the rate of growth. Thrush is a type of yeast infection in the mouth. To decrease the chance of thrush and other systemic reactions, patients are advised to rinse out the mouth with water after each use and to use a spacer or holding chamber attached to the MDI. Ask your doctor about potential side effects in relationship to the goal of adequately controlling asthma.

Long-term oral corticosteroids can have total body (systemic) side effects. Talk with your doctor about how to minimize these while maintaining adequate control of your child's asthma.

Oral corticosteroids may be given in liquid or tablet form and begin to work within a few hours. They are given for a short period of time, such as a few days, to control severe asthma episodes and to speed recovery. These medications may be given for longer periods in patients who have very severe and recurrent asthma attacks. Patients taking corticosteroids must never stop using these medications all at once because this can cause side effects. Rather, their use must be tapered off over a period of a day or two. It is especially important to take these medications exactly as prescribed by your doctor.

Long-acting bronchodilators relax the muscles around the airways, making breathing easier. Their effects last up to 12 hours, and like the inhaled anti-inflammatory agents, they continue to work only if they are taken regularly. These medications can be taken either through a metered-dose inhaler or by mouth, in tablet, capsule, or liquid form. Their side effects may include nervousness, dry mouth, or rapid heartbeat. As with any medications, talk with your doctor about potential side effects.

Leukotriene modifiers are the latest class of medications used to treat asthma. These medications prevent and reduce airway inflammation and constriction of the airway muscles. They also make airways less sensitive to asthma triggers and can reduce the need for short-acting reliever medications. Leukotriene modifiers seem to have fewer side effects than other asthma treatments. Depending on what type of leukotriene modifier is used, side effects may include upset stomach, diarrhea, and changes in liver function tests. As with any new type of medication, frequent, clear communication between you and your doctor is required.

Sometimes asthma medications are combined to provide better treatment than any one used alone can offer. The goals of asthma treatment are to allow restful nighttime sleep, avoid the need for hospital stays, and allow your child to engage in normal play and school activities—in other words, to give him or her a normal life. Many treatment options exist to achieve this goal. The choice of treatment depends on the details of your child's own case.

Be Involved in Your Child's Care

Asthma is an illness that is best understood, rather than feared. If your child has asthma, learn all you can about the disease and work with your child's doctor. This will afford your child the best chance of controlling asthma and allowing him or her to lead a normal, healthy, and happy life.

Asthma Prevalence, Health Care Use, and Mortality Information from the National Center for Health Statistics

Estimates of current asthma prevalence include people who have been diagnosed with asthma by a health professional and who still have asthma. In 2002, 72 people per 1,000 or 20 million people, currently had asthma. Eighty-three per 1,000 children 0–17 years (6.1 million children) had asthma. The current asthma prevalence rate for boys aged 0–17 years (94 per 1,000) was 30% higher than the rate among girls (71 per 1,000).

About 60% of the people who had asthma at the time of the survey had an asthma attack in the previous year. Fifty-eight per 1,000 children 0–17 years (4.2 million children) had an asthma attack in the previous year. The asthma attack prevalence rate for boys aged 0–17 years (68 per 1,000) was 45% higher than the rate among girls (47 per 1,000).

Missed School and Work Days, 2002

Asthma attacks interfere with daily activities, including attending school and going to work. According to the National Health Interview Survey done by the National Center for Health Statistics, among those who reported at least one asthma attack in the previous year:

- children 5–17 years of age missed 14.7 million school days due to asthma

- adults 18 years of age and over who were currently employed missed 11.8 million work days due to asthma

Health Care Use, 2002

Health care use for asthma includes outpatient visits to doctors' offices and hospital outpatient departments, visits to hospital emergency departments (ED), and hospitalizations. In 2002, there were 13.9 million outpatient asthma visits to private physician offices and hospital outpatient departments, or 492 per 10,000 people. Children aged 0–17 years had 5 million visits and an outpatient visit rate of 687 per 10,000; and adults 18 years and older had a rate of 181 per 10,000. There were 1.9 million visits to ED for asthma in 2002, or 67 per 10,000 people. Among children 0–17 years, there were 196,000 hospitalizations (27 per 10,000).

Mortality

In 2002, 4,261 people died from asthma, or 1.5 per 100,000 people. Among children, asthma deaths are rare. In 2002, 187 children aged 0–17 years died from asthma, or 0.3 deaths per 100,000 children compared to 1.9 deaths per 100,000 adults aged 18 or over.

Additional Information

Asthma and Allergy Foundation of America (AAFA)
1233 20ᵗʰ St. NW, Suite 402
Washington, DC 20036
Toll-Free: 800-7-ASTHMA (800-727-8462)
Website: http://www.aafa.org
E-mail: info@aafa.org

Chapter 40

Young People with Cancer

Chapter Contents

Section 40.1

Diagnosis and
Treatment of Childhood Cancer

Excerpted from "Young People with Cancer: A Handbook for Parents,"
National Cancer Institute (NCI), 2001. Reviewed in April 2006 by Dr.
David A. Cooke, M.D., Diplomate, American Board of Internal Medicine.

What Is Cancer?

Cancer is a group of many related diseases that begin in cells, the
body's basic unit of life. To understand cancer, it is helpful to know
what happens when normal cells become cancerous. The body is made
up of many types of cells. Normally, cells grow and divide to produce
more cells only when the body needs them. This orderly process helps
keep the body healthy. Sometimes, however, cells keep dividing when
new cells are not needed. These extra cells form a mass of tissue called
a growth or tumor.

Tumors can be benign or malignant.

- Benign tumors are not cancer. They can often be removed and,
  in most cases, they do not come back. Cells from benign tumors
  do not spread to other parts of the body. Most important, benign
  tumors are rarely a threat to life.

- Malignant tumors are cancer. Cells in these tumors are abnormal and divide without control or order. They can invade and
  damage nearby tissues and organs. Also, cancer cells can break
  away from a malignant tumor and enter the bloodstream or the
  lymphatic system. That is how cancer spreads from the original
  cancer site to form new tumors in other organs. Cancer that has
  spread is called metastatic cancer.

Most cancers are named for the organ or type of cell in which they
begin. When cancer spreads (metastasizes), cancer cells are often found
in nearby or regional lymph nodes (sometimes called lymph glands). If
the cancer has reached these nodes, it means that cancer cells may have

spread to other organs, such as the liver, bones, or brain. When cancer spreads from its original location to another part of the body, the new tumor has the same kind of abnormal cells and the same name as the primary tumor. For example, if lung cancer spreads to the brain, the cancer cells in the brain are actually lung cancer cells. The disease is called metastatic lung cancer (not brain cancer).

Children can get cancer in the same parts of the body as adults do, but some types of cancer are more common in children. The most common form of childhood cancer is leukemia. Leukemia is cancer of the blood. It develops in the bone marrow, which is a spongy substance that fills the inside of the bones and makes blood cells. Other cancers often found in children are brain tumors, childhood lymphomas, Hodgkin disease, Wilms' tumors, neuroblastomas, osteogenic sarcomas, Ewing's sarcomas, retinoblastomas, rhabdomyosarcomas, and hepatoblastomas.

Children's cancers do not always act like, get treated like, or respond like adult cancers. Avoid reading about adult cancer to learn about your child's prognosis. Childhood cancers can occur suddenly, without early symptoms, and have a high rate of cure.

When Your Child Is Diagnosed

After your child's cancer has been diagnosed, a series of tests will be done to help identify your child's specific type of cancer. Called staging, this series of tests is sometimes done during diagnosis. Staging determines how much cancer is in the body and where it is located. To stage solid tumors, the doctor looks at the size of the tumor, the lymph nodes affected, and where it has spread. To stage leukemia, the doctor checks the bone marrow, liver, spleen, and lymph nodes around the sites where the leukemia can hide. Staging must be done to determine the best treatment.

As soon as your child is suspected to have or is diagnosed with cancer, you will face decisions about who will treat your child, whom to ask for a second opinion (if desired or if the diagnosis is not clear), and what the best treatment is. After your child's staging is complete, the treatment team develops a plan that outlines the exact type of treatment, how often your child will receive treatment, and how long it will last.

Talking with Your Child's Doctor

Your child's doctor and the treatment team will give you a lot of details about the type of cancer and possible treatments. Ask your doctor to explain the treatment choices to you. It is important for you to become a partner with your treatment team in fighting your child's cancer. One way for you to be actively involved is by asking questions. You may find it hard to concentrate on what the doctor says, remember everything you want to ask, or remember the answers to your questions. Here are some tips for talking with those who treat your child:

- Write your questions in a notebook and take it to the appointment with you. Record the answers to your questions and other important information.

- Tape record your conversations with your child's health care providers.

- Ask a friend or relative to come with you to the appointment. The friend or relative can help you ask questions and remember the answers.

Questions to Ask the Doctor and Treatment Team

When your child's treatment team gives you information about your child's cancer, you may not remember everything. That is natural. It is a lot of information, and your emotions will get in the way as you try to take it all in. Use the three techniques listed—write, tape record, and/or ask a friend for help—to help you retain the information you need to be an effective partner with your child's treatment team. Make sure you know the answers to these questions:

About the diagnosis:

- What kind of cancer does my child have?

- What is the stage, or extent, of the disease?

- Will any more tests be needed? Will they be painful? How often will they be done?

About treatment choices:

- What are the treatment choices? Which do you recommend for my child? Why?

- Would a clinical trial be right for my child? Why?

- Have you treated other children with this type of cancer? How many?

- What are the chances that the treatment will work?
- Where is the best place for my child to receive treatment? Are there specialists—such as surgeons, radiologists, nurses, anesthesiologists, and others—trained in pediatrics? Can my child have some or all of the treatment in our home town?

About the treatment:

- How long will the treatment last?
- What will be the treatment schedule?
- Whom should we ask about the details of financial matters?
- Will the treatment disrupt my child's school schedule?

About side effects:

- What possible side effects of the treatment can occur, both right away and later?
- What can be done to help if side effects occur?

About the treatment location:

- How long will my child be in the hospital?
- Can any treatment be done at home? Will we need any special equipment?
- Does the hospital have a place where I can stay overnight during my child's treatment?

About school and other activities:

- Is there a child-life worker specialist (a professional who is responsible for making the hospital and treatment experience less scary for the child) to plan play therapy, schoolwork, and other activities?
- When can my child go back to school?
- Are there certain diseases my child cannot be around? Should I have my child and his or her siblings immunized against any diseases?
- Will my child need tutoring?
- Is information available to give to the school system about my child's needs as he or she receives treatment?

Questions Your Child May Ask

Children are naturally curious about their disease and have many questions about cancer and cancer treatment. Your child will expect you to have answers to most questions. Teems may begin to ask questions right after diagnosis or may wait until later. Here are some common questions and some ideas to help you answer them.

Why me?

A teen, like an adult, wonders "Why did I get cancer?" A teen may feel that it is his or her fault, that somehow he or she caused the illness. Make it clear that not even the doctors know exactly what caused the cancer.

Will I get well?

Children often know about family members or friends who died of cancer. As a result, many teens are afraid to ask if they will get well because they fear that the answer will be no. Thus, you might tell your child that cancer is a serious disease, but that treatment—such as medicine, radiation, or an operation—has helped get rid of cancer in other children, and the doctors and nurses are trying their best to cure your child's cancer, too.

What will happen to me?

When your child is first diagnosed with cancer, many new and scary things will happen. It is important to try to get your teen to talk about their concerns. Explain ahead of time about the cancer, treatment, and possible side effects. Discuss what the doctor will do to help if side effects occur. You can also explain that there are many different types of cancer and that even when two children have the same cancer, what happens to one child will not always happen to the other.

Teens should be told about any changes in their treatment schedule or in the type of treatment they receive. This information helps them prepare for visits to the doctor or hospital. Keeping a calendar that shows the days for doctor visits, treatments, or tests helps teens to be involved.

Why do I have to take medicine when I feel okay?

With cancer, your child may feel fine much of the time but need to take medicine often. Children do not understand why they have to take medicine when they feel well. You may want to remind your child of the reason for taking the medicine in the first place.

Treatment

To plan the best treatment, the doctor and treatment team will look at your child's general health, type of cancer, stage of the disease, age, and many other factors. Based on this information, the doctor will prepare a treatment plan that outlines the exact type of treatment, how often your child will receive treatment, and how long it will last. Each child with cancer has a treatment plan that is chosen just for that child; even children with the same type of cancer may receive different treatments. Depending on how your child responds to treatment, the doctor may decide to change the treatment plan or choose another plan.

Before treatment begins, your child's doctor will discuss the treatment plan with you, including the benefits, risks, and side effects. Then you and the treatment team will need to talk with your child about the treatment. After the doctor fully explains the treatment and answers your questions, you will be asked to give your written consent to go ahead with treatment. Depending on your child's age and hospital policy, your child may also be asked to give consent before treatment.

Many parents find it helpful to get a copy of the treatment plan to refer to as the treatment proceeds. It also helps them in arranging their own schedules. Do not be afraid to ask questions or speak up if you feel something is not going right. Your child's doctor is often the best person to answer your questions, but other members of the treatment team can give you information, too. If you feel as though you need extra time with the doctor, schedule a meeting or phone call. Remember, you are part of the treatment team and should be involved in your child's treatment.

Types of Cancer Treatment

The types of treatment used most often to treat cancer are surgery, chemotherapy, radiation therapy, immunotherapy, and bone marrow or peripheral blood stem cell transplantation. Doctors use these treatments to destroy cancer cells. Depending on the type of cancer, children may have one kind of treatment or a combination of treatments. Most children receive a combination of treatments, called combination therapy.

359

Treatments for cancer often cause unwanted or unpleasant side effects such as nausea, hair loss, and diarrhea. Side effects occur because cancer treatment that kills cancer cells can hurt some normal cells, too. As your child begins treatment, you may want to keep the following in mind.

- The kinds of side effects and how bad they will be depend on the kind of drug, the dosage, and the way your child's body reacts.

- The doctor plans treatment so that your child has as few side effects as possible.

- The doctor and treatment team have ways to lessen your child's side effects. Talk with them about things that can be done before, during, and after treatment to make your child comfortable.

- Lowering the treatment dosage slightly to eliminate unpleasant side effects usually will not make the treatment less able to destroy cancer cells or hurt your child's chances of recovery.

- Most side effects go away soon after treatment ends.

Remember that not every child gets every side effect, and some children get few, if any. Also, how serious the side effects are varies from child to child, even among children who are receiving the same treatment. The doctor or treatment team can tell you which, if any, side effects your child is likely to have and how to handle them. If you know what side effects can occur, you can recognize them early.

Hospitalization

Being in the hospital is often scary for any child, especially at first. It is a whole new world to learn about—new people and strange machines, procedures, and routines. Adding a touch of home by having personal things in your child's room can help make the hospital a less scary place. These homey touches can help start a conversation between the hospital staff and your child.

Many hospitals and treatment centers help your family and your child spend as much time together as possible by allowing you to visit anytime and having beds for parents in the child's room or bedrooms nearby.

For teens who are trying to separate themselves from you and be more on their own, being in the hospital may thwart their drive for independence. At a time when young people are normally doing more on their own, cancer makes them rely on you more. As a result, adolescents may make it known, loudly and often, that they are unhappy. They may refuse treatment, break hospital rules, miss outpatient appointments, and rebel in other ways.

Children of any age will often cooperate more if given treatment choices that do not cause problems with their care. Parents can help teens become more independent by allowing them to share the responsibility for their care. Some hospitals also make a special effort to help children cope with illness and being in the hospital, such as allowing teenagers to dress in street clothes whenever possible and to have friends visit. Some hospitals have equipment that allows the child to interact with his or her classmates in their classroom.

Common Medical Procedures

Medical tests and procedures are not only used to diagnose cancer, but also to see how well the treatment is working and to make sure that the treatment is causing as little damage to normal cells as possible. Many of these tests will be repeated from time to time throughout treatment.

Parents and children say that knowing about the tests before they are done helps them to cope. Some of these tests are painful; most are not. For some tests, your child may need to remain still for as long as an hour. Ask your doctor what you and the treatment team can do to help your child become more comfortable during the tests. For procedures that require your child to remain very still, medicines can be given to help your child relax or become sleepy. For tests that can be painful, such as the bone marrow aspiration test and spinal tap, pain medicines are often given. Sometimes a general anesthetic, a drug that causes your child to lose consciousness and all feeling, is given.

Relaxation therapy (methods used to make one feel more relaxed and to feel less pain), guided imagery (using the imagination to create mental pictures), hypnosis (a trance-like state that can be brought on by a person trained in a special technique), music, and other techniques can also help to ease your child's discomfort and fear. When your child is relaxed, the procedures are less painful. Ask your treatment team to help you guide your child through relaxation exercises both before and during the procedures. Often a combination of pain medicine and relaxation techniques is used. Your child will want to be with you during the procedures, and in most situations, that is possible.

When to Call the Doctor

If you have worried about knowing when to call the doctor, you are not alone. Parents want to watch closely for any sign that their child may need to see the doctor but may not be sure what those signs are. They also may worry about bothering the doctor or treatment team. The best approach is to ask the doctor when to call about any problems your child may be having. If you are unsure, this list can be used as a guide for when to call the doctor.

Call the Doctor If...

Your child shows signs of infection.

- Fever (100.4°F or 38°C) or other signs of infection, especially if your child's white count is low. (The doctor will tell you when it is low.) It is important to take your child's temperature with an accurate thermometer.

Your child has trouble eating such as:

- mouth sores that keep your child from eating
- difficulty chewing

Your child has digestive tract problems including:

- vomiting, unless you have been told that your child may vomit after the cancer treatment
- painful urination or bowel movements
- constipation that lasts more than two days
- diarrhea

Your child shows changes in mobility or mood including:

- trouble walking, bending
- trouble talking
- dizziness
- blurred or double vision
- depression or a sudden change in behavior

Your child has troublesome symptoms such as:

- bleeding, including: nosebleeds; red or black bowel movements; pink, red, or brown urine; or many bruises
- severe or continuing headaches
- pain anywhere in the body
- red or swollen areas

Your child needs treatment for other health concerns, such as:

- before your child receives immunizations or dental care, even scheduled vaccinations or regular dental checkups
- before you give your child any over-the-counter medication

Section 40.2

Care for Children and Adolescents with Cancer

Excerpted from "Care for Children and Adolescents with Cancer: Questions and Answers," National Cancer Institute (NCI), November 2005.

Questions and Answers

Survival rates for childhood cancer have risen sharply over the past 25 years. In the United States, more than 75 percent of children with cancer are now alive five years after diagnosis, compared with about 60 percent in the mid-1970s.[1] Much of this dramatic improvement is due to the development of improved therapies at children's cancer centers, where the majority of children with cancer have their treatment.

What are children's cancer centers?

Children's cancer centers are hospitals or units in hospitals that specialize in the diagnosis and treatment of cancer in children and adolescents. Most children's, or pediatric, cancer centers treat patients up to the age of 20.

Why might a family look for a specialized children's cancer center when a child or adolescent is diagnosed with cancer?

Because childhood cancer is relatively rare, it is important to seek treatment in centers that specialize in the treatment of children with cancer. Specialized cancer programs at comprehensive, multidisciplinary cancer centers follow established protocols (step-by-step guidelines for treatment). These protocols are carried out using a team approach. The team of health professionals is involved in designing the appropriate treatment and support program for the child and the child's family. In addition, these centers participate in specially designed and monitored research studies that help develop more effective treatments and address issues of long-term childhood cancer survival.

When children go to a specialized cancer center, does it mean their treatment will be part of a research study?

Not necessarily. Participation in research studies is always voluntary. Parents and patients may choose to receive treatment as part of a clinical trial (research study); only patients and parents who wish to do so take part. However, a large number of children who go to pediatric cancer centers take part in clinical trials. About 70 percent of children with cancer are treated in an NCI-sponsored clinical trial at some point during their illness.

What is a clinical trial or research study?

In cancer research, a clinical trial is a study designed to show how a particular strategy—for instance, a promising anticancer drug, a new diagnostic test, or a possible way to prevent cancer—affects the people who receive it.

Treatment clinical studies fall into three categories:

- Phase I studies evaluate what dose is safe, how a new drug should be given (for example, by mouth, injected into a vein, or injected into the muscle), and how often. Phase I trials usually include a small number of patients and take place at only one or a few locations.

- Phase II studies investigate the safety and effectiveness of the treatment, and study how it affects the human body. Phase II clinical trials usually focus on a particular type of cancer, and include fewer than 100 patients.

- Phase III studies, which usually involve a larger number of patients at many locations, compare the new treatment (or new use of a standard one) with the current standard therapy.

What are the benefits of taking part in a clinical trial?

One advantage is the possibility that a new treatment (or diagnostic test or preventive measure) will turn out to be better than a more established method. Patients who take part in approaches that prove to be better have the first chance to benefit from them. In phase III clinical trials, in which one treatment is compared with another, patients receive either the most advanced and accepted treatment for the kind of cancer they have—known as the standard treatment—or a new treatment that has shown promise of being at least as beneficial as the standard treatment.

People who take part in clinical trials receive specialized care under a very precise set of directions, or protocol. To ensure quality care, highly trained and experienced cancer specialists design, review, and approve each protocol. In addition, all participants in clinical trials are carefully monitored during the study and are followed afterwards. Participants are often included in a network of clinical trials carried out around the country. In this network, doctors and researchers share their ideas and experience, and patients receive the benefit of the shared knowledge.

What are the risks of taking part in a clinical trial?

Clinical trials can involve risks as well as benefits. All cancer treatments have side effects, but treatments being studied may have side effects that are not yet understood as well as the side effects of standard treatments. The potential risks and benefits of each study are explained during the informed consent process, when patients and families discuss all aspects of the study with their doctors or nurses before deciding whether to participate.

What about costs? Do insurance or managed care plans cover treatment at a children's cancer center?

Some health plans cover part or all of the cost of care at children's cancer centers, but benefits vary from plan to plan. Questions or concerns about health care costs should be discussed with a medical social worker or the hospital or clinic billing office. Financial assistance and resources to cover health care costs may be available.

Can children with cancer be treated at the National Cancer Institute?

Children with cancer can receive treatment in clinical trials at the National Institutes of Health (NIH) Clinical Center in Bethesda, Maryland. Two branches of the NCI that study specific types of cancer have their own contact points:

- The Pediatric Oncology Branch (POB) conducts clinical trials for a wide variety of childhood cancers (except brain tumors) at the NIH Clinical Center. To refer children, teenagers, or young adults, call the POB office at 877-624-4878 between 8:30 a.m. and 5:00 p.m. Eastern time. An attending physician will return the call, determine whether the patient is eligible for a research study, and help arrange the referral. More information about the POB can be found at http://home.ccr.cancer.gov/oncology/pediatric/ on the Internet. Attending physicians in the POB are also available to provide a second opinion. The patient, family member, or health care provider can contact the POB to talk about a diagnosis or treatment plan.

- The Neuro-Oncology Branch offers a large number of clinical trials as well as consultation for children with brain tumors. Staff can provide a second opinion for doctors, patients, and family members who are interested in this service. Specialists can either evaluate the patient in person or review the patient's medical records and scans. To find out more about this service, and what information is needed, contact the Neuro-Oncology Branch toll-free at 866-251-9686 between 9:00 a.m. and 5:00 p.m. Eastern time. The Branch's Web site can be found at http://home.ccr.cancer.gov/nob/default.asp on the Internet.

How does a family find a children's cancer center?

A child's pediatrician or family doctor often can provide a referral to a children's cancer center. Families and health professionals also can call the NCI's Cancer Information Service (CIS) to learn about children's cancer centers that belong to the Children's Oncology Group (COG). All of the cancer centers that participate in these Groups have met strict standards of excellence for childhood cancer care. A directory of COG institutions by state is also available at http://www.curesearch.org/resources/cog.aspx on the Internet.

How do families cope with practical issues like getting to a treatment center and finding a place to stay near the center?

Many families receive helpful information from their doctors and nurses. Treatment centers often have social work departments that can provide assistance. In addition, various organizations offer support to families, including help with transportation, lodging, and financial assistance.

Selected Reference

1. Ries LAG, Eisner MP, Kosary CL, et al. (eds). *SEER Cancer Statistics Review, 1975–2002*, National Cancer Institute. Bethesda, MD, 2005 (http://seer.cancer.gov/csr/1975_2002).

Section 40.3

Follow-Up Care and Survivorship of Childhood Cancer

"Follow-Up Care: Questions and Answers," National Cancer Institute (NCI), September 2004; and an excerpt from "Living Beyond Cancer: Finding a New Balance: President's Cancer Panel 2003–2004 Annual Report: Executive Summary," National Cancer Institute (NCI), May 2004.

It is natural for anyone who has completed cancer treatment to be concerned about what the future holds. Many people are concerned about the way they look and feel, and about whether the cancer will recur (come back). They wonder what they can do to keep the cancer from coming back. They also want to know how often to see the doctor for follow-up appointments, and what tests they should have. Understanding what to expect after cancer treatment can help patients and their loved ones plan for follow-up care, make lifestyle changes, and make decisions about quality of life and finances.

What does follow-up care involve, and why is it important?

Follow-up care involves regular medical checkups that include a review of a patient's medical history and a physical exam. Imaging procedures (methods of producing pictures of areas inside the body); endoscopy (the use of a thin, lighted tube to examine organs inside the body); or lab tests may be part of follow-up care for certain cancers. Physical therapy, occupational or vocational therapy, pain management, support groups, or home care may also be included in the follow-up care plan.

Follow-up care is important because it helps to identify changes in health. The main purpose of follow-up care is to check for the return of cancer in the primary site (recurrence), or the spread of cancer to another part of the body (metastasis). Follow-up care can also help to identify the development of a second cancer, unknown or unusual treatment side effects, and late effects of cancer treatments (side effects that develop months or years after treatment).

It is important to note that cancer recurrences are not always detected during follow-up visits. Many times, recurrences are suspected or found by patients themselves between scheduled checkups. It is important for patients to be aware of changes in their health, and report any problems to their doctor. The doctor can determine whether the problems are related to the cancer, the treatment the patient received, or an unrelated health problem.

How are follow-up care schedules planned?

Ongoing health needs are not the same for everyone. Follow-up care is individualized based on the type of cancer, the type of treatment received, and the person's overall health. In general, people return to the doctor for follow-up appointments every three to four months during the first two to three years after treatment, and once or twice a year after that.

At these follow-up appointments, the doctor may recommend tests to check for recurrence or to screen for other types of cancer. In many cases, it is not clear that follow-up tests improve survival or quality of life. This is why it is important for the doctor to help determine what follow-up care plan is appropriate. The doctor may not need to perform any tests if the person appears to be in good physical condition and does not have any symptoms. It is important for the patient to talk with the doctor about any questions or concerns related to the follow-up care schedule.

When planning a follow-up care schedule, patients should consider who will provide the follow-up care and other medical care. They should think about selecting a doctor with whom they feel comfortable. This may be the same doctor who provided the person's cancer treatment. For other medical care, people can continue to see a family doctor or medical specialist as needed.

Some people might not have a choice in who provides their follow-up care. Some insurance plans pay for follow-up care only with certain doctors, and for a set number of visits. Patients may want to check their medical coverage plan to see what restrictions, if any, apply to their follow-up care.

Do some doctors or clinics specialize in follow-up care?

Very few comprehensive cancer centers and academic medical centers have clinics devoted to the follow-up care of adult cancer patients. However, a number of clinics provide follow-up care for pediatric cancer survivors. Patients can contact local comprehensive cancer centers or academic medical centers to see if follow-up care clinics exist in their area.

What questions should people ask their doctor about follow-up care?

People may want to ask the doctor these questions about follow-up care:

- How often should I have a routine visit?
- What follow-up tests, if any, should I have?
- How often will I need these tests?
- What symptoms should I watch for?
- If I develop any of these symptoms, whom should I call?

Many patients find it helpful to write these questions down and take notes, or tape their discussions with the doctor to refer to at a later time.

How can patients deal with their emotions during follow-up care?

It is common to experience stress, depression, and anxiety after cancer treatment. Many people find it best to talk about their feelings with

369

family and friends, health professionals, other patients, and counselors such as clergy and psychotherapists. Being part of a support group may be another effective outlet for people to share their feelings. Relaxation techniques such as imagery and slow rhythmic breathing can also help to ease negative thoughts or feelings. Reaching out to others by participating in volunteer activities is also an effective way for a person who has completed cancer treatment to feel stronger and more in control. However, people who continue to experience emotional distress should talk to their doctor about a referral for further evaluation of what may be causing or contributing to their distress, and how to deal with it.

What kinds of medical records and information should patients keep?

It is important for people to keep records of their health history. Patients may not always see the same doctor for their follow-up care, so having this information available to share with another doctor can be helpful. It is important to keep track of the following types of information:

- specific type of cancer (diagnosis)

- date(s) of cancer diagnosis

- details of all cancer treatment, including the places and dates where treatment was received (for example, type and dates of all surgeries; names and doses of all drugs; sites and total amounts of radiation therapy)

- contact information for all doctors and other health professionals involved in treatment and follow-up care

- complications that occurred after treatment

- information on supportive care received (for example, pain or nausea medication, emotional support, and nutritional supplements)

What other services may be useful during follow-up care?

Other services that may be helpful during follow-up care include financial aid and housing for patients receiving follow-up care. Information about services after cancer treatment is available from national cancer organizations, hospitals, local churches or synagogues, the Young Men's Christian Association (YMCA) or Young Women's Christian Association (YWCA), or local or county government agencies. To get the most from any of these services, it is important to think about what questions to ask before calling. Many people find it helpful to write out their questions, and to take notes during the conversation. It is also important to find out about eligibility requirements for services.

Issues Affecting Cancer Survivors: Information from the President's Cancer Panel, 2003

For the nearly ten million Americans now living with a cancer history, life after cancer means finding a new balance—one that celebrates the triumph and relief of completing treatment, recognizes changes or losses the disease has wrought, and assimilates revised perspectives, newfound strengths, and lingering uncertainties. Typically, few signposts exist to guide these highly personal journeys into a familiar but forever changed world.

Life after cancer treatment may hold diverse and often unexpected challenges. These challenges may be influenced by numerous factors, including the survivor's age at the time of diagnosis, the type and severity of both the cancer and its treatment, the duration of an individual's survival, financial and geographic access to needed follow-up care, employment and educational issues, information needs, and cultural, spiritual, literacy, and language differences. The impact of many of these factors, and the issues that arise from them, is magnified among many survivors from minority and other underserved populations.

Issues Affecting Cancer Survivors across the Life Span

Both the testimony and additional data gathered suggested that several issues affect cancer survivors and their families regardless of whether the survivor was diagnosed as a child, an adolescent or young adult, in adulthood, or in older age:

- Many survivors leave treatment with neither adequate documentation of the care they received nor a written description of recommended follow-up care and resources for obtaining that care. The lack of a national electronic health record system is an impediment to continuity and quality of care for cancer survivors.

- Cancer survivors and their families need better information about existing laws and regulations that may protect their employment, insurance, and assets.

371

- Privacy provisions of the Health Insurance Portability and Accountability Act (HIPAA) are inhibiting needed research on survivor issues and blocking appropriate information sharing among providers and between providers and the patient's caregivers.

- Education about cancer, cancer treatment, and survivorship needs is inadequate. The general public, newly diagnosed patients and their caregivers, post-treatment survivors, and health care providers all have significant unmet information needs. Understanding of clinical trials also is limited among all of these groups.

- Many survivors, caregivers, and family members need, but are not receiving, psychosocial assistance and support, both during treatment and in the months and years that follow. Family caregivers increasingly are becoming medical care providers in the home, but are not receiving adequate training and ongoing support for this role.

- The risk of infertility associated with cancer treatment and opportunities for preserving reproductive capacity are not being conveyed fully to newly diagnosed cancer patients of reproductive age or to the parents of children diagnosed with cancer prior to selecting or initiating treatment. For many, access to available fertility preservation options is limited by cost.

- Existing insurance systems in the United States are a significant impediment to appropriate care for people with a cancer history. The link between employment and insurance particularly disadvantages cancer survivors, who risk losing both their employment and insurance during extensive treatment. Lower income, young adult, and near elderly survivors are particularly vulnerable to becoming uninsured. Coverage for psychosocial care and follow-up care is inadequate even under most comprehensive health plans or Medicare.

Survivors Diagnosed as Children

Five issues of special importance to survivors diagnosed before age 15 were identified:

1. Survivors of cancer diagnosed in childhood may need special assistance to re-enter the classroom setting successfully and

may require accommodations to learning difficulties resulting from their disease or its treatment. Parents of these survivors may need assistance advocating for their children in the school system.

2. Some survivors of childhood cancers have social development and psychosocial issues that require attention years after treatment ends. These issues may include depression, social problems due to missing typical childhood experiences, and difficulty integrating the cancer experience as a part of the individual's life.

3. Many survivors of childhood cancers are not being transitioned appropriately from pediatric care to adult health care settings and receive inadequate assistance in coordinating their follow-up care. Issues include inadequate transfer of information between pediatric oncologists and primary care providers, particularly if the child received treatment away from home, and lack of understanding among primary care providers of the follow-up care needs of childhood cancer survivors.

4. Caregivers and siblings of children with cancer have longer-term psychosocial needs that are not being met. Both parents and siblings are vulnerable to post-traumatic stress disorder. Support groups and services available during the treatment period are far less available post-treatment, particularly when the patient was treated away from home.

5. Continued research is needed on the long-term effects of cancer treatment on survivors of pediatric cancers. Limited follow-up of pediatric patients, even those treated on clinical trials, is a major barrier to better understanding late treatment effects experienced by this population. Specialized late effects clinics may prove useful for addressing this issue, but require further development and evaluation.

Survivors Diagnosed as Adolescents or Young Adults

In addition to concerns common to survivors of all ages, people diagnosed between the ages of 15 and 29 have other distinct needs:

*   Adolescent and young adult cancer survivors—sometimes called the orphaned cohort—are a vastly understudied population. Because they often relocate to attend college or obtain employment, follow-up on this population has been particularly difficult.

- Diagnosis and treatment during this crucial developmental period often results in a range of psychosocial issues, including problems with depression, limited social skills, difficulty planning for the future and establishing independence, and coping with neurocognitive problems resulting from cancer treatment. Body image and fertility issues may be a significant impediment to developing intimate relationships.

- Similar to childhood cancer survivors, adolescents and young adults treated in the pediatric setting are not being transitioned effectively to care in the adult setting.

- Adolescent and young adult cancer survivors, particularly those with disabilities requiring accommodation, may find themselves at a disadvantage when competing for jobs, and may be starting adulthood burdened by significant treatment-related debt. In addition, once terminated from their parents' health insurance policies, they are highly likely to become uninsured and lose access to follow-up care.

Psychosocial and Support Needs

Family members, primary care providers, cancer specialists, and others who are close to or provide medical care to adolescent and young adult survivors should be made aware that depression, anxiety, or other psychosocial issues may affect the survivor long after treatment ends and should be instructed on how to intervene should the survivor experience such difficulties.

Adolescent and young adult survivors should be taught self-advocacy skills that may be needed to secure accommodations for learning differences resulting from cancer or its treatment. Physicians and other providers should act as advocates for survivors when necessary.

Additional Help and Information

Association of Cancer Online Resources (ACOR)
173 Duane St., Suite 3A
New York, NY 10013-3334
Phone: 212-226-5525
Website: http://www.acor.org

The Association of Cancer Online Resources (ACOR), a cancer information system that offers access to electronic mailing lists and Web sites, provides a list of long-term follow-up care clinics for children and adolescents treated for cancer. This list is on ACOR's Pediatric Oncology Resource Center Web page at: http://www.acor.org/ped-onc/treatment/surclinics.html

Candlelighters Childhood Cancer Foundation
National Office
P.O. Box 498
Kensington, MD 20895-0498
Toll-Free: 800-366-CCCF (800-366-2223)
Phone: 301-962-3520
Fax: 301-962-3521
Website: http://www.candlelighters.org
E-mail: staff@candlelighters.org

Candlelighters is an international organization of parents whose children have or have had cancer. It offers information and assistance to families through a national parent information service, newsletters, and other publications. It also has local chapters in many towns and cities around the United States, which can be important sources of practical information and support for families.

Leukemia and Lymphoma Society
Information Resource Center
1311 Mamaroneck Ave.
White Plains, NY 10605-5221
Toll-Free: 800-955-4572
Fax: 914-949-6691
Website: http://www.leukemia-lymphoma.org

The Leukemia and Lymphoma Society offers financial assistance and consultation services for referrals to other means of local support are offered by chapters of the Leukemia and Lymphoma Society to patients with leukemia, lymphomas, and myeloma. Educational materials for patients and family members are provided through local chapters and the Home Office.

National Cancer Institute (NCI)
Cancer Information Service
Toll-Free: 800-4-CANCER (800-422-6237)
TTY: 800-332-8615

Website: http://www.cancer.gov
Live online assistance:
https://cissecure.nci.nih.gov/livehelp/welcome.asp

A list of National Cancer Institute (NCI)-designated cancer centers is available in the fact sheet "The National Cancer Institute Cancer Centers Program" on the Internet at: http://www.cancer.gov/cancertopics/factsheet/NCI/cancer-centers

National Children's Cancer Society
1015 Locust St., Suite 600
St. Louis, MO 63101
Toll-Free: 800-5-FAMILY (800-532-6459)
Phone: 314-241-1600 (Program Services)
Fax: 314-241-1996
Website: http://www.children-cancer.com

The National Children's Cancer Society. This independent, national organization provides a broad range of services, including financial and in-kind assistance, advocacy, support services, and education and prevention programs.

Ronald McDonald House Charities
One Kroc Drive
Oak Brook, IL 60523
Phone: 630-623-7048
Fax: 630-623-7488
Website: http://www.rmhc.com

Ronald McDonald House Charities. Many major cities have Ronald McDonald Houses where out-of-town families can stay while their children are being treated for a serious illness. The room rates are economical.

Chapter 41

Type 1 (Juvenile) Diabetes

Diabetes is a chronic disease in which the body does not make or properly use insulin, a hormone that is needed to convert glucose and other food into energy. People with diabetes have increased blood glucose levels due to an absence of insulin, or failure to respond to insulin's effects (insulin resistance). Inadequate insulin results in high concentrations of glucose that build up in the blood and spill into the urine, causing an obligate urinary excretion of glucose. As a result, the body loses its main source of fuel.

Type 1 diabetes is an autoimmune disease in which the immune system destroys the insulin-producing beta cells of the pancreas that regulate blood glucose. Type 1 diabetes has an acute onset, with children and adolescents usually able to pinpoint when symptoms began. Onset can occur at any age, but it most often occurs in children and young adults. Since the pancreas can no longer produce insulin, people with type 1 diabetes require daily injections of insulin for life. Children with type 1 diabetes are at risk for long-term complications (damage to cardiovascular system, kidneys, eyes, nerves, blood vessels, gums, and teeth).

Type 1 diabetes accounts for five to ten percent of all diagnosed cases of diabetes, but is the leading cause of diabetes in children. A diabetes management plan for young people includes insulin therapy, self-monitoring of blood glucose, healthy eating, and physical activity. The plan is designed to ensure proper growth and prevention of

Excerpted from "Overview of Diabetes in Children and Adolescents," National Diabetes Education Program, January 2006.

hypoglycemia. New management strategies are helping children with type 1 diabetes live long and healthy lives.

Symptoms. The symptoms of type 1 diabetes usually develop over a short period of time. They include increased thirst and urination, constant hunger, weight loss, and blurred vision. Children also may feel very tired. If not diagnosed and treated with insulin, the individual with type 1 diabetes can lapse into a life-threatening diabetic coma, known as diabetic ketoacidosis or DKA. Often, children will present with vomiting, a sign of DKA, and mistakenly be diagnosed as having gastroenteritis. New-onset diabetes can be differentiated from a gastrointestinal (GI) infection by the frequent urination that accompanies continued vomiting as opposed to decreased urination due to dehydration if the vomiting is caused by a GI infection.

Risk Factors. A combination of genetic and environmental factors put people at increased risk for type 1 diabetes. Researchers are working to identify these factors and to stop the autoimmune process that destroys the pancreas.

Co-morbidities. Autoimmune diseases such as celiac disease and autoimmune thyroiditis are associated with type 1 diabetes.

Statistics

Diabetes is one of the most common chronic diseases in school-aged children. In the United States, about 176,500 people under 20 years of age have diabetes. About one in every 400 to 600 children has type 1 diabetes. Each year, more than 13,000 children are diagnosed with type 1 diabetes. The incidence of type 1 is about 7 per 100,000 per year in children ages four and under; 15 per 100,000 per year in children 5 to 9 years; and about 22 per 100,000 per year in those 10 to 14 years of age. About 75 percent of all newly diagnosed cases of type 1 diabetes occur in individuals younger than 18 years of age.

Identifying Children with Type 1 Diabetes

The rate of beta cell destruction in type 1 diabetes is quite variable—rapid in some individuals (mainly infants and children) and slow in others (mainly adults). Children and adolescents may present with ketoacidosis as the first indication of the disease. Others may have modest fasting hyperglycemia that rapidly changes to severe hyperglycemia and/or ketoacidosis in the presence of infection or other stress.

Treatment Strategies

The basic elements of type 1 diabetes management are insulin administration, nutrition management, physical activity, blood glucose testing, and the avoidance of hypoglycemia. Algorithms are used for insulin dosing based on blood glucose level and food intake. Children receiving fixed insulin doses of intermediate- and rapid-acting insulin must have food given at the time of peak action of the insulin. Children receiving a long-acting insulin analogue or using an insulin pump receive a rapid-acting insulin analogue just before a meal, with the amount of pre-meal insulin based on carbohydrate content of the meal using an insulin/carbohydrate ratio and a sliding scale for hyperglycemia. Further adjustment of insulin or food intake may be made based on anticipation of special circumstances such as increased exercise. Children on these regimens are expected to check their blood glucose levels routinely before meals and at bedtime.

There is no single recipe to manage diabetes that fits all children. Blood glucose targets, frequency of blood glucose testing, type, dose and frequency of insulin, use of insulin injections or a pump, and details of nutrition management, all may vary among individuals. The family and diabetes care team determine the regimen that best suits each child's individual characteristics and circumstances.

Blood Glucose Goals

To control diabetes and prevent complications, blood glucose levels must be managed as close to a normal range as is safely possible (70 to 100 mg/dl before eating). Families should work with their health care team to set target blood glucose levels appropriate for the child.

The American Diabetes Association has developed recommendations for blood glucose goals for young people with type 1 diabetes. Key concepts in setting glycemic goals:

- Goals should be individualized and lower goals may be reasonable based on benefit: risk assessment.

- Blood glucose goals should be higher than those listed above in children with frequent hypoglycemia or hypoglycemia unawareness.

- Postprandial blood glucose values should be measured when there is a disparity between preprandial blood glucose values and A1C levels.

Table 41.1. Optimal plasma blood glucose and A1C goals for type 1 diabetes by age group

Values by Age (Years)	Plasma Blood Glucose Goal Range (mg/dl)		A1C Percent	Rationale
	Before Meals	Bedtime/ Overnight		
Toddlers and preschoolers under age 6	100–180	110–200	less than or equal to 8.5 but greater than or equal to 7.5	High risk and vulnerability to hypoglycemia
School age, ages 6 to 12	90–180	100–180	less than 8	Risks of hypogly-cemia and rela tively low risk of complications prior to puberty
Adolescents and young adults, ages 13 to 19	90–130	90–150	less than 7.5*	Risk of hypogly-cemia Developmental and psychological issues

*A lower goal (less than 7.0) is reasonable if it can be achieved without excessive hypoglycemia.

Hypoglycemia

Diabetes treatment can sometimes cause blood glucose levels to drop too low, with resultant hypoglycemia. Taking too much insulin, missing a meal or snack, or exercising too much may cause hypoglycemia. A child can become irritable, shaky, and confused. When blood glucose levels fall very low, loss of consciousness or seizures may develop.

When hypoglycemia is recognized, the child should drink or eat a concentrated sugar to raise the blood glucose value to greater than 80 mg/dl. Once the blood glucose is over 80, the child can eat food containing protein to maintain blood glucose levels in the normal range. The concentrated sugar will increase blood glucose levels and cause resolution of symptoms quickly, avoiding over-treatment of lows. If the child is unable to eat or drink, a glucose gel may be administered to the buccal mucosa of the cheek or glucagon may be injected.

Hyperglycemia

Causes of hyperglycemia include forgetting to take medications on time, eating too much, and getting too little exercise. Being ill also can raise blood glucose levels. Over time, hyperglycemia can cause damage to the eyes, kidneys, nerves, blood vessels, gums, and teeth. Sick-day management rules, including assessment for ketosis with every illness, must be established for children with type 1 diabetes. Families need to be taught what to do for vomiting and for ketosis to prevent severe hyperglycemia and ketoacidosis.

Monitoring Complications and Reducing Cardiovascular Disease Risk

The following recommendations are based on the American Diabetes Association's Standards of Medical Care.

Retinopathy. Although retinopathy most commonly occurs after the onset of puberty and after 5–10 years of diabetes duration, it has been reported in prepubertal children and with diabetes duration of only 1–2 years. Referrals should be made to eye care professionals with expertise in diabetic retinopathy, an understanding of the risk for retinopathy in the pediatric population, as well as experience in counseling the pediatric patient and family on the importance of early prevention/intervention. The first ophthalmologic examination should be obtained once the child is ten years of age or older and has had diabetes for 3–5 years. After the initial examination, annual routine follow-up is generally recommended. Less frequent examinations may be acceptable on the advice of an eye care professional.

Nephropathy. To reduce the risk and/or slow the progression of nephropathy, optimize glucose and blood pressure control. Annual screening for microalbuminuria should be initiated once the child is ten years of age and has had diabetes for five years. Screening may be done with a random spot urine sample analyzed for microalbumin-to-creatinine ratio. Confirmed, persistently elevated microalbumin levels should be treated with an angiotensin-converting enzyme (ACE) inhibitor, titrated to normalization of microalbumin excretion if possible.

Neuropathy. Although it is unclear whether foot examinations are important in children and adolescents, annual foot examinations are

381

painless, inexpensive, and provide an opportunity for education about foot care. The risk for foot complications is increased in people who have had diabetes over ten years.

Lipids. In children older than two years of age with a family history of total cholesterol over 240 mg/dl, or a cardiovascular disease (CVD) event before age 55, or if family history is unknown, perform a lipid profile after diagnosis of diabetes and when glucose control has been established. If family history is not a concern, then perform a lipid profile at puberty. Based on data obtained from studies in adults, having diabetes is equivalent to having had a heart attack, making diabetes a key risk factor for future cardiovascular disease.

Pubertal children should have a lipid profile at the time of diagnosis after glucose control has been established. If lipid values fall within the accepted risk levels (low density lipoprotein (LDL) less than 100 mg/dl), repeat lipid profile every five years.

The goal for LDL-cholesterol (LDL-C) in children and adolescents with diabetes is less than 100 mg/dl (2.60 mmol/l). If the LDL-cholesterol is greater than 100 mg/dl, the child should be treated with an exercise plan and a Step 2 American Heart Association diet. If, after six months of diet and exercise, the LDL-C level remains above 160 mg/dl, pharmacologic agents should be given. If, the LDL-C is between 130 and 160 mg/dl, pharmacologic therapy should be considered. Statins are the agents of choice. Weight loss, increased physical activity, and improvement in glycemic control often result in improvements in lipid levels.

Blood pressure. Careful control of hypertension in children is critical. Hypertension in childhood is defined as an average systolic or diastolic blood pressure greater than 95th percentile for age, sex, and height measured on at least three separate days. Normal blood pressure levels for age, sex, and height, appropriate methods for measurement, and treatment recommendations are available online at: www.nhlbi.nih.gov/health/prof/heart/hbp/hbp_ped.pdf. CE inhibitors are the agents of choice in children with microalbuminuria. They have beneficial effects on slowing progression or preventing diabetic nephropathy.

Visiting the Health Care Team

Because most newly diagnosed cases of type 1 diabetes occur in individuals younger than 18 years of age, and more children and teens are now getting type 2 diabetes, care of this group requires integration of diabetes management with the complicated physical and emotional growth needs of children, adolescents, and their families, as well as with their emerging autonomy and independence.

Diabetes care for children should be provided by a team that can deal with these special medical, educational, nutritional, and behavioral issues. The team usually consists of a physician, diabetes educator, dietitian, social worker or psychologist, along with the patient and family. Children should be seen by the team at diagnosis and in follow-up, as agreed upon by the primary care provider and the diabetes team. The following schedule of care is based on the American Diabetes Association's Standards of Medical Care, published in 2005.

At Diagnosis

- Establish the goals of care and required treatment.

- Check lipids in children with a significant family history. In children with no significant family history, check lipids at puberty and if normal, repeat profile every five years.

- Begin diabetes self-management education about healthy eating habits, daily physical activity, and insulin/medication administration, and self-monitoring of blood glucose levels if appropriate. A solid educational base is needed so that the individual and family can become increasingly independent in self-management of diabetes. Diabetes educators play an important role in this aspect of management.

- Provide nutritional therapy by an individual experienced with the nutritional needs of the growing child and the behavioral issues that have an impact on adolescent diets.

- Conduct a psychosocial assessment to identify emotional and behavioral disorders.

Each Quarterly Visit

Most young people with diabetes are seen by the health care team every three months. At each visit, the following should be monitored or examined:

- A1C, an indicator of average blood glucose control
- growth (height and weight)
- BMI (body mass index)

- blood pressure
- injection sites
- self-testing blood glucose records
- psychosocial assessment

Annually

- evaluate nutrition therapy
- provide ophthalmologic examination—less often on the advice of an eye care professional (The first ophthalmologic examination should be obtained once the child is age ten or older and has had diabetes for 3 to 5 years.)
- check for microalbuminuria (once the child is ten years old and has had diabetes for five years)
- perform thyroid function test (for children with type 1 diabetes)
- administer influenza vaccination
- examine feet

Helping Children Manage Diabetes

The health care provider team, in partnership with the young person with diabetes and caregivers, can develop a personal diabetes plan for the child that puts a daily schedule in place to keep diabetes under control. The plan shows the child how to follow a healthy meal plan, get regular physical activity, check blood glucose levels, take insulin or oral medication as prescribed, and manage hyperglycemia and hypoglycemia.

Follow a Healthy Meal Plan

Young people with diabetes need to follow a meal plan developed by a registered dietitian, diabetes educator, or physician. For children with type 1 diabetes, the meal plan must ensure proper nutrition for growth. A meal plan also helps keep blood glucose levels in the target range. Children or adolescents and their families can learn how different types of food—especially carbohydrates such as breads, pasta, and rice—can affect blood glucose levels. Portion sizes, the right amount of calories for the child's age, and ideas for healthy food choices at meal and snack time also should be discussed including reduction in soda and juice consumption.

Get Regular Physical Activity

Children with diabetes need regular physical activity, ideally a total of 60 minutes each day. In children with type 1 diabetes, the most common problem encountered during physical activity is hypoglycemia. If possible, a child or a teen should check blood glucose levels before beginning a game or a sport. If blood glucose levels are too low, the child should not by physically active until the low blood glucose level has been treated.

Check Blood Glucose Levels Regularly

Young people with diabetes should know the acceptable range for their blood glucose. Children, particularly those using insulin should check blood glucose values regularly with a blood glucose meter, preferably one with a built-in memory. A health care team member can teach a child how to use a blood glucose meter properly and how often to use it. Children should keep a journal or other records of blood glucose results to discuss with their health care team. This information helps providers make any needed changes to the child's or teen's personal diabetes plan.

Take All Diabetes Medication as Prescribed

Parents, caregivers, school nurses, and others can help a child or teen learn how to take medications as prescribed. For type 1 diabetes, a child or teen takes insulin at prescribed times each day via multiple injections or an insulin pump. It is important to stress that all medication should be balanced with food and activity every day.

Special Issues

Diabetes presents unique issues for young people with the disease. Simple things, such as going to a birthday party, playing sports, or staying overnight with friends, need careful planning. Checking blood glucose, making correct food choices, and taking insulin or oral medication can make school-age children feel different from their classmates and this can be particularly bothersome for teens.

For any child or teen with diabetes, learning to cope with the disease is a big task. Dealing with a chronic illness such as diabetes may cause emotional and behavioral challenges, sometimes leading to depression. Talking to a social worker or psychologist may help young people and their families learn to adjust to the lifestyle changes needed to stay healthy.

Family Support

Managing diabetes in children and adolescents is most effective when the entire family gets involved. Diabetes education should involve family members. Families can be encouraged to share concerns with physicians, diabetes educators, dietitians, and other health care providers to get their help in the day-to-day management of diabetes. Extended family members, teachers, school nurses, counselors, coaches, day care providers, and other resources in the community can provide information, support, guidance, and help with coping skills. These individuals also may be knowledgeable about resources for health education, financial services, social services, mental health counseling, transportation, and home visits.

Diabetes is stressful for both the children and their families. Parents should be alert for signs of depression or eating disorders and seek appropriate treatment. While all parents should talk to their children about avoiding tobacco, alcohol, and other drugs, this is particularly important for children with diabetes. Smoking and diabetes each independently increase the risk of cardiovascular disease and people with diabetes who smoke have a greatly increased risk of heart disease and circulatory problems. Binge drinking can cause hyperglycemia acutely, followed by an increased risk of hypoglycemia. The symptoms of intoxication are very similar to the symptoms of hypoglycemia, and thus, may result in delay of treatment of hypoglycemia with potentially disastrous consequences.

Transition to Independence

Children with diabetes—depending on their age and level of maturity—will learn to take over much of their care. Most school-age children can recognize symptoms of hypoglycemia and monitor blood glucose levels. They also participate in nutrition decisions. They often can give their own insulin injections but may not be able to draw up the dose accurately in a syringe until a developmental age of 11 to 12 years.

Adolescents often have the motor and cognitive skills to perform all diabetes-related tasks and determine insulin doses based on blood glucose levels and food intake. This is a time, however, when peer acceptance is important, risk-taking behaviors common, and rebellion against authority is part of teens' search for independence. Thus, adolescents must be supervised in their diabetes tasks and allowed gradual independence with the understanding that the independence will be continued only if they adhere to the diabetes regimen and succeed in maintaining reasonable metabolic control. During mid-adolescence, the family and health care team should stress to teens the importance of checking blood glucose levels prior to driving a car to avoid hypoglycemia while driving.

Diabetes at School

School principals, administrators, nurses, teachers, coaches, bus drivers, health care, and lunch-room staff all play a role in helping students with diabetes succeed.

Several Federal and some State laws provide protections to children with disabilities, including diabetes. These laws help ensure that all students with diabetes are educated in a medically safe environment and have the same access to educational opportunities as their peers—in public and some private schools. Students with diabetes are entitled to accommodations and modifications necessary for them to stay healthy at school. Accommodations may need to be made in the classroom, with physical education, on field trips, and/or for after-school activities. Written plans outlining each student's diabetes management help students, their families, school staff, and the student's health care providers know what is expected of them. These expectations should be laid out in written documents, such as a:

- Diabetes Medical Management Plan, developed by the student's personal health care team and family;

- Quick Reference Emergency Plan, which describes how to recognize hypoglycemia and hyperglycemia and what to do as soon as signs or symptoms of these conditions are observed;

- Education plan, such as the Section 504 Plan or Individualized Education Program (IEP);

- Care Plan or Individual Health Plan generated by the school nurse that provides instructions to faculty and staff.

The school nurse is the most appropriate person to coordinate care for students with diabetes. Each student with diabetes should have a written plan, developed by the school nurse, incorporating physician orders, parent requests, and tailored to the specific developmental, physical, cognitive, and skill ability of the child. The nurse will conduct a nursing assessment of the student and develop a nursing care plan, taking into consideration the child's cognitive, emotional, and physical status as well as the medical orders contained in the Diabetes Medical Management Plan. A team approach to developing the care plan, involving the student, parent, health care provider, key school personnel, and school nurse, is the most effective way to ensure safe and effective diabetes management during the school day.

The nursing care plan would also identify school employees assigned to provide care to an individual student, under the direction of the school nurse, when allowed by state nurse practice acts. The school nurse is responsible for training, monitoring, and supervising these school personnel. The school nurse will promote and encourage independence and self-care consistent with the student's ability, skill, maturity, and developmental level.

Camps and Support Groups

Local peer groups and camps for children and teens with diabetes can provide positive role models and group activities. Peer encouragement often helps children perform diabetes-related tasks that they had been afraid to do previously and encourages independence in diabetes management. Talking with other children who have diabetes helps young people feel less isolated and less alone in having to deal with the demands of diabetes. They have the opportunity to discuss issues they share in common that others in their peer group cannot understand, and they can share solutions to problems that they have encountered. Often, these programs challenge children physically and teach them how to deal with increased exercise, reinforcing the fact that diabetes should not limit them in their ability to perform strenuous physical activity.

Additional Information

National Diabetes Education Program (NDEP)
One Diabetes Way
Bethesda, MD 20814-9692
Toll-Free: 800-438-5383
Phone: 301-496-3583
Website: http://www.ndep.nih.gov
E-mail: ndep@mail.nih.gov

National Diabetes
Information Clearinghouse
1 Information Way
Bethesda, MD 20892-3560
Toll-Free: 800-860-8747
Fax: 703-738-4929
Website: http://diabetes.niddk.nih.gov
E-mail: ndic@info.niddk.nih.gov

Centers for Disease Control
and Prevention (CDC)
INFO Contact Center
Toll-Free: 800-232-4636
Toll-Free TTY: 888-232-6348
E-mail: cdcinfo@cdc.gov
Website: http://www.cdc.gov/diabetes

American Association
of Diabetes Educators
100 W. Monroe, Suite 400
Chicago, IL 60603
Toll-Free: 800-338-3633
Fax: 312-424-2427
Website: http://www.aadenet.org

American Diabetes Association
1701 N. Beauregard St.
Alexandria, VA 22311
Toll-Free: 800-DIABETES (800-342-2383)
Website: http://www.diabetes.org
E-mail: AskADA@diabetes.org

Juvenile Diabetes Research
Foundation International
120 Wall Street
New York, NY 10005-4001
Toll-Free: 800-223-1138 or 800-533-2873
Fax: 212-785-9595
Website: http://www.jdf.org
E-mail: info@jdrf.org

Chapter 42

Type 2 Diabetes

Diabetes means that your blood sugar, or glucose, is too high. Glucose comes from the food you eat and is also made in your liver and muscles. Your blood always has some glucose in it because your body needs glucose for energy, but too much glucose in the blood is not good for your health.

An organ called the pancreas controls the amount of glucose in the blood. The pancreas makes insulin which helps glucose get from food into your cells. Cells take the glucose and make it into energy you need for life.

In a person with diabetes, the pancreas makes little or no insulin or the cells do not use insulin very well. So glucose builds up in the blood and cannot get into your cells. Your blood glucose gets too high and diabetes can then damage your body.

In type 2 diabetes, the pancreas still makes some insulin but the cells cannot use it very well. Type 2 used to be called adult-onset diabetes, but now more kids are getting type 2 diabetes.

How do you manage diabetes?

The key to taking care of diabetes is to keep your blood glucose as close to normal as possible. The best way is to eat healthy foods, get exercise every day, stay at a healthy weight, take your medicine, and

This chapter includes: "Tips for Kids with Type 2 Diabetes," National Diabetes Education Program (NDEP), NIH Publication No. 03-5295, August 2005; and "Dealing with the Ups and Downs of Diabetes," NDEP, NIH Publication No. 04-5558, August 2005.

check your blood glucose to see how you are doing. Kids with type 2 diabetes may need to take insulin or pills to help the body's supply of insulin work better.

Your doctor will tell you what blood glucose level is good for you and will teach you how to use a meter to check it. Your goal is to keep your blood glucose as close to this level as you can.

Carbohydrates are a good source of energy for our bodies. If you eat too many carbs at one time, your blood glucose may go too high. Many foods contain carbs. Whole grain foods, nonfat or low-fat milk, fresh fruits, and vegetables are better carbohydrate choices than white bread, whole milk, sweetened fruit drinks, soda pop, potato chips, sweets, and desserts. Learn to eat the right amount at meals and snack times to keep your blood glucose in balance.

Eat small servings of food and be active to prevent weight gain and to keep your blood glucose in a healthy range. Illness and stress also can make your blood glucose go up. Things that make your blood glucose go down are insulin and exercise.

Why do you get type 2 diabetes?

Being overweight increases the risk of getting type 2 diabetes. Kids who are not active or who have a family member with diabetes are more likely to get it. Some racial and ethnic groups have a greater chance of getting diabetes including: American Indians, African Americans, Hispanics/Latinos, Asian Americans, and Pacific Islanders. You do not get diabetes from eating too much sugar.

Why do you need to take care of your diabetes?

After several years, diabetes can lead to health problems. Blood vessels get damaged and cause heart attacks in young people. Damage to organs in your body can cause blindness, kidney failure, loss of legs or feet, and gum problems or loss of teeth.

The good news is that when you take care of your diabetes, you can avoid these problems. How? Eat healthy foods, be active every day, stay at a healthy weight, take your medicine, and check your blood glucose. Do not let diabetes stop you. You can do all the things your friends do and live a long and healthy life.

Dealing with the Ups and Downs of Diabetes

Many teens deal with type 2 diabetes every day. Most of the time, it is not a problem for them. But sometimes, they just want it to go away. Do you ever—

- Ask: Why me?
- Think you're the only one who feels sad, mad, alone, afraid, or different?
- Get tired of others teasing you if you are overweight?
- Blame yourself or your family for your diabetes?

All of these feelings are normal. Lots of teens who have diabetes feel the same way. It is okay to get angry, feel sorry for yourself, or think you are different every now and then. But then you need to take charge and do something to feel better. Remember that everyone feels down sometimes. You are not alone.

Still down?

Reach out for help. Talk to someone in your family or where you worship, an older friend, a school counselor, or your doctor or diabetes educator. It might help to write down your feelings in a journal. If you still feel down or sad, ask your parents to help you find a counselor. It is okay to ask for help.

Stay Cool.

There are many people who care about you and who want to help you stay healthy and happy. Your health care team (doctor, diabetes educator, social worker, nurse, and dietitian) can help you learn how to eat right, be more active, and feel good about yourself. Stay in touch with them. Let your health care team know how you feel and what you need.

Mom, Dad, Get with It!

It is easier to manage diabetes when the whole family works at it with you. What's healthy for you is healthy for everyone in your family.

Get everyone eating well. Ask your family to eat the same healthy foods you eat—fruits, vegetables, whole grain breads, and low-fat meats, milk, cheese, and snacks such as popcorn without butter. Ask them to keep healthy foods in the house, and not to tempt you with cookies, cake, candy, and soda.

Get everyone moving by being more active. Play hard. Shoot hoops, play ball, ride bikes, go for a walk—together. Being active helps you to lower stress and become healthier.

Let Your School Know What's Up.

Let people at your school know you have type 2 diabetes and that you need to eat healthy foods, take your meals or medicine on time, and be active. Include the teachers, nurses, bus drivers, counselors, coach, and cafeteria lunch room staff. Do not let diabetes stop you. You can do the things everyone else does.

Still My Friend?

Ever worry that your friends get wrong ideas about diabetes?

- Tell them that you have diabetes. You do not have to keep it a secret. The more people know about diabetes the more they will understand. Explain that your body needs help to use the food you eat.

- Be sure everyone knows that no one can catch diabetes from you.

- Good friends help each other out. If you have friends who help you choose healthy foods when you are all eating out, hang on to them.

- If kids tease you about your diabetes or your weight, the best thing is to just walk away.

Want to Meet Other Teens Who Feel Like You Do?

- Look for a hospital, clinic, or health center near you that offers programs for teens with type 2 diabetes.

- Head for a diabetes or weight loss summer camp. You will do all the things that other campers do: swim, hike, dance, and more. But the best part is that everyone has diabetes or is trying to lose weight just like you.

- Find a support group near you. Meetings can be a lot of fun and you will meet others who are dealing with the same things you are.

- Find a pen pal or e-mail buddy.

Action!

It's time for you to do something about your diabetes care.

- Set goals to target what you will do. Start small and work your way up. For example: "I will cut down on sodas and drink water instead." When that is going well, take the next step. Add another goal—"I will dance or bike ride a couple of times a week." Then add a new goal—"I will eat smaller servings of cookies, burgers, and fries."

- Try to make each new goal just a bit harder. After you shoot hoops twice a week, try adding another activity on three other days. Raise the goal until you reach a level that works for you.

- Avoid goals that will be too hard to meet. For example, rather than saying you will never eat a burger or candy bar again; say you will eat only one a week.

- Reward yourself when you reach your goal. Do something or buy something you like.

- Tell your family or friends about your goals. Maybe they will be active with you or help out some other way.

- Choose goals that you can really meet. Write down your top three goals. Put in the date when you set the goal and when you met it.

Got It

Over time, you will feel good about yourself if you manage your diabetes by eating healthy foods, being more active, and working towards a healthier weight. It is up to you. Do not blame things on your diabetes. Take it one step at a time and soon you will see progress.

Additional Information

American Association of Diabetes Educators
100 W. Monroe, Suite 400
Chicago, IL 60603
Toll-Free: 800-338-3633
Fax: 312-424-2427
Website: http://www.aadenet.org

American Diabetes Association (ADA)
1701 N. Beauregard St.
Alexandria, VA 22311
Toll-Free: 800-DIABETES (800-342-2383)
Website: http://www.diabetes.org
Youth Website: http://www.diabetes.org/youthzone
E-mail: AskADA@diabetes.org

Find your local ADA at: http://www.diabetes.org/local

Children with Diabetes/Diabetes123
5689 Chancery Place
Hamilton, OH 45011
Website: http://www.childrenwithdiabetes.com/kids
E-mail: info@childrenwithdiabetes.com

Juvenile Diabetes Research Foundation International
120 Wall Street
New York, NY 10005-4001
Toll-Free: 800-223-1138 or 800-533-2873
Fax: 212-785-9595
Website: http://kids.jdrf.org
E-mail: info@idrf.org

National Diabetes Education Program (NDEP)
One Diabetes Way
Bethesda, MD 20814-9692
Toll-Free: 800-438-5383
Phone: 301-496-3583
Website: http://www.ndep.nih.gov
E-mail: ndep@mail.nih.gov

National Diabetes Information Clearinghouse
1 Information Way
Bethesda, MD 20892-3560
Toll-Free: 800-860-8747
Fax: 703-738-4929
Website: http://diabetes.niddk.nih.gov
E-mail: ndic@info.niddk.nih.gov

Chapter 43

Growth Problems
in Adolescence

Do you feel like the smallest person in your class? Guys and girls who are shorter may feel out of sync with their peers—just as guys who mature earlier may feel strange if they shave first or girls who get their periods before their friends may feel awkward. In most cases, teens who are small are probably just physically maturing a little bit more slowly than their friends. Or, maybe their parents are smaller and they take after them.

Occasionally, though, there's a medical reason why some people grow more slowly than usual. Read on to find out more about some growth disorders and what doctors can do to help.

What's Normal and What's Not

Kids and teens grow and go through puberty at different times. For girls, puberty usually begins between ages 8 and 13. For guys it often begins a bit later—between 10 and 15. Girls become more rounded in the hips and their breasts begin to develop. Usually, about two years after their breasts begin to develop, girls begin to menstruate, or get their periods. Guys' penises and testicles grow larger and both guys and girls grow hair in their pubic areas and under their arms. Guys

This information was provided by TeensHealth, one of the largest resources online for medically reviewed health information written for parents, kids, and teens. For more articles like this one, visit www.TeensHealth.org, or www.KidsHealth.org. © 2004 The Nemours Center for Children's Health Media, a division of The Nemours Foundation.

get more muscular, begin to grow hair on their faces, and their voices get deeper.

Some teens develop a lot earlier than their friends (called precocious puberty), whereas others develop much later than other people of the same age (called delayed puberty).

There are lots of reasons why kids and teens may not grow as fast as their peers. If you're short, you may just have familial (genetic) short stature. In other words, short parents tend to have short children. If a doctor finds you have no growth disorder and you're growing steadily and sexually maturing at the usual expected age, then you can probably expect to grow to a normal size, although you may be somewhat shorter than average.

Some teens have constitutional growth delay. These teens grow at a normal rate when they are younger kids, but they lag behind and don't start their pubertal development and their growth spurt until after most of their peers. People who have constitutional growth delay are often referred to as late bloomers. If a doctor suspects constitutional growth delay in a kid or teen, he or she might take x-rays of bones and compare them with x-rays of what's considered average for their age. Teens with constitutional growth delay tend to have bones that look younger than what's expected for their age. These teens will have a late growth spurt and continue growing and developing until an older age. They usually catch up with their peers by the time they are young adults.

Not getting adequate amounts of protein, calories, and other nutrients in your diet can also cause growth to slow, as well as a number of other chronic medical conditions such as kidney, heart, lung, and intestinal diseases. People with sickle cell anemia may also grow and develop more slowly. Following the treatment plan worked out with a doctor can help teens with health conditions achieve a more normal growth pattern.

What Are Growth Disorders?

There are other reasons why teens may have growth problems, though. Growth is controlled by the hormones the body produces. Many diseases of the endocrine system, which is made up of the glands that produce hormones, can affect growth.

Hormones are secreted by the endocrine glands and carried throughout the body in the bloodstream. The hypothalamus (part of the brain) controls the pituitary gland, which in turn releases some of the hormones that control growth and sexual development. Estrogen and testosterone are important hormones that drive sexual development and function and also play a role in growth.

Hypothyroidism can cause slow growth because the thyroid gland isn't producing enough thyroid hormone, which is necessary to support normal growth. A major symptom of hypothyroidism is feeling tired or sluggish. A blood test of a person's thyroid levels can show if he or she has this disorder, which can develop at any time in life and is common in teen girls and women of childbearing age.

Some diseases aren't caused by the hormones, but they can impact the body's ability to produce the hormones needed to grow and develop. For example, Turner syndrome is a genetic condition (due to a problem with a person's genes) that occurs in girls. It is caused by a missing or abnormal X chromosome. Girls with Turner syndrome tend to be short and don't usually undergo normal sexual development because their ovaries (organs in the lower abdomen that produce eggs and female hormones) don't mature and function normally.

Another condition that can lead to significantly short stature is dwarfism. Dwarfism results from abnormal growth of the bones and cartilage in the body. In many forms of dwarfism the person has abnormal body proportions, such as noticeably short limbs. Most cases of dwarfism are genetic.

Growth Hormone Deficiency

One growth disorder that is specific to the hormones that govern growth is called growth hormone deficiency (or GH deficiency). This condition involves the pituitary gland, the small gland located at the base of the brain that produces growth hormone and other hormones. If the pituitary gland doesn't produce enough hormones for normal growth, growth slows down or stops.

GH deficiency can occur at any age, and the most common sign in kids and teens is a slowing of growth to less than two inches (five centimeters) a year. Kids with this disorder usually have normal body proportions—in other words, their bodies look normal, just smaller. Growth hormone deficiency does not affect intelligence or brain function.

The cause of growth hormone deficiency can be an underdeveloped, damaged, or malfunctioning pituitary gland or hypothalamus, which can happen before or during birth or can be caused later by an accident or trauma or certain diseases. Tumors near the pituitary gland, like craniopharyngioma (pronounced: kray-nee-o-far-un-jee-o-muh), can also damage the hypothalamus and pituitary gland and affect growth. In most cases, though, the cause of growth hormone deficiency is simply unexplained.

Growth hormone deficiency usually affects only one person in a family and isn't generally passed on from parents to children.

What Do Doctors Do?

Your doctor has probably been charting your growth since you were born to make sure there is a growth curve showing steady growth in weight and height. If this curve flattens out, a doctor usually does a thorough physical exam and may order special blood tests and x-rays of the bones.

Your doctor will also look at growth patterns in your family. Teens with familial short stature have inherited this trait from their parents. And teens with constitutional growth delay often have close relatives who were also late bloomers.

Growth conditions like familial short stature or constitutional growth delay usually don't require any special treatment. Extra vitamins or special diets won't make a person with one of these conditions grow any taller or faster. Occasionally, though, doctors will give hormone treatment—usually testosterone—to guys with constitutional growth delay who are having a rough time waiting for puberty to kick in. The treatments can temporarily increase growth and development until the guy starts producing puberty hormones on his own.

If a doctor finds that a person has growth hormone deficiency, it can be treated by replacing the missing hormone. The replacement hormone is produced in a laboratory and is given as a daily shot. Taking the hormone by mouth doesn't work because the hormone is destroyed by the stomach's digestive juices. Depending on when the diagnosis is made, treatment usually lasts for several years—until the growth areas of the bones close (after that, no more growth can occur).

It can take weeks or months to notice the effects of growth hormone replacement, but most kids will grow two to five times faster during the first year of treatment than they were growing beforehand. The rate of growth after that is usually somewhat slower, about 3 to 4 inches (7.6 to 10.2 centimeters) per year.

Recently, growth hormone treatment has been approved for some kids and teens who are not growth hormone deficient but who appear to be headed for a very short adult height (under 5 feet, 4 inches [1.6 meters] for boys and under 4 feet, 11 inches [1.5 meters] for girls). This treatment can help increase the person's final height by about 2 to 3 inches (5 to 7.6 centimeters).

Growth disorders that are caused by other conditions can also be treated. Girls with Turner syndrome can benefit from growth hormone and estrogen therapy. Thyroid medication can help restore a normal growth rate in kids and teens with hypothyroidism. In most cases, growth will also improve with specific treatment of chronic medical conditions that are slowing a teen's growth.

Dealing with Growth Disorders

It can be tough having a growth disorder as a teen because it can affect a person's body image and self-esteem. Talking with a mental health professional is one way some people deal with feelings and concerns about their growth. Your doctor can also be a good resource for advice on your growth pattern. And, although no one has much control over the changes taking place in their bodies during puberty, you can do what you can to keep your body in top shape by eating a healthy diet, getting enough sleep, and exercising.

Chapter 44

Infectious Mononucleosis and Epstein-Barr Virus

Epstein-Barr virus, frequently referred to as EBV, is a member of the herpesvirus family and one of the most common human viruses. The virus occurs worldwide, and most people become infected with EBV sometime during their lives. In the United States, as many as 95% of adults between 35 and 40 years of age have been infected. Infants become susceptible to EBV as soon as maternal antibody protection (present at birth) disappears. Many children become infected with EBV, and these infections usually cause no symptoms or are indistinguishable from the other mild, brief illnesses of childhood. In the United States and in other developed countries, many persons are not infected with EBV in their childhood years. When infection with EBV occurs during adolescence or young adulthood, it causes infectious mononucleosis 35% to 50% of the time.

Symptoms of infectious mononucleosis include: fever, sore throat, swollen lymph glands, and sometimes, a swollen spleen or liver involvement. Heart problems or involvement of the central nervous system occur only rarely, and infectious mononucleosis is almost never fatal. There are no known associations between active EBV infection and problems during pregnancy, such as miscarriages or birth defects. Although the symptoms of infectious mononucleosis usually resolve in one or two months, EBV remains dormant or latent in a few cells in the throat and blood for the rest of the person's life. Periodically, the virus

"Epstein-Barr Virus and Infectious Mononucleosis," Centers for Disease Control and Prevention (CDC), September 13, 2005.

can reactivate and is commonly found in the saliva of infected persons. This reactivation usually occurs without symptoms of illness.

EBV also establishes a lifelong dormant infection in some cells of the body's immune system. A late event in a very few carriers of this virus is the emergence of Burkitt lymphoma and nasopharyngeal carcinoma—two rare cancers that are not normally found in the United States. EBV appears to play an important role in these malignancies, but is probably not the sole cause of disease.

Most individuals exposed to people with infectious mononucleosis have previously been infected with EBV and are not at risk for infectious mononucleosis. In addition, transmission of EBV requires intimate contact with the saliva (found in the mouth) of an infected person. Transmission of this virus through the air or blood does not normally occur. The incubation period, or the time from infection to appearance of symptoms, ranges from four to six weeks. Persons with infectious mononucleosis may be able to spread the infection to others for a period of weeks. However, no special precautions or isolation procedures are recommended, since the virus is also found frequently in the saliva of healthy people. In fact, many healthy people can carry and spread the virus intermittently for life. These people are usually the primary reservoir for person-to-person transmission. For this reason, transmission of the virus is almost impossible to prevent.

The clinical diagnosis of infectious mononucleosis is suggested on the basis of the symptoms of fever, sore throat, swollen lymph glands, and the age of the patient. Usually, laboratory tests are needed for confirmation. Serologic results for persons with infectious mononucleosis include an elevated white blood cell count, an increased percentage of certain atypical white blood cells, and a positive reaction to a mono spot test.

There is no specific treatment for infectious mononucleosis, other than treating the symptoms. No antiviral drugs or vaccines are available. Some physicians have prescribed a five-day course of steroids to control the swelling of the throat and tonsils. The use of steroids has also been reported to decrease the overall length and severity of illness, but these reports have not been published.

It is important to note that symptoms related to infectious mononucleosis caused by EBV infection seldom last for more than four months. When such an illness lasts more than six months, it is frequently called chronic EBV infection. However, valid laboratory evidence for continued active EBV infection is seldom found in these patients. The illness should be investigated further to determine if it meets the criteria for chronic fatigue syndrome (CFS). This process includes ruling out other causes of chronic illness or fatigue.

Diagnosis of EBV Infections

In most cases of infectious mononucleosis, the clinical diagnosis can be made from the characteristic triad of fever, pharyngitis, and lymphadenopathy lasting for one to four weeks. Serologic test results include a normal to moderately elevated white blood cell count, an increased total number of lymphocytes, greater than 10% atypical lymphocytes, and a positive reaction to a mono spot test. In patients with symptoms compatible with infectious mononucleosis, a positive Paul-Bunnell heterophile antibody test result is diagnostic, and no further testing is necessary. Moderate-to-high levels of heterophile antibodies are seen during the first month of illness and decrease rapidly after week four. False-positive results may be found in a small number of patients, and false-negative results may be obtained in 10% to 15% of patients, primarily in children younger than ten years of age. True outbreaks of infectious mononucleosis are extremely rare.

When mono spot or heterophile test results are negative, additional laboratory testing may be needed to differentiate EBV infections from a mononucleosis-like illness induced by Cytomegalovirus, adenovirus, or *Toxoplasma gondii*. Direct detection of EBV in blood or lymphoid tissues is a research tool and is not available for routine diagnosis. Instead, serologic testing is the method of choice for diagnosing primary infection.

EBV-Specific Laboratory Tests

Laboratory tests are not always foolproof. For various reasons, false-positive and false-negative results can occur for any test. However, the laboratory tests for EBV are for the most part accurate and specific. In most cases, a distinction can be made as to whether a person is susceptible to EBV, has had a recent infection, has had infection in the past, or has a reactivated EBV infection.

Even when EBV antibody tests, such as the early antigen test, suggest that reactivated infection is present, this result does not necessarily indicate that a patient's current medical condition is caused by EBV infection. A number of healthy people with no symptoms have antibodies to the EBV early antigen for years after their initial EBV infection.

Therefore, interpretation of laboratory results is somewhat complex and should be left to physicians who are familiar with EBV testing and who have access to the entire clinical picture of a person. To determine if EBV infection is associated with a current illness, consult with an experienced physician.

Additional Information about EBV Antibody Tests and Interpretation

Antibody tests for EBV can measure the presence and/or the concentration of at least six specific EBV antibodies. By evaluating the results of these different tests, the stage of EBV infection can be determined. However, these tests are expensive and not usually needed for the diagnosis of infectious mononucleosis.

Chapter 45

Juvenile Rheumatoid Arthritis

Arthritis means joint inflammation and refers to a group of diseases that cause pain, swelling, stiffness, and loss of motion in the joints. While arthritis usually refers to wear and tear degeneration of the joints that occurs with aging, arthritis includes many other kinds of diseases. Arthritis is a more general term that refers to the more than 100 rheumatic diseases that may affect the joints but can also cause pain, swelling, and stiffness in other supporting structures of the body such as muscles, tendons, ligaments, and bones. Most of these other kinds of arthritis involve an abnormality of the immune system that causes it to attack and damage the joints. Some rheumatic diseases can affect other parts of the body, including various internal organs. Children can develop almost all types of arthritis that affect adults, but the most common type that affects children is juvenile rheumatoid arthritis (JRA).

Juvenile rheumatoid arthritis (JRA) is arthritis that causes joint inflammation and stiffness for more than six weeks in a child of 16 years of age or less. In JRA, immune system cells attack the joints for unknown reasons. This inflammation causes redness, swelling, warmth, and soreness in the joints, although many children with JRA do not complain of joint pain. Any joint can be affected and

"Questions and Answers about Juvenile Rheumatoid Arthritis," National Institute of Arthritis and Musculoskeletal and Skin Diseases (NIAMS), NIH Publication No. 01–4942, July 2001. Updated in April 2006 by Dr. David A Cooke, M.D., Diplomate, American Board of Internal Medicine.

inflammation may limit the mobility of affected joints. One type of JRA can also affect the internal organs. Doctors classify JRA into three types by the number of joints involved, the symptoms, and the presence or absence of certain antibodies found by a blood test. (Antibodies are special proteins made by the immune system.) These classifications help the doctor determine how the disease will progress and whether the internal organs or skin are affected.

Pauciarticular (PAW-see-are-TICK-you-lar) means that four or fewer joints are affected. Pauciarticular is the most common form of JRA; about half of all children with JRA have this type. Pauciarticular disease typically affects large joints, such as the knees. Girls under age eight are most likely to develop this type of JRA.

Some children have special kinds of antibodies in the blood. One is called antinuclear antibody (ANA) and one is called rheumatoid factor (RF). Eye disease affects about 20 to 30 percent of children with pauciarticular JRA. Up to 80 percent of those with eye disease also test positive for ANA and the disease tends to develop at a particularly early age in these children. Regular examinations by an ophthalmologist (a doctor who specializes in eye diseases) are necessary to prevent serious eye problems such as iritis (inflammation of the iris, the colored part of the eye) or uveitis (inflammation of the uvea, or the inner eye). Some children with pauciarticular disease outgrow arthritis by adulthood, although eye problems can continue and joint symptoms may recur in some people.

Polyarticular. About 30 percent of all children with JRA have polyarticular disease. In polyarticular disease, five or more joints are affected. The small joints, such as those in the hands and feet, are most commonly involved, but the disease may also affect large joints. Polyarticular JRA often is symmetrical; that is, it affects the same joint on both sides of the body. Some children with polyarticular disease have an antibody in their blood called IgM rheumatoid factor (RF). These children often have a more severe form of the disease, which doctors consider to be similar in many ways to adult rheumatoid arthritis.

Systemic. Besides joint swelling, the systemic form of JRA is characterized by fever and a light skin rash, and may also affect internal organs such as the heart, liver, spleen, and lymph nodes. Doctors sometimes call it Still disease. Almost all children with this type of JRA test negative for both RF and ANA. The systemic form affects 20 percent of all children with JRA. A small percentage of these children develop arthritis in many joints and can have severe arthritis that continues into adulthood.

What Causes Juvenile Rheumatoid Arthritis?

JRA is an autoimmune disorder, which means that the body mistakenly identifies some of its own cells and tissues as foreign. The immune system, which normally helps to fight off harmful, foreign substances such as bacteria or viruses, begins to attack healthy cells and tissues. The result is inflammation—marked by redness, heat, pain, and swelling. Doctors do not know why the immune system goes awry in children who develop JRA. Scientists suspect that it is a two-step process. First, something in a child's genetic makeup gives them a tendency to develop JRA; then an environmental factor, such as a virus, triggers the development of JRA.

What Are the Symptoms and Signs of Juvenile Rheumatoid Arthritis?

The most common symptom of all types of JRA is persistent joint swelling, pain, and stiffness that typically is worse in the morning or after a nap. The pain may limit movement of the affected joint although many children, especially younger ones, will not complain of pain. JRA commonly affects the knees and joints in the hands and feet. One of the earliest signs of JRA may be limping in the morning because of an affected knee. Besides joint symptoms, children with systemic JRA have a high fever and a light skin rash. The rash and fever may appear and disappear very quickly. Systemic JRA also may cause the lymph nodes located in the neck and other parts of the body to swell. In some cases (less than half), internal organs including the heart and, very rarely, the lungs may be involved.

Eye inflammation is a potentially severe complication that sometimes occurs in children with pauciarticular JRA. Eye diseases such as iritis and uveitis often are not present until some time after a child first develops JRA.

Typically, there are periods when the symptoms of JRA get better or go away (remissions) and times when symptoms are worse (flare-ups). JRA is different in each child—some may have just one or two flare-ups and never have symptoms again, while others experience many flare-ups or even have symptoms that never go away.

Some children with JRA may have growth problems. Depending on the severity of the disease and the joints involved, growth in affected joints may be too fast or too slow, causing one leg or arm to be longer than the other. Overall growth may also be slowed. Doctors are exploring the use of growth hormones to treat this problem. JRA also may cause joints to grow unevenly or to one side.

How Is Juvenile Rheumatoid Arthritis Diagnosed?

Doctors usually suspect JRA, along with several other possible conditions, when they see children with persistent joint pain or swelling, unexplained skin rashes and fever, swelling of lymph nodes, or inflammation of internal organs. A diagnosis of JRA also is considered in children with an unexplained limp or excessive clumsiness.

No one test can be used to diagnose JRA. A doctor diagnoses JRA by carefully examining the patient and considering the patient's medical history, the results of laboratory tests, and x-rays that help rule out other conditions.

Symptoms. One important consideration in diagnosing JRA is the length of time that symptoms have been present. Joint swelling or pain must last for at least six weeks for the doctor to consider a diagnosis of JRA. Because this factor is so important, it may be useful to keep a record of the symptoms, when they first appeared, and when they are worse or better.

Laboratory tests, usually blood tests, cannot by themselves provide the doctor with a clear diagnosis. But these tests can be used to help rule out other conditions and to help classify the type of JRA that a patient has. Blood may be taken to test for RF and ANA and to determine the erythrocyte sedimentation rate (ESR).

- ANA is found in the blood more often than RF, and both are found in only a small portion of JRA patients. The RF test helps the doctor tell the difference among the three types of JRA.

- ESR is a test that measures how quickly red blood cells fall to the bottom of a test tube. Some people with rheumatic disease have an elevated ESR or sed rate (cells fall quickly to the bottom of the test tube), showing that there is inflammation in the body. Not all children with active joint inflammation have an elevated ESR.

X-rays are needed if the doctor suspects injury to the bone or unusual bone development. Early in the disease, some x-rays can show cartilage damage. In general, x-rays are more useful later in the disease, when bones may be affected.

Other diseases. Because there are many causes of joint pain and swelling, the doctor must rule out other conditions before diagnosing JRA. These include physical injury, bacterial or viral infection, Lyme disease, inflammatory bowel disease, lupus, dermatomyositis, and some forms of cancer. The doctor may use additional laboratory tests to help rule out these and other possible conditions.

Treatment of Juvenile Rheumatoid Arthritis

The special expertise of rheumatologists in caring for patients with JRA is extremely valuable. Pediatric rheumatologists are trained in both pediatrics and rheumatology and are best equipped to deal with the complex problems of children with arthritis and other rheumatic diseases. However, there are very few such specialists, and some areas of the country have none at all. In such circumstances, a team approach involving the child's pediatrician and a rheumatologist with experience in both adult and pediatric rheumatic disease provides optimal care for children with arthritis. Other important members of the team include physical therapists and occupational therapists.

The main goals of treatment are to preserve a high level of physical and social functioning and maintain a good quality of life. To achieve these goals, doctors recommend treatments to reduce swelling; maintain full movement in the affected joints; relieve pain; and identify, treat, and prevent complications. Most children with JRA need medication and physical therapy to reach these goals.

Several types of medication are available to treat JRA:

- Nonsteroidal anti-inflammatory drugs (NSAIDs)—Aspirin, ibuprofen (Motrin, Advil, Nuprin), and naproxen or naproxen sodium (Naprosyn, Aleve) are examples of NSAIDs. They often are the first type of medication used. Most doctors do not treat children with aspirin because of the possibility that it will cause bleeding problems, stomach upset, liver problems, or Reye syndrome. But for some children, aspirin in the correct dose (measured by blood test) can control JRA symptoms effectively with few serious side effects. If the doctor prefers not to use aspirin, other NSAIDs are available. For example, in addition to those mentioned, diclofenac and tolmetin are available with a doctor's prescription. Studies show that these medications are as effective as aspirin with fewer side effects. An upset stomach is the most common complaint. Any side effects should be reported to the doctor, who may change the type or amount of medication.

411

- Disease-modifying anti-rheumatic drugs (DMARDs)—If NSAIDs do not relieve symptoms of JRA, the doctor is likely to prescribe this type of medication. DMARDs slow the progression of JRA, but because they take weeks or months to relieve symptoms, they often are taken with an NSAID. Various types of DMARDs are available. Doctors are likely to use one type of DMARD, methotrexate, for children with JRA. Also, researchers have learned that methotrexate is safe and effective for some children with rheumatoid arthritis whose symptoms are not relieved by other medications. Because only small doses of methotrexate are needed to relieve arthritis symptoms, potentially dangerous side effects rarely occur. The most serious complication is liver damage, but it can be avoided with regular blood screening tests and doctor followup. Careful monitoring for side effects is important for people taking methotrexate. When side effects are noticed early, the doctor can reduce the dose and eliminate side effects.

- Corticosteroids—In children with very severe JRA, stronger medicines may be needed to stop serious symptoms such as inflammation of the sac around the heart (pericarditis). Corticosteroids like prednisone may be added to the treatment plan to control severe symptoms. This medication can be given either intravenously (directly into the vein) or by mouth. Corticosteroids can interfere with a child's normal growth and can cause other side effects, such as a round face, weakened bones, and increased susceptibility to infections. Once the medication controls severe symptoms, the doctor may reduce the dose gradually and eventually stop it completely. Because it can be dangerous to stop taking corticosteroids suddenly, it is important that the patient carefully follow the doctor's instructions about how to take or reduce the dose.

- Biologic agents—Children with polyarticular JRA who have gotten little relief from other drugs may be given one of a new class of drug treatments called biologic agents. These medications target specific hormones produced by the immune system that are responsible for some of the symptoms of JRA. Etanercept (Enbrel), for example, blocks the actions of tumor necrosis factor, a naturally occurring protein in the body that helps cause inflammation. Several other drugs of this type are now available, and new agents are being developed quite rapidly. These drugs lack many of the risks and side effects of other treatments; however, they do suppress the immune system and can lead to severe infections, so they must be used very cautiously.

- Physical therapy—Exercise is an important part of a child's treatment plan. It can help to maintain muscle tone and pre-serve and recover the range of motion of the joints. A physiatrist (rehabilitation specialist) or a physical therapist can design an appropriate exercise program for a person with JRA. The specialist also may recommend using splints and other devices to help maintain normal bone and joint growth.

- Complementary and alternative medicine—Many adults seek alternative ways of treating arthritis, such as special diets or supplements. No research to date shows that they help and most of these treatments have never been tested for safety. Some people have tried acupuncture, in which thin needles are inserted at specific points in the body. Others have tried glu-cosamine and chondroitin sulfate, two natural substances found in and around cartilage cells, for osteoarthritis of the knee. Some alternative or complementary approaches may help a child to cope with or reduce some of the stress of living with a chronic illness. If the doctor feels the approach has value and will not harm the child, it can be incorporated into the treat-ment plan. Be aware that some alternative treatments can be harmful, or interfere with other kinds of medical treatments. In any case, it is important not to neglect regular health care or treatment of serious symptoms and to discuss with your doctor any alternative treatments you may be using or considering.

How can the family help a child live well with JRA?

JRA affects the entire family who must cope with the special chal-lenges of this disease. JRA can strain a child's participation in social and after-school activities and make school work more difficult. There are several things that family members can do to help the child do well physically and emotionally.

- Treat the child as normally as possible.

- Ensure that the child receives appropriate medical care and follows the doctor's instructions. Many treatment options are available, and because JRA is different in each child, what works for one may not work for another. If the medications that the doctor prescribes do not relieve symptoms or if they cause unpleasant side effects, patients and parents should discuss other choices with their doctor. A person with JRA can be more active when symptoms are controlled.

413

- Encourage exercise and physical therapy for the child. For many young people, exercise and physical therapy play important roles in managing JRA. Parents can arrange for children to participate in activities that the doctor recommends. During symptom-free periods, many doctors suggest playing team sports or doing other activities to help keep the joints strong and flexible and to provide play time with other children and encourage appropriate social development.

- Work closely with the school to develop a suitable plan for the child and to educate the teacher and the child's classmates about JRA. Some children with JRA may be absent from school for prolonged periods and need to have the teacher send assignments home. Some minor changes such as an extra set of books, or leaving class a few minutes early to get to the next class on time can be a great help. With proper attention, most children progress normally through school.

- Explain to the child that getting JRA is nobody's fault. Some children believe that JRA is a punishment for something they did.

- Consider joining a support group. The American Juvenile Arthritis Organization runs support groups for people with JRA and their families. Support group meetings provide the chance to talk to other young people and parents of children with JRA and may help a child and the family cope with the condition.

- Work with therapists or social workers to adapt more easily to the lifestyle change JRA may bring.

Do children with JRA have to limit activities?

Although pain sometimes limits physical activity, exercise is important to reduce the symptoms of JRA and maintain function and range of motion of the joints. Most children with JRA can take part fully in physical activities and sports when their symptoms are under control. However, during a disease flare-up, the doctor may advise limiting certain activities depending on the joints involved. Once the flare-up is over, a child can start regular activities again.

Swimming is particularly useful because it uses many joints and muscles without putting weight on the joints. A doctor or physical therapist can recommend exercises and activities.

Additional Information

**National Institute of Arthritis and
Musculoskeletal and Skin Diseases
(NIAMS) Information Clearinghouse**
1 AMS Circle
Bethesda, MD 20892-3675
Toll-Free: 877-22-NIAMS (64267)
Phone: 301-495-4484
TTY: 301-565-2966
Fax: 301-718-6366
Website: http://www.niams.nih.gov
E-mail: niamsinfo@mail.nih.gov

American Academy of Orthopaedic Surgeons
6300 N. River Rd.
Rosemont, IL 60018-4262
Toll-Free: 800-346-2267
Phone: 847-823-7186
Fax: 847-823-8125
Website: http://www.aaos.org

American College of Rheumatology
1800 Century Place, Suite 250
Atlanta, GA 30345-4300
Phone: 404-633-3777
Fax: 404-633-1870
Website: http://www.rheumatology.org

American Juvenile Arthritis Organization
1330 W. Peachtree St., Suite 100
Atlanta, GA 30309
Toll-Free: 800-568-4045
Phone: 404-965-7538
Website: http://www.arthritis.org
E-mail: help@arthritis.org

Chapter 46

Meningitis

Meningococcal Vaccines: Protecting You from Bacterial Meningitis

Meningitis is an infection of the fluid surrounding the brain and the spinal cord. Meningitis is usually caused by a virus or bacterial infection. Bacterial meningitis is usually more severe than viral meningitis. For bacterial meningitis, it is also important to know which type of bacteria is causing the meningitis. Vaccines are available to help protect against some forms bacterial meningitis.

Neisseria meningitidis is one type of bacteria that causes both meningitis and a serious blood infection called meningococcal disease. Anyone can get meningococcal disease. It is most common in infants less than one year of age and people with certain medical conditions, such as someone who has had their spleen removed. College freshmen who live in dormitories also have an increased risk of getting meningococcal disease.

Meningococcal infections can be treated with drugs such as penicillin. Still, about one out of every ten people who get the disease may die from it, and many others are affected for life. They may lose their arms or legs, become deaf, have problems with their nervous systems, become mentally impaired, or suffer seizures or strokes. This is why preventing the disease through use of meningococcal vaccines is important for people at highest risk.

"Meningococcal Vaccines," Centers for Disease Control and Prevention (CDC), September 30, 2005.

Meningococcal Vaccines

MCV-4 (meningococcal conjugate vaccine) was:

- licensed for use in the United States in early 2005
- licensed for people age 11 to 55 years of age
- expected to provide longer-lasting protection from meningococcal disease
- considered to be better at preventing the spread of disease from person to person

MPSV-4 (meningococcal polysaccharide vaccine) has been:

- used in the United States since the 1970s
- licensed for children older than two years of age as well as adolescents and adults

Both vaccines are known to protect more than 90 percent of those who get the vaccine; and to prevent four types of meningococcal disease, including two of the three types most common in the United States and a type that causes epidemics in Africa. Meningococcal vaccines cannot prevent all types of the disease, but they do protect many people who might become sick if they did not get the vaccine.

Who Should Get the New Vaccine, MCV-4?

Adolescents who should get the MCV-4 vaccine include:

- eleven to twelve year-olds at their routine preadolescent check-up
- those entering high school, if not previously vaccinated
- other adolescents who want to lower their risk of meningococcal disease

Anyone who has an elevated risk of meningococcal disease should get the MCV-4 vaccine, including:

- college freshmen living in dormitories
- microbiologists who are routinely exposed to isolates of *N. meningitides*
- military recruits

- people who travel to, or live in countries where meningococcal disease is very common

- anyone whose spleen has been damaged or removed and persons with certain other immune system disorders

- persons advised to receive vaccination during an outbreak

Who Should Not Get the New Vaccine?

- Anyone who has ever had a severe (life-threatening) allergic reaction to a previous dose of either meningococcal vaccine should not get another dose.

- Anyone who has a severe (life threatening) allergy to any vaccine component should not get the vaccine. Tell your doctor if you have any severe allergies.

- Anyone who is moderately or severely ill at the time the shot is scheduled should probably wait until they recover. Ask your doctor or nurse. People with a mild illness can usually get the vaccine.

- Meningococcal vaccines may be given to pregnant women. However, MCV-4 is a new vaccine and has not been studied in pregnant women as much as MPSV-4.

Chapter 47

Scoliosis in Adolescents

Scoliosis is a musculoskeletal disorder in which there is a sideways curvature of the spine, or backbone. The bones that make up the spine are called vertebrae. Some people who have scoliosis require treatment. Other people, who have milder curves, may only need to visit their doctor for periodic observation.

Who Gets Scoliosis?

People of all ages can have scoliosis, but this chapter focuses on children and adolescents. Of every 1,000 children, three to five develop spinal curves that are considered large enough to need treatment. Adolescent idiopathic scoliosis (scoliosis of unknown cause) is the most common type and occurs after the age of ten. Girls are more likely than boys to have this type of scoliosis. Since scoliosis can run in families, a child who has a parent, brother, or sister with idiopathic scoliosis should be checked regularly for scoliosis by the family physician.

Idiopathic scoliosis can also occur in children younger than ten years of age, but is very rare. Early onset or infantile idiopathic scoliosis occurs in children less than three years old. It is more common in Europe than in the United States. Juvenile idiopathic scoliosis occurs in children between the ages of three and ten.

"Questions and Answers about Scoliosis in Children and Adolescents," National Institute of Arthritis and Musculoskeletal and Skin Diseases (NIAMS), NIH Publication No. 01–4862, July 2001. Updated in April 2006 by Dr. David A. Cooke, MD, Diplomate, American Board of Internal Medicine.

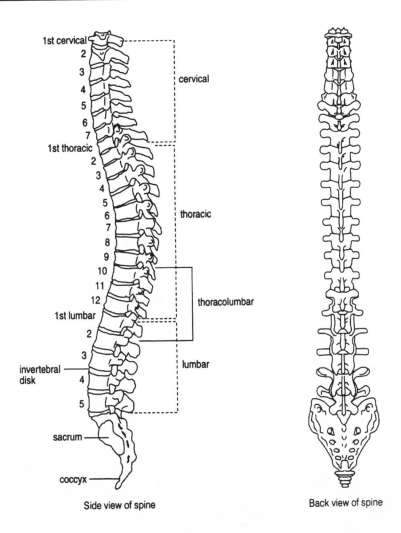

1st cervical
2
3
4
5
6
7
1st thoracic
2
3
4
5
6
7
8
9
10
11
12
1st lumbar
2
3
4
5

cervical

thoracic

thoracolumbar

lumbar

invertebral disk

sacrum

coccyx

Side view of spine

Back view of spine

Figure 47.1. *Normal Spine*

What Causes Scoliosis?

In 80 to 85 percent of people, the cause of scoliosis is unknown; this is called idiopathic scoliosis. Before concluding that a person has idiopathic scoliosis, the doctor looks for other possible causes, such as injury or infection. Causes of curves are classified as either non-structural or structural.

- Nonstructural (functional) scoliosis—A structurally normal spine that appears curved. This is a temporary, changing curve. It is caused by an underlying condition such as a difference in leg length, muscle spasms, or inflammatory conditions such as appendicitis. Doctors treat this type of scoliosis by correcting the underlying problem.

- Structural scoliosis—A fixed curve that doctors treat case by case. Sometimes structural scoliosis is one part of a syndrome or disease, such as Marfan syndrome—an inherited connective tissue disorder. In other cases, it occurs by itself. Structural scoliosis can be caused by neuromuscular diseases (such as cerebral palsy, poliomyelitis, or muscular dystrophy), birth defects (such as hemivertebra, in which one side of a vertebra fails to form normally before birth), injury, certain infections, tumors (such as those caused by neurofibromatosis—a birth defect sometimes associated with benign tumors on the spinal column), metabolic diseases, connective tissue disorders, rheumatic diseases, or unknown factors (idiopathic scoliosis).

How Does the Doctor Diagnose Scoliosis?

The doctor takes the following steps to evaluate a patient for scoliosis:

- Medical history—The doctor talks to the patient and the patient's parent(s), and reviews the patient's records to look for medical problems that might be causing the spine to curve, for example, birth defects, trauma, or other disorders that can be associated with scoliosis.

- Physical examination—The doctor looks at the patient's back, chest, pelvis, legs, feet, and skin. The doctor checks if the patient's shoulders are level, whether the head is centered, and whether opposite sides of the body look level. The doctor also examines the back muscles while the patient is bending forward to see if one side of the rib cage is higher than the other. If there is a significant asymmetry (difference between opposite sides of the body), the doctor will refer the patient to an orthopaedic spine specialist (a doctor who has experience treating people with scoliosis). Certain changes in the skin, such as so-called café au lait (coffee-with-milk-colored) spots, can suggest that the scoliosis is caused by a birth defect.

- X-ray evaluation—Patients with significant spinal curves, unusual back pain, or signs of involvement of the central nervous system (brain and spinal cord) such as bowel and bladder control problems need to have an x-ray. The x-ray should be done with the patient standing with his or her back to the x-ray machine. The view is of the entire spine on one long (36-inch) film. Occasionally, doctors ask for more tests to see if there are other problems.

- Curve measurement—The doctor measures the curve on the x-ray image. He or she finds the vertebrae at the beginning and end of the curve and measures the angle of the curve. Curves that are greater than 20 degrees require treatment.

Doctors group curves of the spine by their location, shape, pattern, and cause. They use this information to decide how best to treat the scoliosis.

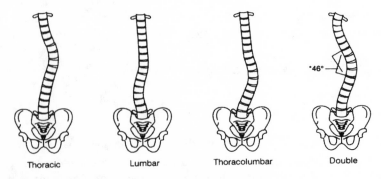

Figure 47.2. Curve Patterns of the Spine

- Location—To identify a curve's location, doctors find the apex of the curve (the vertebra within the curve that is the most off-center)—the location of the apex is the location of the curve. A thoracic curve has its apex in the thoracic area (the part of the spine to which the ribs attach). A lumbar curve has its apex in the lower back. A thoracolumbar curve has its apex where the thoracic and lumbar vertebrae join.

- Shape—The curve usually is S- or C-shaped.

- Pattern—Curves frequently follow patterns that have been studied in previous patients. The larger the curve is, the more likely it will progress (depending on the amount of growth remaining).

Does Scoliosis Have to Be Treated? What Are the Treatments?

Many children who are sent to the doctor by a school scoliosis screening program have very mild spinal curves that do not need treatment. When a child does need treatment, the doctor may send him or her to an orthopaedic spine specialist.

The doctor will suggest the best treatment for each patient based on the patient's age, how much more he or she is likely to grow, the degree and pattern of the curve, and the type of scoliosis. The doctor may recommend observation, bracing, or surgery.

- Observation—Doctors follow patients without treatment and re-examine them every four to six months when the patient is still growing (is skeletally immature) and has an idiopathic curve of less than 25 degrees.

- Bracing—As a child nears the end of growth, the indications for bracing will depend on how the curve affects the child's appearance, whether the curve is getting worse, and the size of the curve. Doctors advise patients to wear a brace to stop a curve from getting any worse when the patient:

  - is still growing and has an idiopathic curve that is more than 25 to 30 degrees;

  - has at least two years of growth remaining, has an idiopathic curve that is between 20 and 29 degrees, and, if a girl, has not had her first menstrual period; or

  - is still growing and has an idiopathic curve between 20 and 29 degrees that is getting worse.

- Surgery—Doctors advise patients to have surgery to correct a curve or stop it from worsening when the patient is still growing, has a curve that is more than 45 degrees, and has a curve that is getting worse.

Are There Other Ways to Treat Scoliosis?

Some people have tried other ways to treat scoliosis, including manipulation by a chiropractor, electrical stimulation, dietary supplements, and corrective exercises. Studies of these treatments have not shown them to cure scoliosis, or to prevent worsening of the curvature.

Which Brace Is Best?

The decision about which brace to wear depends on the type of curve and whether the patient will follow the doctor's directions about how many hours a day to wear the brace.

There are two main types of braces. Braces can be custom-made or can be made from a prefabricated mold. All must be selected for the specific curve problem and fitted to each patient. To have their intended effect (to keep a curve from getting worse), braces must be worn every day for the full number of hours prescribed by the doctor until the child stops growing.

- Milwaukee brace—Patients can wear this brace to correct any curve in the spine. This brace has a neck ring.

- Thoracolumbosacral orthosis (TLSO)—Patients can wear this brace to correct curves whose apex is at or below the eighth thoracic vertebra. The TLSO is an underarm brace, which means that it fits under the arm and around the rib cage, lower back, and hips.

If the Doctor Recommends Surgery, Which Procedure Is Best?

Many surgical techniques can be used to correct the curves of scoliosis. The main surgical procedure is correction, stabilization, and fusion of the curve. Fusion is the joining of two or more vertebrae. Surgeons can choose different ways to straighten the spine and also different implants to keep the spine stable after surgery. (Implants are devices that remain in the patient after surgery to keep the spine aligned.) The decision about the type of implant will depend on the cost; the size of the implant, which depends on the size of the patient; the shape of the implant; its safety; and the experience of the surgeon. Each patient should discuss his or her options with at least two experienced surgeons.

Can People with Scoliosis Exercise?

Although exercise programs have not been shown to affect the natural history of scoliosis, exercise is encouraged in patients with scoliosis to minimize any potential decrease in functional ability over time. It is very important for all people, including those with scoliosis, to exercise and remain physically fit. Girls have a higher risk than boys of developing osteoporosis (a disorder that results in weak bones that can break easily) later in life. The risk of osteoporosis is reduced in women who exercise regularly all their lives; and weight-bearing exercise, such as walking, running, soccer, and gymnastics, increases bone density and helps prevent osteoporosis. For boys and girls, exercising and participating in sports also improves their general sense of well-being.

Additional Information

American Physical Therapy Association
1111 N. Fairfax St.
Alexandria, VA 22314-1488
Toll-Free: 800-999-2782
Phone: 703-684-2782
TDD: 703-683-6748
Fax: 703-684-7343
Website: http://www.apta.org

National Institute of Arthritis and Musculoskeletal and Skin Diseases (NIAMS) Information Clearinghouse
1 AMS Circle
Bethesda, MD 20892-3675
Toll-Free: 877-22-NIAMS (64267)
Phone: 301-495-4484
TTY: 301-565-2966
Fax: 301-718-6366
Website: http://www.niams.nih.gov
E-mail: niamsinfo@mail.nih.gov

National Scoliosis Foundation
5 Cabot Place
Stoughton, MA 02072
Toll-Free: 800-673-6922
Fax: 617-341-8333
Website: http://www.scoliosis.org
E-mail: nsf@scoliosis.org

Scoliosis Association, Inc.
P.O. Box 811705
Boca Raton, FL 33481-1705
Toll-Free: 800-800-0669
Phone: 561-994-4435
Fax: 561-994-2455
Website: http://www.scoliosis-assoc.org

Scoliosis Research Society

555 E. Wells St., Suite 1100
Milwaukee, WI 53202-3823
Phone: 414-289-9107
Fax: 414-276-3349
Website: http://www.srs.org
E-mail: info@srs.org

Chapter 48

Chronic Illnesses: Tips for Students, Families, and Schools

Chronic illnesses affect at least 10 to 15 percent of American children. Responding to the needs of students with chronic conditions, such as asthma, allergies, diabetes, and epilepsy (also known as seizure disorders), in the school setting requires a comprehensive, coordinated, and systematic approach. Students with chronic health conditions can function to their maximum potential if their needs are met. The benefits to students can include better attendance, improved alertness and physical stamina, fewer symptoms, fewer restrictions on participation in physical activities and special activities such as field trips, and fewer medical emergencies. Schools can work together with parents, students, health care providers, and the community to provide a safe and supportive educational environment for students with chronic illnesses and to ensure that students with chronic illnesses have the same educational opportunities as do other students.

Family's Responsibilities

- Notify the school of the student's health management needs and diagnosis when appropriate. Notify schools as early as possible and whenever the student's health needs change.

- Provide a written description of the student's health needs at school, including authorizations for medication administration

"Students with Chronic Illnesses: Guidance for Families, Schools, and Students," National Heart, Lung, and Blood Institute (NHLBI), 2002.

and emergency treatment, signed by the student's health care provider.

- Participate in the development of a school plan to implement the student's health needs:

  - Meet with the school team to develop a plan to accommodate the student's needs in all school settings.

  - Authorize appropriate exchange of information between school health program staff and the student's personal health care providers.

  - Communicate significant changes in the student's needs or health status promptly to appropriate school staff.

- Provide an adequate supply of student's medication, in pharmacy-labeled containers, and other supplies to the designated school staff, and replace medications and supplies as needed. This supply should remain at school.

- Provide the school a means of contacting you or another responsible person at all times in case of an emergency or medical problem.

- Educate the student to develop age-appropriate self-care skills.

- Promote good general health, personal care, nutrition, and physical activity.

School District's Responsibilities

- Develop and implement districtwide guidelines and protocols applicable to chronic illnesses generally and specific protocols for asthma, allergies, diabetes, epilepsy (seizure disorders), and other common chronic illnesses of students.

- Guidelines should include safe, coordinated practices (as age and skill level appropriate) that enable the student to successfully manage his or her health in the classroom and at all school-related activities.

- Protocols should be consistent with established standards of care for students with chronic illnesses and Federal laws that provide protection to students with disabilities, including ensuring confidentiality of student health care information and appropriate information sharing.

- Protocols should address education of all members of the school environment about chronic illnesses, including a component addressing the promotion of acceptance and the elimination of stigma surrounding chronic illnesses.

- Develop, coordinate, and implement necessary training programs for staff that will be responsible for chronic illness care tasks at school and school-related activities.

- Monitor schools for compliance with chronic illness care protocols.

- Meet with parents, school personnel, and health care providers to address issues of concern about the provision of care to students with chronic illnesses by school district staff.

School's Responsibilities

- Identify students with chronic conditions, and review their health records as submitted by families and health care providers.

- Arrange a meeting to discuss health accommodations and educational aids and services that the student may need and to develop a 504 Plan, Individualized Education Program (IEP), or other school plan, as appropriate. The participants should include the family, student (if appropriate), school health staff, 504/IEP coordinator (as applicable), individuals trained to assist the student, and the teacher who has primary responsibility for the student. Health care provider input may be provided in person or in writing.

- Provide nondiscriminatory opportunities to students with disabilities. Be knowledgeable about and ensure compliance with applicable Federal laws, including Americans with Disabilities Act (ADA), Individuals with Disabilities Education Act (IDEA), Section 504, and Family Educational Rights and Privacy Act of 1974 (FERPA). Be knowledgeable about any State or local laws or district policies that affect the implementation of students' rights under Federal law.

- Clarify the roles and obligations of specific school staff, and provide education and communication systems necessary to ensure that students' health and educational needs are met in a safe and coordinated manner.

- Implement strategies that reduce disruption in the student's school activities, including physical education, recess, offsite events, extracurricular activities, and field trips.

- Communicate with families regularly and as authorized with the student's health care providers.

- Ensure that the student receives prescribed medications in a safe, reliable, and effective manner and has access to needed medication at all times during the school day and at school-related activities.

- Be prepared to handle health needs and emergencies and to ensure that there is a staff member available who is properly trained to administer medications or other immediate care during the school day and at all school-related activities, regardless of time or location.

- Ensure that all staff who interact with the student on a regular basis receive appropriate guidance and training on routine needs, precautions, and emergency actions.

- Provide appropriate health education to students and staff.

- Provide a safe and healthy school environment.

- Ensure that case management is provided as needed.

- Ensure proper record keeping, including appropriate measures to both protect confidentiality and to share information.

- Promote a supportive learning environment that views students with chronic illnesses the same as other students except to respond to health needs.

- Promote good general health, personal care, nutrition, and physical activity.

Student's Responsibilities

- Notify an adult about concerns and needs in managing his or her symptoms or the school environment.

- Participate in the care and management of his or her health as appropriate to his or her developmental level.

Part Seven

Abuse and Violence Affects Adolescent Health

Chapter 49

Youth Violence: A National Problem

A National Problem

Violent injury and death disproportionately affect children, adolescents, and young adults in the United States. Homicide is the second leading cause of death among young people ages 15 to 19. Among African American youths in that age group, homicide is the leading killer. Just as alarming as the number of young people dying from violence is the number of young people who are committing violent acts.

Violence does not have to be fatal to greatly affect individuals and communities. Violence-related injuries can leave emotional and physical scars that remain with victims long after the violent event has occurred. The rates of nonfatal victimization for rape, sexual assault, robbery, and aggravated assault are higher among people under age 25 than among other age groups.

Facts about Youth Violence

Occurrence

- In 2003, 5,570 young people ages 10 to 24 were murdered—an average of 15 each day. Of these victims, 82% were killed with firearms (CDC 2006).

This chapter includes: Excerpts from "Youth Violence: A National Problem," Centers for Disease Control and Prevention (CDC), November 30, 2005; "Youth Violence: Fact Sheet," CDC, October 13, 2005; and "Youth Violence Warning Signs," CDC National Youth Violence Prevention Resource Center, November 2003.

- Although high-profile school shootings have increased public concern for student safety, school-associated violent deaths account for less than 1% of homicides among school-aged children and youth (Anderson et al. 2001).

- In 2004, more than 750,000 young people ages 10 to 24 were treated in emergency departments for injuries sustained due to violence (CDC 2006).

- In a nationwide survey of high school students (CDC 2004):

  - 33% reported being in a physical fight one or more times in the 12 months preceding the survey.

  - 17% reported carrying a weapon (e.g., gun, knife, or club) on one or more of the 30 days preceding the survey.

- An estimated 30% of 6th to 10th graders in the United States were involved in bullying as a bully, a target of bullying, or both (Nansel et al. 2001).

Consequences

- Direct and indirect costs of youth violence (for example, medical, lost productivity, quality of life) exceed $158 billion every year (Children's Safety Network Economics and Data Analysis Resource Center 2000).

- In a nationwide survey of high school students, about 6% reported not going to school on one or more days in the 30 days preceding the survey because they felt unsafe at school or on their way to and from school (CDC 2004).

- In addition to causing injury and death, youth violence affects communities by increasing the cost of health care, reducing productivity, decreasing property values, and disrupting social services (Mercy et al. 2002).

Groups at Risk

- Among 10 to 24 year olds, homicide is the leading cause of death for African Americans, the second leading cause of death for Hispanics, and the third leading cause of death for American Indians, Alaska Natives, and Asian/Pacific Islanders (CDC 2006).

- Of the 5,570 homicides reported in 2003 among 10 to 24 year olds, 86% were males and 14% were females (CDC 2005).

- Male students are more likely to be involved in a physical fight than female students (41% vs. 25%; CDC 2004).

Risk Factors

Research on youth violence has increased our understanding of factors that make some populations more vulnerable to victimization and perpetration. Many risk factors are the same, in part, because of the overlap among victims and perpetrators of violence.

Risk factors increase the likelihood that a young person will become violent. However, risk factors are not direct causes of youth violence; instead, risk factors contribute to youth violence (Mercy et al. 2002; DHHS 2001).

Research associates the following risk factors with perpetration of youth violence (DHHS 2001; Lipsey and Derzon 1998; Resnick et al. 2004):

Individual Risk Factors

- history of violent victimization or involvement
- attention deficits, hyperactivity, or learning disorders
- history of early aggressive behavior
- involvement with drugs, alcohol, or tobacco
- low intelligence quotient (IQ)
- poor behavioral control
- deficits in social cognitive or information-processing abilities
- high emotional distress
- history of treatment for emotional problems
- antisocial beliefs and attitudes
- exposure to violence and conflict in the family

Family Risk Factors

- authoritarian child rearing attitudes
- harsh, lax, or inconsistent disciplinary practices
- low parental involvement
- low emotional attachment to parents or caregivers
- low parental education and income

- parental substance abuse or criminality
- poor family functioning
- poor monitoring and supervision of children

Peer / School Risk Factors

- association with delinquent peers
- involvement in gangs
- social rejection by peers
- lack of involvement in conventional activities
- poor academic performance
- low commitment to school and school failure

Community Risk Factors

- diminished economic opportunities
- high concentrations of poor residents
- high level of transiency
- high level of family disruption
- low levels of community participation
- socially disorganized neighborhoods

Protective Factors

Protective factors buffer young people from risks of becoming violent. These factors exist at various levels. To date, protective factors have not been studied as extensively or rigorously as risk factors. However, identifying and understanding protective factors are equally as important as researching risk factors.

Most research is preliminary. Studies propose the following protective factors (DHHS 2001; Resnick et al. 2004):

Individual Protective Factors

- intolerant attitude toward deviance
- high IQ or high grade point average
- positive social orientation
- religiosity

Family Protective Factors

- connectedness to family or adults outside of the family
- ability to discuss problems with parents
- perceived parental expectations about school performance are high
- frequent shared activities with parents
- consistent presence of parent during at least one of the following: when awakening, when arriving home from school, at evening mealtime, and when going to bed
- involvement in social activities

Peer / School Protective Factors

- commitment to school
- involvement in social activities

References

Anderson MA, Kaufman J, Simon TR, Barrios L, Paulozzi L, Ryan G, et al. School-associated violent deaths in the United States, 1994–1999. *Journal of the American Medical Association* 2001;286:2695–702.

Centers for Disease Control and Prevention, National Center for Injury Prevention and Control. Web-based Injury Statistics Query and Reporting System (WISQARS) [online]. (2006) [cited 2006 Feb 8]. Available from: http://www.cdc.gov/ncipc/wisqars.

Centers for Disease Control and Prevention. Youth risk behavior surveillance—United States, 2003. *MMWR* 2004;53(SS02):1–96.

Children's Safety Network Economics and Data Analysis Resource Center. *State costs of violence perpetrated by youth*. Available from: http://www.edarc.org/pubs/tables/youth-viol.htm.

Department of Health and Human Services (DHHS). *Youth violence: a report of the Surgeon General* [online]; 2001. Available from http://www.surgeongeneral.gov/library/youthviolence/toc.html.

Lipsey MW, Derzon JH. Predictors of violent and serious delinquency in adolescence and early adulthood: a synthesis of longitudinal research. In: Loeber R, Farrington DP, editors. *Serious and violent juvenile offenders: risk factors and successful interventions.* Thousand Oaks (CA): Sage Publications; 1998. p. 86–105.

Mercy J, Butchart A, Farrington D, Cerdá M. Youth violence. In: Krug E, Dahlberg LL, Mercy JA, et al., editors. *The world report on violence and health.* Geneva (Switzerland): World Health Organization; 2002. p. 25–56.

Nansel TR, Overpeck M, Pilla RS, Ruan WJ, Simons-Morton B, Scheidt P. Bullying behaviors among US youth: prevalence and association with psychosocial adjustment. *Journal of the American Medical Association* 2001;285(16):2094–100.

Resnick MD, Ireland M, Borowsky I. Youth violence perpetration: what protects? What predicts? Findings from the National Longitudinal Study of Adolescent Health. *Journal of Adolescent Health* 2004; 35:424.e1–e10.

Youth Violence Warning Signs

Researchers have identified a number of warning signs that suggest that a child may be at risk for violent behavior. The presence of one or more of the following increases the risk of violent or dangerous behavior:

- past violent or aggressive behavior (including uncontrollable angry outbursts)
- access to guns or other weapons
- bringing a weapon to school
- past suicide attempts or threats
- family history of violent behavior or suicide attempts
- blaming others and/or unwilling to accept responsibility for one's own actions
- recent experience of humiliation, shame, loss, or rejection
- bullying or intimidating peers or younger children
- a pattern of threats
- being a victim of abuse or neglect (physical, sexual, or emotional)
- witnessing abuse or violence in the home

- themes of death or depression repeatedly evident in conversation, written expressions, reading selections, or artwork

- preoccupation with themes and acts of violence in television shows, movies, music, magazines, comics, books, video games, and Internet sites

- mental illness, such as depression, mania, psychosis, or bipolar disorder

- use of alcohol or illicit drugs

- disciplinary problems at school or in the community (delinquent behavior)

- past destruction of property or vandalism

- cruelty to animals

- fire-setting behavior

- poor peer relationships and/or social isolation

- involvement with cults or gangs

- little or no supervision or support from parents or other caring adult

Source: American Academy of Child and Adolescent Psychiatry. (2002). *Children and Threats: When Are They Serious?* Facts for Families Series.

Typically, the greater the number of these warning signs present, the greater the risk. It is important to realize, however, that many children exhibit these warning signs and never resort to violence. Even so, these signs can be a cue that something is wrong, and the individual needs help.

Additional Information

CDC National Center for Injury Prevention and Control
Mailstop K65
4770 Buford Highway NE
Atlanta, GA 30341-3724
Toll-Free: 800-CDC-INFO (800-232-4636)
Website: http://www.cdc.gov
E-mail: cdcinfo@cdc.gov

Chapter 50

Abuse and Neglect Defined

Child abuse and neglect are defined by both Federal and State law. The Child Abuse Prevention and Treatment Act (CAPTA) is the Federal legislation that provides minimum standards for the definition of child abuse and neglect that States must incorporate in their statutory definitions. Under CAPTA, child abuse and neglect means, at a minimum:

- Any recent act or failure to act on the part of a parent or caretaker, which results in death, serious physical or emotional harm, sexual abuse, or exploitation, or an act or failure to act which presents an imminent risk of serious harm.[1]

The term sexual abuse includes:

- The employment, use, persuasion, inducement, enticement, or coercion of any child to engage in, or assist any other person to engage in, any sexually explicit conduct or simulation of such conduct for the purpose of producing a visual depiction of such conduct; or

- The rape, and in cases of caretaker or interfamilial relationships, statutory rape, molestation, prostitution, or other form of sexual exploitation of children, or incest with children.[2]

"Definitions of Child Abuse and Neglect," National Clearinghouse on Child Abuse and Neglect Information, 2005.

Types of Abuse

Each State, U.S. territory, and the District of Columbia provides its own definitions of child abuse and neglect. As applied to reporting statutes, these definitions determine the grounds for State intervention in the protection of a child's[3] well-being. Definitions vary among States. For example, some States define child abuse and neglect as a single concept, while others provide separate definitions for physical abuse, neglect, sexual abuse, and/or emotional abuse.

Physical Abuse

All States and territories provide definitions for physical abuse. The term is generally defined as any nonaccidental physical injury to the child, and can include striking, kicking, burning, or biting the child, or any action that results in a physical impairment of the child.

Substance Abuse

Substance abuse is an element of the definition of child abuse or neglect in some States.[4] Circumstances that can be considered abuse or neglect include:

- manufacture of a controlled substance in the presence of child or on the premises occupied by a child[5]

- allowing a child to be present where the chemicals or equipment for the manufacture of controlled substances are used or stored[6]

- selling, distributing, or giving drugs or alcohol to a child[7]

- use of a controlled substance by a caregiver that impairs the caregiver's ability to adequately care for the child[8]

- exposure of the child to drug paraphernalia,[9] the criminal sale or distribution of drugs,[10] or drug-related activity[11]

Neglect

Neglect is also addressed in the statutes of all States and territories, either in a separate definition, or as a type of abuse. Neglect is frequently defined in terms of deprivation of adequate food, clothing, shelter, or medical care. Several States distinguish between failure to provide based on the financial inability to do so and the failure to provide for no apparent financial reason. The latter constitutes neglect.

Sexual Abuse/Exploitation

All States include sexual abuse in their definitions. Some States refer in general terms to sexual abuse, while others specify various acts as sexual abuse. Sexual exploitation is an element of the definition of sexual abuse in most jurisdictions. Sexual exploitation includes allowing the child to engage in prostitution or in the production of child pornography.

Emotional Abuse

All States and territories except Georgia and Washington include emotional maltreatment as part of their definitions of abuse or neglect. Approximately[12] 22 States,[13] the District of Columbia, the Northern Mariana Islands, and Puerto Rico provide specific definitions of emotional abuse or mental injury to a child. Typical language used in these definitions is "injury to the psychological capacity or emotional stability of the child as evidenced by an observable or substantial change in behavior, emotional response, or cognition," or as evidenced by "anxiety, depression, withdrawal, or aggressive behavior."

Abandonment

Many States and territories now provide definitions for child abandonment in their reporting laws. Approximately 18 States[14] and the District of Columbia include abandonment in their definition of neglect, while 13 States,[15] American Samoa, Guam, Puerto Rico, and the Virgin Islands provide separate definitions for establishing abandonment. In general, it is considered abandonment of the child when the parent's identity or whereabouts are unknown, the child has been left by the parent in circumstances where the child suffers serious harm, or the parent has failed to maintain contact with the child or to provide reasonable support for a specified period of time.

Standards for Reporting

The standard for what constitutes an abusive act varies among the States. Many States define abuse in terms of harm or threatened harm to a child's health or welfare. Other standards commonly seen include acts or omissions, recklessly fails or refuses to act, willfully causes or permits, and failure to provide. These standards guide mandatory reporters in their decision on whether to make a report to child protective services.

Persons Responsible for the Child

In addition to defining the acts or omissions that constitute child abuse or neglect, several statutes provide specific definitions of the persons who are reportable under the civil child abuse reporting laws to child protective services as perpetrators of abuse and neglect. These are persons who have some relationship or regular responsibility for the child. This generally includes parents, guardians, foster parents, relatives, or other caretakers responsible for the child's welfare.

Exceptions

A number of States provide exceptions in their reporting laws, which exempt certain acts or omissions from their statutory definitions of child abuse and neglect. For instance, in six States[16] and the District of Columbia, financial inability to provide for a child is exempted from the definition of neglect. In 14 States,[17] the District of Columbia, American Samoa, and the Northern Mariana Islands, physical discipline of a child, as long as it is reasonable and causes no bodily injury to the child, is an exception to the definition of abuse.

The Child Abuse Prevention and Treatment Act Amendments of 1996 added new provisions specifying that nothing in the Act be construed as establishing a Federal requirement that a parent or legal guardian provide any medical service or treatment that is against the religious beliefs of the parent or legal guardian. At the State level, civil child abuse reporting laws may provide an exception to the definition of child abuse and neglect for parents who choose not to seek medical care for their children due to religious beliefs.

Approximately 30 States,[18] the District of Columbia, and Guam provide an exemption from the definition of neglect for parents who choose not to seek medical care for their children due to religious beliefs, while three States[19] specifically provide an exception for Christian Science treatment. However, 17 of these States[20] authorize the court to order medical treatment for the child when the child's condition warrants intervention, and four States[21] require mandated reporters to report instances when a child is not receiving medical care so that an investigation can be made.

References

1. 42 U.S.C.A. § 5106g(2) (West Supp. 1998)
2. 42 U.S.C.A. § 5106g(4) (West Supp. 1998)

3. The term child means a person who has not attained the age of 18 years.

4. For a more complete discussion of this issue, see the Clearinghouse publication *Parental Drug Use as Child Abuse*, at http://nccanch.acf.hhs.gov/general/legal/statutes/drugexposed.cfm.

5. Colorado, Indiana, Iowa, Montana, South Dakota, Tennessee, and Virginia

6. Arizona and New Mexico

7. Florida, Hawaii, Illinois, Minnesota, and Texas

8. Kentucky, New York, Rhode Island, and Texas

9. North Dakota

10. Montana and Virginia

11. District of Columbia

12. The word approximately is used to stress the fact that the States frequently amend their laws, so this information is current only through January 2005.

13. Alaska, Arizona, Arkansas, California, Colorado, Florida, Idaho, Kentucky, Maine, Maryland, Minnesota, Montana, Nevada, New York, Ohio, Pennsylvania, Rhode Island, South Carolina, Tennessee, Vermont, Wisconsin, and Wyoming

14. Colorado, Connecticut, Florida, Illinois, Kentucky, Louisiana, Minnesota, Nevada, New Jersey, North Carolina, Oklahoma, Rhode Island, South Dakota, Texas, Vermont, Virginia, West Virginia, and Wyoming

15. Arizona, Arkansas, Idaho, Indiana, Kansas, Maine, Montana, New Hampshire, New Mexico, New York, North Dakota, Ohio, and South Carolina

16. Arkansas, Florida, Louisiana, Pennsylvania, West Virginia, and Wisconsin

17. Arkansas, Colorado, Florida, Georgia, Indiana, Minnesota, Mississippi, Missouri, Ohio, Oklahoma, Oregon, South Carolina, Texas, and Washington

18. Alabama, Alaska, California, Colorado, Delaware, Florida, Georgia, Idaho, Illinois, Indiana, Iowa, Kansas, Kentucky, Louisiana, Maine, Michigan, Minnesota, Mississippi, Missouri,

Montana, Nevada, New Hampshire, New Jersey, New Mexico, Ohio, Oklahoma, Pennsylvania, Vermont, Virginia, and Wyoming

19. Arizona, Connecticut, and Washington

20. Alabama, Colorado, Florida, Idaho, Indiana, Iowa, Kansas, Kentucky, Louisiana, Michigan, Minnesota, Missouri, Montana, Nevada, Ohio, Oklahoma, and Pennsylvania

21. Michigan, Missouri, Ohio, and Oklahoma

Additional Information

National Clearinghouse on Child Abuse and Neglect Information

Children's Bureau/ACYF
1250 Maryland Ave. SW, 8th Floor
Washington, DC 20024
Toll-Free: 800-394-3366
Phone: 703-385-7565
Fax: 703-385-3206
Website: http://nccanch.acf.hhs.gov
E-mail: nccanch@caliber.com

Chapter 51

Bullying Is a Major Concern for Students

What We Know about Bullying

Bullying is aggressive behavior that is intentional and that involves an imbalance of power or strength. Typically, it is repeated over time. A child who is being bullied has a hard time defending himself or herself.

Bullying can take many forms, such as hitting or punching (physical bullying); teasing or name calling (verbal bullying); intimidation using gestures or social exclusion (nonverbal bullying or emotional bullying); and sending insulting messages by e-mail (cyberbullying).

Prevalence of Bullying

- Studies show that between 15–25 percent of U.S. students are bullied with some frequency (sometimes or more often) while 15–20 percent report that they bully others with some frequency.

- Recent statistics show that although school violence has declined four percent during the past several years, the incidence of behaviors such as bullying has increased by five percent between 1999 and 2001.

This chapter includes: Excerpts from "What We Know about Bullying," Health Resources and Services Administration (HRSA), 2005; "Why Should Adults Care about Bullying," HRSA, 2005; and "What Can Students and Youth Do to Lend a Hand?" HRSA, 2004.

- Bullying has been identified as a major concern by schools across the U.S.

- In surveys of third through eighth graders in 14 Massachusetts schools, nearly half who had been frequently bullied reported that the bullying had lasted six months or longer.

- Research indicates that children with disabilities or special needs may be at a higher risk of being bullied than other children.

Bullying and Gender

- By self-report, boys are more likely than girls to bully others.

- Girls frequently report being bullied by both boys and girls, but boys report that they are most often bullied only by other boys.

- Verbal bullying is the most frequent form of bullying experienced by both boys and girls. Boys are more likely to be physically bullied by their peers; girls are more likely to report being targets of rumor spreading and sexual comments. Girls are more likely to bully each other using social exclusion.

- Use of derogatory speculation about sexual orientation is so common that many parents do not think of telling their children that it could be hurtful.

Consequences of Bullying

- Stresses of being bullied can interfere with student's engagement and learning in school.

- Children and youth who are bullied are more likely than other children to be depressed, lonely, anxious, have low self-esteem, feel unwell, and think about suicide.

- Students who are bullied may fear going to school, using the bathroom, and riding on the school bus.

- In a survey of third through eighth graders in 14 Massachusetts schools, more than 14 percent reported that they were often afraid of being bullied.

- Research shows that bullying can be a sign of other serious antisocial or violent behavior. Children and youth who frequently bully their peers are more likely than others to get into frequent fights, be injured in a fight, vandalize or steal property, drink alcohol, smoke, be truant from school, drop out of school, and carry a weapon.

- Bullying also has an impact on other students at school who are bystanders to bullying. Bullying creates a climate of fear and disrespect in schools and has a negative impact on student learning.

Adult Response to Bullying

- Adults are often unaware of bullying problems. In one study, 70 percent of teachers believed that teachers intervene almost always in bullying situations; only 25 percent of students agreed with this assessment.

- Twenty-five percent of teachers see nothing wrong with bullying or putdowns and consequently intervene in only four percent of bullying incidents.

- Students often feel that adult intervention is infrequent and unhelpful and they often fear that telling adults will only bring more harassment from bullies.

- In a survey of students in 14 elementary and middle schools in Massachusetts, more than 30 percent believed that adults did little or nothing to help in bullying incidents.

What Adults Can Do

There are a number of reasons why adults should be concerned about bullying among children and youth.

1. Many children are involved in bullying, and most are extremely concerned about it.

   - Studies show that between 15–25% of U.S. students are bullied with some frequency (sometimes or more often) while 15–20% admit that they bully others with some frequency.

   - Not only is bullying prevalent, but children and youth report being extremely concerned about it. In a 2003 Harris poll of 8–17 year-old girls, commissioned by the Girl Scouts of the USA, bullying topped girls' list of concerns regarding their safety. When asked what they worried about the most, the most common response was being socially ostracized—being teased or made fun of. [*Feeling Safe: What Girls Say* by Judy Schoenberg, Ed.M., Toija Riggins, Ph.D., and Kimberlee Salmond, M.P.P. (New York, NY: Girl Scouts of the USA, 2003). 114 pp. (Executive Summary, 23 pp.)]

2. Bullying can seriously affect the mental health, academic work, and physical health of children who are targeted.

   • Children who are bullied are more likely than other children to have lower self-esteem; higher rates of depression, loneliness, anxiety, and suicidal thoughts. They also are more likely to want to avoid attending school and have higher school absenteeism rates.

   • Recent research on the health-related effects of bullying indicates that victims of frequent bullying are more likely to experience headaches, sleeping problems, and stomach ailments.

   • Some emotional scars can be long-lasting. Research suggests that adults who were bullied as children are more likely than their non-bullied peers to be depressed and have low self-esteem as adults.

3. Children who bully are more likely than other children to be engaged in other antisocial, violent, or troubling behavior. Findings from research in the U.S. and abroad indicate that children who bully are more likely to:

   • get into frequent fights
   • be injured in a fight
   • steal, vandalize property
   • drink alcohol
   • smoke
   • be truant, drop out of school
   • report poorer academic achievement
   • perceive a negative climate at school
   • carry a weapon

4. Bullying can negatively affect children who observe bullying going on around them—even if they are not targeted themselves.

- Children who are bystanders to bullying can feel fearful (Maybe I'll be targeted next.), guilty (I should do something to stop this, but I'm afraid to.), and distracted from school work.

- Bullying can contribute to a negative social climate at school.

5. Bullying is a form of victimization or abuse, and it is wrong. Children should be able to attend school or take part in community activities without fear of being harassed, assaulted, belittled, or excluded.

What Can Students and Youth Do to Lend a Hand?

Bullying happens when someone hurts or scares another person on purpose. The person being bullied has a hard time defending himself or herself. Usually, bullying happens over and over.

Sometimes bullying is easy to notice, such as with hitting or name-calling, and other times it is hard to see, such as with leaving a person out or saying mean things behind someone's back. Both boys and girls bully, and both boys and girls get bullied. Bullying is not fair, and it hurts.

What do you do when you see someone being bullied at school?

Ask yourself: Is it my job to help? Think about how you might feel if the bullying was happening to you. You and other kids can lend a hand, even when you aren't close friends with the kids who are bullied. Your school will be a better place if you help stop bullying. And making your school a better place is everyone's job.

What can I do?

Think about what may work for you:

- Do not just stand there—say something.

- Kids who bully may think they are being funny or cool. If you feel safe, tell the person to stop the bullying behavior. Say you do not like it and that it is not funny.

453

- Do not bully back. It will not help if you use mean names or actions, and it could make things worse.

What if I do not feel safe telling a bully to stop?

That is okay. No one should put themselves in an unsafe situation. Think of other ways you can lend a hand when bullying happens.

- Say kind words to the child who is being bullied, such as "I am sorry about what happened," and "I do not like it." Help them understand that it is not his or her fault. Be a friend. Invite that student to do things with you, such as sit together at lunch or work together on a project. Everyone needs a friend.

- Tell the student who is being bullied to talk to someone about what happened. Offer to help by going along.

- Pay attention to the other kids who see the bullying. (These people are called bystanders.) Are any of them laughing or joining in with the bullying? If yes, these kids are part of the problem. Let those students know that they are not helping. Don't be one of them.

- Tell an adult. (This is important.) Chances are, the kid who is being bullied needs help from an adult. The kid who is doing the bullying probably does, too. Often, the bullying does not get reported. If you need help telling, take a friend along. But, who should you tell? Think about who you could tell in your school:

  - teacher (which one would you talk to?)
  - school counselor
  - cafeteria or playground aid
  - school nurse
  - principal
  - bus driver
  - other adults you feel comfortable telling

Why do kids not tell when they see bullying?

- They may not want others to think they are tattling.
- They may be afraid that the kids who bully will pick on them next.

- They may think that their friends will make fun of them for trying to help.

Telling is very important. Reporting that someone is getting bullied or hurt in some other way is not tattling. Adults at school can help. Ask them to help keep you safe after telling. Explain to your friends that bullying is not fair and encourage them to join in helping.

What if the bullying does not happen at school?

- If there is an adult around, report the bullying to an adult (your youth group leader, minister, or sports coach).

- No matter where the bullying happens, you should talk to your parents about bullying that you see or know about. Ask them for their ideas about how to help.

Additional Information

Stop Bullying Now
Website: http://www.stopbullyingnow.hrsa.gov
E-mail: comments@hrsa.gov

Chapter 52

Online Abuse of Adolescents

Chapter Contents

Section 52.1

Sexual Solicitations of Teens

This section includes: Excerpts from "Youth Internet Safety Survey," U.S. Department of Justice, December 28, 2004; and excerpts from "A Parent's Guide to Internet Safety," Federal Bureau of Investigation (FBI), 2000. Despite the date of this document, the guidelines described are still deemed pertinent.

Youth Internet Safety Survey

The research done by Dr. David Finkelhor, Director of the Crimes Against Children Research Center at the University of New Hampshire on Internet victimization of youth provides the best profile of this problem to date. Crimes Against Children Research Center staff interviewed a nationally representative sample of 1,501 youth, aged 10 to 17, who used the Internet regularly. Regular use was defined as using the Internet at least once a month for the past six months on a computer at home, at school, in a library, at someone else's home, or in some other place.

The survey looked at four types of online victimization of youth, which Finkelhor defined as:

- Sexual solicitation and approaches: Requests to engage in sexual activities, sexual talk, or to give personal sexual information that were unwanted, or whether wanted or not, requests made by an adult.

- Aggressive sexual solicitation: Sexual solicitations involving offline contact with the perpetrator through mail, by telephone, or in person, or attempts or requests for offline contact.

- Unwanted exposure to sexual material: When online opening e-mail or e-mail links, and not seeking or expecting sexual material, being exposed to pictures of naked people or people having sex.

- Harassment: Threats or other offensive content (not sexual solicitation) sent online to the youth or posted online for others to see.

458

The survey also explored Internet safety practices used by youth and their families, what factors may put some youth more at risk for victimization than others, and the families' knowledge of how to report online solicitations and harassment.

Statistical Findings

The survey results offered the following statistical highlights:

- One in five youth received a sexual approach or solicitation over the Internet in the past year.

- One in 33 youth received an aggressive sexual solicitation in the past year. This means a predator asked a young person to meet somewhere, called a young person on the phone, and/or sent the young person correspondence, money, or gifts through the U.S. Postal Service.

- One in four youth had an unwanted exposure in the past year to pictures of naked people or people having sex.

- One in 17 youth was threatened or harassed in the past year.

- Most young people who reported these incidents were not very disturbed about them, but a few found them distressing.

- Only a fraction of all episodes were reported to authorities such as the police, an Internet service provider, or a hotline.

- About 25 percent of the youth who encountered a sexual approach or solicitation told a parent. Almost 40 percent of those reporting an unwanted exposure to sexual material told a parent.

- Only 17 percent of youth and 11 percent of parents could name a specific authority, such as the Federal Bureau of Investigation (FBI), CyberTipline, or an Internet service provider, to which they could report an Internet crime, although more indicated they were vaguely aware of such authorities.

- In households with home Internet access, one-third of parents said they had filtering or blocking software on their computers.

Other Findings

The survey results confirm what is already known: although the Internet is a wonderfully fun and educational tool, it can also be very dangerous. According to the survey, one in five youth who regularly use the Internet received sexual solicitations or approaches during a one-year period. The survey also found that offenses and offenders are more diverse than previously thought. In addition to pedophiles, other predators use the Internet. Nearly half (48 percent) of the offenders were other youth, and one-fourth of the aggressive episodes were initiated by females. Further, 77 percent of targeted youth were age 14 or older—not an age characteristically targeted by pedophiles. Although the youth stopped most solicitations by leaving the Web site, logging off, or blocking the sender, the survey confirmed current thinking that some youth are particularly vulnerable to online advances.

Most youth reported not being distressed by sexual exposures online. However, a significant 23 percent reported being very or extremely upset, 20 percent reported being very or extremely embarrassed, and 20 percent reported at least one symptom of stress. These findings point to the need for more research on the effects on youth of unwanted exposure to sexual materials and the indicators of potentially exploitative adult-youth relationships.

The large number of solicitations that went unreported by youth and families was of particular interest. This underreporting is attributed to feelings of embarrassment or guilt, ignorance that the incident was a reportable act, ignorance of how to report it, and perhaps resignation to a certain level of inappropriate behavior in the world.

Possibly due to the nature and small sample size of the survey, there were no reported incidences of traveler cases. The survey also revealed no incidences of completed Internet seduction or sexual exploitation, including trafficking of child pornography. Despite the findings of this survey, law enforcement agencies report increasing incidents of Internet crimes against children.

Among the many findings of Finkelhor's survey, the most significant is that we are only beginning to realize the extent of the complex and increasingly prevalent phenomenon of Internet-based crimes against children. We have much to learn about the magnitude of the problem, the characteristics of its victims and perpetrators, its impact on children, and strategies for prevention and intervention.

A Parent's Guide to Internet Safety

What are signs that your child might be at risk online?

- Your child spends large amounts of time online, especially at night. Children online are at the greatest risk during the evening hours.

- You find pornography on your child's computer.

- Your child receives phone calls from men you do not know or is making calls, sometimes long distance, to numbers you do not recognize.

- Your child receives mail, gifts, or packages from someone you do not know.

- Your child turns the computer monitor off or quickly changes the screen on the monitor when you come into the room.

- Your child becomes withdrawn from the family.

- Your child is using an online account belonging to someone else. Even if you do not subscribe to an online service or Internet service, your child may meet an offender while online at a friend's house or the library.

What should you do if you suspect your child is communicating with a sexual predator online?

- Consider talking openly with your child about your suspicions. Tell them about the dangers of computer-sex offenders.

- Review what is on your child's computer. Pornography or any kind of sexual communication can be a warning sign.

- Use the Caller ID service to determine who is calling your child. Most telephone companies that offer Caller ID also offer a service that allows you to block your number from appearing on someone else's Caller ID.

- Devices can be purchased that show telephone numbers that have been dialed from your home phone. Additionally, the last number called from your home phone can be retrieved provided that the telephone is equipped with a redial feature.

- Monitor your child's access to all types of live electronic communications (such as chat rooms, instant messages, Internet Relay Chat), and monitor your child's e-mail. Computer-sex offenders almost always meet potential victims via chat rooms. After meeting a child online, they will continue to communicate electronically often via e-mail.

Should any of the following situations arise in your household, via the Internet, or online service, you should immediately contact your

461

local or state law enforcement agency, the FBI, and the National Center for Missing and Exploited Children:

1. Your child or anyone in the household has received child pornography.

2. Your child has been sexually solicited by someone who knows that your child is under 18 years of age.

3. Your child has received sexually explicit images from someone that knows your child is under the age of 18.

If one of these scenarios occurs, keep the computer turned off in order to preserve any evidence for future law enforcement use. Unless directed to do so by the law enforcement agency, you should not attempt to copy any of the images and/or text found on the computer.

What can you do to minimize the chances of an online exploiter victimizing your child?

- Communicate, and talk to your child about sexual victimization and potential online danger.

- Spend time with your children online. Have them teach you about their favorite online destinations.

- Keep the computer in a common room in the house, not in your child's bedroom. It is much more difficult for a computer-sex offender to communicate with a child when the computer screen is visible to a parent or another member of the household.

- Utilize parental controls provided by your service provider and/or blocking software. While electronic chat can be a great place for children to make new friends and discuss various topics of interest, it is also prowled by computer-sex offenders. Use of chat rooms, in particular, should be heavily monitored. While parents should utilize these mechanisms, they should not totally rely on them.

- Always maintain access to your child's online account and randomly check his/her e-mail. Be aware that your child could be contacted through the U.S. mail. Be up front with your child about your access and reasons why.

- Teach your child the responsible use of the resources online. There is much more to the online experience than chat rooms.

- Find out what computer safeguards are utilized by your child's school, the public library, and at the homes of your child's friends. These are all places, outside your normal supervision, where your child could encounter an online predator.

- Understand, even if your child was a willing participant in any form of sexual exploitation, that he/she is not at fault and is the victim. The offender always bears the complete responsibility for his or her actions.

- Instruct your children:

  - to never arrange a face-to-face meeting with someone they met online;

  - to never upload (post) pictures of themselves onto the Internet or online service to people they do not personally know;

  - to never give out identifying information such as their name, home address, school name, or telephone number;

  - to never download pictures from an unknown source, as there is a good chance there could be sexually explicit images;

  - to never respond to messages or bulletin board postings that are suggestive, obscene, belligerent, or harassing;

  - that whatever they are told online may or may not be true.

My child has received an e-mail advertising a pornographic website, what should I do?

Generally, advertising an adult, pornographic website that is sent to an e-mail address does not violate federal law or the current laws of most states. In some states it may be a violation of law if the sender knows the recipient is under the age of 18. Such advertising can be reported to your service provider and, if known, the service provider of the originator. It can also be reported to your state and federal legislators, so they can be made aware of the extent of the problem.

Is any service safer than the others?

Sex offenders have contacted children via most of the major online services and the Internet. The most important factors in keeping your child safe online are the utilization of appropriate blocking software and/or parental controls, along with open, honest discussions with your child, monitoring his/her online activity, and following the tips in this chapter.

Should I just forbid my child from going online?

There are dangers in every part of our society. By educating your children to these dangers and taking appropriate steps to protect them, they can benefit from the wealth of information now available online.

Section 52.2

Student Cyberbullying

"Why Should Adults Care about Bullying: Cyberbullying," Health Resources and Services Administration (HRSA), 2005.

Bullying is aggressive behavior that is intentional and involves an imbalance of power or strength. Usually, it is repeated over time. Traditionally, bullying has involved actions such as hitting or punching (physical bullying), teasing or name-calling (verbal bullying), or intimidation through gestures or social exclusion. In recent years, technology has given children and youth a new means of bullying each other—cyberbullying.

Cyberbullying, which is sometimes referred to as online social cruelty or electronic bullying, can involve:

- sending mean, vulgar, or threatening messages or images

- posting sensitive, private information about another person

- pretending to be someone else in order to make that person look bad

- intentionally excluding someone from an online group (Willard, 2005)

Children and youth can cyberbully each other through e-mails, instant messaging, text or digital imaging messages sent on cell phones, web pages, web logs (blogs), chat rooms or discussion groups, and other information communication technologies.

How common is cyberbullying?

Although very little research has been conducted on cyberbullying, studies have found that:

* Eighteen percent of students in grades 6–8 said they had been cyberbullied at least once in the last couple of months; and 6% said it had happened to them two or more times (Kowalski et al., 2005).

* Eleven percent of students in grades 6–8 said they had cyberbullied another person at least once in the last couple of months, and 2% said they had done it two or more times (Kowalski et al., 2005).

* Nineteen percent of regular Internet users between the ages of 10 and 17 reported being involved in online aggression; 15% had been aggressors, and 7% had been targets (3% were both aggressors and targets) (Ybarra and Mitchell, 2004).

Who are the victims and perpetrators of cyberbullying?

In a recent study of students in grades 6–8 (Kowalski et al., 2005):

* Girls were about twice as likely as boys to be victims and perpetrators of cyberbullying.

* Of those students who had been cyberbullied relatively frequently (at least twice in the last couple of months):

  * 62% said that they had been cyberbullied by another student at school

  * 46% had been cyberbullied by a friend

  * 55% didn't know who had cyberbullied them

* Of those students who admitted cyberbullying others relatively frequently, 60% had cyberbullied another student at school, and 56% had cyberbullied a friend.

What are the most common methods of cyberbullying?

In a recent study of students in grades 6–8 (Kowalski et al., 2005), the most common way that children and youth reported being cyberbullied was through instant messaging. Somewhat less common ways involved the use of chat rooms, e-mails, and messages posted on websites.

How does cyberbullying differ from other traditional forms of bullying?

Although there is little research yet on cyberbullying among children and youth, available research and experience suggest that cyberbullying may differ from more traditional forms of bullying in a number of ways (Willard, 2005), including:

- Cyberbullying can occur any time of the day or night.

- Cyberbullying messages and images can be distributed quickly to a very wide audience.

- Children and youth can be anonymous when cyberbullying, which makes it difficult (and sometimes impossible) to trace them.

What can adults do to prevent and address cyberbullying?

Adults seldom are present in the online environments frequented by children and youth. Therefore, it is extremely important that adults pay close attention to the cyberbullying and the activities of children and youth when using these new technologies.

Tips for Dealing with Cyberbullying That Your Child Has Experienced

Because cyberbullying can range from rude comments to lies, impersonations, and threats, your responses may depend on the nature and severity of the cyberbullying. Here are some actions that you may want to take after-the-fact.

- Strongly encourage your child not to respond to the cyberbullying.

- Do not erase the messages or pictures. Save these as evidence.

- Try to identify the individual doing the cyberbullying. Even if the cyberbully is anonymous (for example, is using a fake name or someone else's identity) there may be a way to track them through your Internet Service Provider (ISP). If the cyberbullying is criminal (or if you suspect that it may be), contact the police and ask them to do the tracking.

- Sending inappropriate language may violate the Terms and Conditions of e-mail services, Internet Service Providers, websites, and cell phone companies. Consider contacting these providers and filing a complaint.

- If the cyberbullying is coming through e-mail or a cell phone, it may be possible to block future contact from the cyberbully. Of course, the cyberbully may assume a different identity and continue the bullying.

- Contact your school. If the cyberbullying is occurring through your school district's Internet system, school administrators have an obligation to intervene. Even if the cyberbullying is occurring off campus, make your school administrators aware of the problem. They may be able to help you resolve the cyberbullying or be watchful for face-to-face bullying.

- Consider contacting the cyberbully's parents. These parents may be very concerned to learn that their child has been cyberbullying others, and they may effectively put a stop to the bullying. On the other hand, these parents may react very badly to your contacting them. So, proceed cautiously. If you decide to contact a cyberbully's parents, communicate with them in writing—not face-to-face. Present proof of the cyberbullying (for example, copies of an e-mail message) and ask them to make sure the cyberbullying stops.

- Consider contacting an attorney in cases of serious cyberbullying. In some circumstances, civil law permits victims to sue a bully or his or her parents in order to recover damages.

- Contact the police if cyberbullying involves acts such as:
  - threats of violence
  - extortion
  - obscene or harassing phone calls or text messages
  - harassment, stalking, or hate crimes
  - child pornography

If you are uncertain if cyberbullying violates your jurisdiction's criminal laws, contact your local police, who will advise you.

Suggestions for Educators

• Educate your students, teachers, and other staff members about cyberbullying, its dangers, and what to do if someone is cyberbullied.

• Be sure that your school's anti-bullying rules and policies address cyberbullying.

• Closely monitor students' use of computers at school.

• Use filtering and tracking software on all computers, but do not rely solely on this software to screen out cyberbullying and other problematic online behavior.

• Investigate reports of cyberbullying immediately. If cyberbullying occurs through the school district's Internet system, you are obligated to take action. If the cyberbullying occurs off-campus, consider what actions you might take to help address the bullying:

  • Notify parents of victims and parents of cyberbullies of known or suspected cyberbullying.

  • Notify the police if the known or suspected cyberbullying involves a threat.

  • Closely monitor the behavior of the affected students at school for possible bullying.

  • Talk with all students about the harms caused by cyberbullying. Remember—cyberbullying that occurs off-campus can travel like wildfire among your students and can affect how they behave and relate to each other at school.

  • Investigate to see if the victim(s) of cyberbullying could use some support from a school counselor or school-based mental health professional.

• Contact the police if cyberbullying involves acts such as:

  • threats of violence

  • extortion

- obscene or harassing phone calls or text messages
- harassment, stalking, or hate crimes
- child pornography

Willard, N. (2005). *A parent's guide to cyberbullying and cyberthreats.* Center for Safe and Responsible Internet Use.

Kowalski, R., Limber, S. P. Scheck, A., Redfearn, M., Allen, J., Calloway, A., Farris, J., Finnegan, K., Keith, M., Kerr, S., Singer, L., Spearman, J., Tripp, L., and Vernon, L. (2005, August). *Electronic bullying among school-aged children and youth.* Paper presented at the annual meeting of the American Psychological Association. Washington, DC.

Ybarra, M. L., and Mitchell, K. J. (2004). Online aggressors/targets, aggressors, and targets: a comparison of associated youth characteristics. *Journal of Child Psychology and Psychiatry*, 45, 1308–1316.

Section 52.3

Guidelines for Internet Safety

"Stop-Think-Click: 7 Practices for Safer Computing," U.S. Federal Trade Commission (FTC), September 2005.

With awareness as your safety net, you can minimize the chance of an Internet mishap. Being on guard online helps you protect your information, your computer, even yourself. To be safer and more secure online, adopt these practices.

Protect Your Personal Information

It is valuable. Why? To an identity thief, your personal information can provide instant access to your financial accounts, your credit record, and other assets.

- If you are asked for your personal information—your name, e-mail or home address, phone number, account numbers, or Social Security number—find out how it is going to be used and how it will be protected before you share it. If you have children, teach them to not give out your last name, your home address, or your phone number on the Internet.

- If you get an e-mail or pop-up message asking for personal information, do not reply or click on the link in the message. The safest course of action is not to respond to requests for your personal or financial information. If you believe there may be a need for such information by a company with whom you have an account or placed an order, contact that company directly in a way you know to be genuine. In any case, do not send your personal information via e-mail because e-mail is not a secure transmission method.

- If you are shopping online, do not provide your personal or financial information through a company's website until you have checked for indicators that the site is secure, such as a lock icon on the browser's status bar or a website URL that begins https: (the "s" stands for secure). Unfortunately, no indicator is foolproof; some scammers have forged security icons.

- Read website privacy policies. They should explain what personal information the website collects, how the information is used, and whether it is provided to third parties. The privacy policy also should tell you whether you have the right to see what information the website has about you and what security measures the company takes to protect your information. If you do not see a privacy policy—or if you cannot understand it—consider doing business elsewhere.

Know Who You Are Dealing With

Know what you are getting into. There are dishonest people in the bricks and mortar world and on the Internet. It is remarkably simple for online scammers to impersonate a legitimate business, so you need to know whom you are dealing with. If you are shopping online, check out the seller before you buy. A legitimate business or individual seller should give you a physical address and a working telephone number at which they can be contacted in case you have problems.

Anti-Virus Software and Firewalls

Use anti-virus software and a firewall, and update both regularly. Dealing with anti-virus and firewall protection may sound about as exciting as flossing your teeth, but it is just as important as a preventive measure. Having intense dental treatment is never fun; neither is dealing with the effects of a preventable computer virus.

Operating System and Web Browser Set Up

Be sure to set up your operating system and Web browser software properly, and update them regularly. Hackers also take advantage of Web browsers (like Internet Explorer or Netscape) and operating system software (like Windows or Linux) that are unsecured. Lessen your risk by changing the settings in your browser or operating system and increasing your online security. Check the "tools" or "options" menus for built-in security features. If you need help understanding your choices, use your "help" function.

Your operating system also may offer free software patches that close holes in the system that hackers could exploit. In fact, some common operating systems can be set to automatically retrieve and install patches for you. If your system does not do this, bookmark the website for your system's manufacturer so you can regularly visit and update your system with defenses against the latest attacks. Updating can be as simple as one click. Your e-mail software may help you avoid viruses by giving you the ability to filter certain types of spam. It's up to you to activate the filter.

If you are not using your computer for an extended period, turn it off or unplug it from the phone or cable line. When it is off, the computer does not send or receive information from the Internet and is not vulnerable to hackers.

Protect Passwords

Keep your passwords in a secure place, and out of plain view. Do not share your passwords on the Internet, over e-mail, or on the phone. Your Internet Service Provider (ISP) should never ask for your password.

In addition, hackers may try to figure out your passwords to gain access to your computer. You can make it tougher for them by:

- Using passwords that have at least eight characters and include numbers or symbols.

471

- Avoiding common words: some hackers use programs that can try every word in the dictionary.

- Not using your personal information, your login name, or adjacent keys on the keyboard as passwords.

- Changing your passwords regularly (at a minimum, every 90 days).

- Not using the same password for each online account you access.

One way to create a strong password is to think of a memorable phrase and use the first letter of each word as your password, converting some letters into numbers that resemble letters. For example, "How much wood could a woodchuck chuck" would become HmWc@wC.

Back Up Important Files

If you follow these tips, you are more likely to be secure online, free of interference from hackers, viruses, and spammers. But no system is completely secure. If you have important files stored on your computer, copy them onto a removable disc, and store them in a safe place.

If Something Goes Wrong

Hacking or Computer Virus

If your computer gets hacked or infected by a virus:

- Immediately unplug the phone or cable line from your machine. Then scan your entire computer with fully updated anti-virus software, and update your firewall.

- Take steps to minimize the chances of another incident.

- Alert the appropriate authorities by contacting:

  - your ISP and the hacker's ISP (if you can tell what it is). You can usually find an ISP's e-mail address on its website. Include information on the incident from your firewall's log file. By alerting the ISP to the problem on its system, you can help it prevent similar problems in the future.

  - the Federal Bureau of Investigation's (FBI) Internet Crime Complaint Center at http://www.ic3.gov. To fight computer criminals, they need to hear from you.

Internet Fraud

If a scammer takes advantage of you through an Internet auction, when you are shopping online, or in any other way, report it to the Federal Trade Commission's Onguard Online at http://onguardonline.gov/index.html. The FTC enters Internet, identity theft, and other fraud-related complaints into Consumer Sentinel, a secure, online database available to hundreds of civil and criminal law enforcement agencies in the U.S. and abroad.

Deceptive Spam

If you get deceptive spam, including e-mail phishing for your information, forward it to spam@uce.gov. Be sure to include the full header of the e-mail, including all routing information. You also may report phishing e-mail to http://www.antiphishing.org where the Anti-Phishing Working Group, a consortium of ISPs, security vendors, financial institutions and law enforcement agencies, uses these reports to fight phishing.

Divulged Personal Information

If you believe you have mistakenly given your personal information to a fraudster, identity theft can be reported to the FTC at http://www.consumer.gov/idtheft.

Parents

Parental controls are provided by most ISPs, or are sold as separate software. Remember that no software can substitute for parental supervision. Talk to your kids about safe computing practices, as well as the things they are seeing and doing online.

Chapter 53

Teen Dating Violence

Teen life, with its fads, crushes, clashes, and breakups, seems to be a world away from abusive relationships. Yet, there can be a dark side to all of the social drama. Many teens go through the same types of abuse—sexual, physical, and emotional—that some adults go through.

Dating violence is a pattern of violent and abusive behavior that someone uses against a girlfriend or boyfriend.[1] There is no single definition for dating violence, but the American Bar Association provides these statements to help us better understand dating violence among teens:

- Dating violence occurs in a dating relationship when one person uses physical, emotional, or sexual abuse to gain power and to keep control over the other person.[1]

- Dating violence is a pattern of physical, sexual, and emotional abuse by one partner to gain power and control over the other partner—the dynamics are the same for teens and adults.[1]

Before violence starts, a teen may experience criticisms and demands from his or her boyfriend or girlfriend. For example, a teen

---

This chapter includes: "Dating Violence Common among Teens," Substance Abuse and Mental Health Services Administration (SAMHSA), 2005; and "Confronting Teens Involved in Dating Violence," National Youth Violence Prevention Resource Center of the Centers for Disease Control and Prevention (CDC), 2003.

might tell their partner what clothes to wear and whom they can hang out with. Teens may be confused by these demands and may not know how to deal with a dating partner's mind games. Threats and rage may be followed by vows of love and pleas for forgiveness. Yet, over time, the violence can get worse.

Teens may be afraid to break up with their partners out of fear that their partner will hurt them or will harm himself or herself. A teen may want to be there to help a boyfriend or girlfriend, may hope that things will get better, or simply may not realize what can happen. Teen victims may begin to believe—wrongly—that they deserve the abuse.

If you have a teen who is dating, be alert for signs of abuse, both physical and emotional. Outward signs include:

- bruises and injuries
- changing the way he or she looks or dresses
- dropping old friends
- giving up things he or she cares about

New friends as well as changes in attitudes, styles, hobbies, and school activities are common in young people. Still, they can be clues that a teen is being controlled by a boyfriend or girlfriend.

Emotional abuse is harder to see than physical abuse since it happens over time and can take several forms, including:

- name-calling
- put downs
- blame
- threats
- envy
- anger
- attempts to control a partner's dress, activities, and friendships[2]

A young person who suffers emotional abuse may become insecure, destructive, angry, or withdrawn. He or she also may abuse alcohol or drugs.

If a child has been exposed to domestic violence at home, it increases the chance that he or she will take on the role of either an abuser or a victim in his or her own relationships. Abuse can seem normal to youth who witness it in their own homes.

If you believe that your child is being abused, talk to your teen. Ask questions, set limits, and offer advice. You may want to seek help from counselors, community health agencies, and domestic violence or crisis centers. These and other resources can provide you with information and guidance about how to help your teen.

Keep in mind that your child may find it hard to talk about stress from a dating relationship. So, do not show anger or push so hard that he or she pulls away. Instead, let your teen know that you respect their views and are there for him or her. Tell your teen that you care about him or her and want him or her to be safe.

If you believe that your child is abusing his dating partner, confront your teen about it and seek expert help.

If You Think Your Child Is a Victim of Dating Violence

If you suspect your child is in a violent relationship, ask your child about the relationship. Be specific about why you are concerned. If your child chooses to talk with you, listen quietly, without judging. If your child does not want to discuss it with you, encourage your child to talk with another trusted adult and provide the names of people and organizations that can help. This could be a relative, friend of the family, clergy member, teacher, school counselor, coach or even the police. A local domestic violence program or the National Domestic Violence Hotline (800-799-7233) can tell you if there is a program or support group in your community.

If your child does open up to you, focus your response on your child's needs and feelings and your concern for his/her well-being. Do not criticize or attack the abusive partner. Your child will need to make the actual decision to end the abusive relationship, not you. Ask: What can I do to help you? Encourage your child to talk with a counselor who specializes in teen dating violence, and continue to support your child by being loving, open, and non-judgmental. Whether your teen is ready to leave the abusive partner or not, it is important to encourage your teen to think about ways to stay safe, for example, by making sure friends are around so that he or she is not alone with the partner.

If You Think Your Child Is Hurting Their Girlfriend or Boyfriend

If you suspect that your child is hurting someone in a dating relationship, it is important to talk with your child about your concerns. Before you talk with your child, have specific examples in mind. Listen to what your child has to say, and make it clear that you love and support him or her. You have a responsibility, however, to make it clear that the behavior is unacceptable and must stop. Do not let your child deny or minimize the violence or to make excuses. Help him/her to recognize that violence is not an acceptable way to solve problems. Offer to help him/her to locate community resources that can provide counseling. If your child's behavior is truly dangerous, you may have to make the difficult decision to report your teen's violence to law enforcement.

References

1. American Bar Association. *What Is Teen Dating Violence?* last referenced 3/11/04.

2. Washington State PTA, 1998. *Every Teen Counts*, last referenced 3/11/04.

Additional Resources

Washington State Office of the Attorney General, 2004. *Teen Dating Violence, FAQ: Relationship Violence—Help for Parents*, last referenced 4/12/05.

The National Women's Health Information Center, 2004. *Violence Against Women: Dating Violence,* last referenced 4/12/05.

Additional Information

National Domestic Violence Hotline
Toll-Free: 800-799-7233
Toll-Free TTY: 800-787-3224

Chapter 54

What You Should Know about Sexual Assault

Facts about Sexual Violence

Sexual violence is a serious problem that affects millions of people every year. Its victims are at increased risk of being abused again.

Statistics about sexual violence vary due to differences in how it is defined and how data is collected. Sexual violence data usually come from police, clinical settings, nongovernmental organizations, and survey research.

Available data greatly underestimate the true magnitude of the problem. Rape is one of the most underreported crimes. According to the Department of Justice, in 2002, only 39% of rapes and sexual assaults were reported to law enforcement officials (DOJ 2003). While not an exhaustive list, here are some statistics on the occurrence of sexual violence.

- About two out of 1000 children in the United States were confirmed by child protective service agencies as having experienced sexual assault in 2003.

- Nationwide, about 9% of high school students reported that they had been forced to have sexual intercourse.

Excerpts from "Sexual Violence Fact Sheet," Centers for Disease Control and Prevention (CDC), March 2006; and "Frequently Asked Questions about Sexual Assault," National Women's Health Information Center (NWHIC), January 2005.

- Female high school students are more likely than male students to report sexual assault (11.9% vs. 6.1%).

- Nationwide, 12.3% of Black high school students, 10.4% of Hispanic high school students, and 7.3% of White high school students reported that they had been forced to have sexual intercourse.

- Among college students nationwide, between 20% and 25% of women reported experiencing completed or attempted rape.

Consequences

Sexual violence can have very harmful and lasting consequences for victims, families, and communities including:

- Women who experience both sexual and physical abuse are significantly more likely to have sexually transmitted diseases (STD).

- Over 32,000 pregnancies result from rape every year.

- Immediate psychological consequences include: shock, denial, fear, confusion, anxiety, withdrawal, guilt, nervousness, distrust of others, symptoms of post-traumatic stress disorder, emotional detachment, sleep disturbances, flashbacks, and mental replay of assault.

- Mental chronic psychological consequences include: depression, attempted or completed suicide, alienation, post-traumatic stress disorder, unhealthy diet-related behaviors, fasting, vomiting, abusing diet pills, and overeating.

- Strained relationships with the victim's family, friends, and intimate partners.

- Less emotional support from friends and family.

- Less frequent contact with friends and relatives.

- Lower likelihood of marriage.

- Engaging in high-risk sexual behavior.

- Using or abusing harmful substances.

Groups at Risk

Certain groups are at risk for intimate partner violence (IPV) victimization or perpetration.

- Women are more likely to be victims of sexual violence than men: 78% of the victims of rape and sexual assault are women and 22% are men.

- Sexual violence starts very early in life. More than half of all rapes of women (54%) occur before age 18; 22% of these rapes occur before age 12. For men, 75% of all rapes occur before age 18, and 48% occur before age 12.

- Prevalence of IPV varies among race. American Indian and Alaskan Native women are significantly more likely (34%) to report being raped than African American women (19%) or White women (18%).

- Women in college who use drugs, attend a university with high drinking rates, belong in a sorority, and drank heavily in high school are at greater risk for rape while intoxicated.

Perpetration

- Most perpetrators of sexual violence are men. Among acts of sexual violence committed against women since the age of 18, 100% of rapes, 92% of physical assaults, and 97% of stalking acts were perpetrated by men. Sexual violence against men is also mainly male violence: 70% of rapes, 86% of physical assaults, and 65% of stalking acts were perpetrated by men.

Frequently Asked Questions about Sexual Assault

What is sexual assault?

Sexual assault and abuse is any type of sexual activity that you do not agree to, including:

- inappropriate touching
- vaginal, anal, or oral penetration
- sexual intercourse that you say no to
- rape
- attempted rape
- child molestation

Sexual assault can be verbal, visual, or anything that forces a person to join in unwanted sexual contact or attention. Examples of this are voyeurism (when someone watches private sexual acts), exhibitionism (when someone exposes him/herself in public), incest (sexual contact between family members), and sexual harassment. It can happen in different situations, by a stranger in an isolated place, on a date, or in the home by someone you know.

Rape is a common form of sexual assault. It is committed in many situations—on a date, by a friend or an acquaintance, or when you think you are alone. Educate yourself on date rape drugs. They can be slipped into a drink when a victim is not looking. Never leave your drink unattended—no matter where you are. Try to always be aware of your surroundings. Date rape drugs make a person unable to resist assault and can cause memory loss so the victim does not know what happened.

What do I do if I have been sexually assaulted?

Take steps right away if you have been sexually assaulted.

- Get away from the attacker to a safe place as fast as you can. Then call 911 or the police.

- Call a friend or family member you trust. You also can call a crisis center or a hotline to talk with a counselor. One hotline is the National Sexual Assault Hotline at 800-656-HOPE (4673). Feelings of shame, guilt, fear, and shock are normal. It is important to get counseling from a trusted professional.

- Do not wash, comb, or clean any part of your body. Do not change clothes if possible, so the hospital staff can collect evidence. Do not touch or change anything at the scene of the assault.

- Go to your nearest hospital emergency room as soon as possible. You need to be examined, treated for any injuries, and screened for possible sexually transmitted diseases (STDs) or pregnancy. The doctor will collect evidence using a rape kit for fibers, hairs, saliva, semen, or clothing that the attacker may have left behind.

- You or the hospital staff can call the police from the emergency room to file a report.

- Ask the hospital staff about possible support groups you can attend right away.

How can I protect myself from being sexually assaulted?

There are things you can do to reduce your chances of being sexually assaulted. Follow these tips from the National Crime Prevention Council.

- Be aware of your surroundings—who is out there and what is going on.

- Walk with confidence. The more confident you look, the stronger you appear.

- Do not let drugs or alcohol cloud your judgment.

- Be assertive—do not let anyone violate your space.

- Trust your instincts. If you feel uncomfortable in your surroundings, leave.

- Do not prop open self-locking doors.

- Lock your door and your windows, even if you leave for just a few minutes.

- Watch your keys. Do not lend them. Do not leave them. Do not lose them. And do not put your name and address on the key ring.

- Watch out for unwanted visitors. Know who is on the other side of the door before you open it.

- Be wary of isolated spots, like underground garages, offices after business hours, and apartment laundry rooms.

- Avoid walking or jogging alone, especially at night. Vary your route. Stay in well-traveled, well-lit areas.

- Have your key ready to use before you reach the door—home, car, or work.

- Park in well-lit areas and lock the car, even if you will only be gone a few minutes.

- Drive on well-traveled streets, with doors and windows locked.

- Never hitchhike or pick up a hitchhiker.

- Keep your car in good shape with plenty of gas in the tank.

- In case of car trouble, call for help on your cellular phone. If you do not have a phone, put the hood up, lock the doors, and put a banner in the rear mirror that says, "Help. Call police."

How can I help someone who has been sexually assaulted?

You can help someone who is abused or who has been assaulted by listening and offering comfort. Go with her or him to the police, the hospital, or to counseling. Reinforce the message that she or he is not at fault and that it is natural to feel angry and ashamed.

Crisis Help Hotlines

National Domestic Violence
Toll-Free: 800-799-7233; Toll-Free TDD: 800-787-3224

National Sexual Assault Hotline
Toll-Free: 800-656-4673

If you are sexually assaulted, it is not your fault. Do not be afraid to ask for help or support. Help is available. There are many organizations and hotlines in every state and territory. These crisis centers and agencies work hard to stop assaults and help victims. You can obtain the numbers of local shelters, counseling services, and legal assistance in your phone book, or call the crisis hotlines listed for assistance.

Additional Information

Division of Violence Prevention
CDC National Center for Injury Prevention and Control
Website: http://www.cdc.gov/ncipc/dvp/dvp.htm

National Center for Victims of Crime
2000 M Street NW, Suite 480
Washington, DC 20036
Toll-Free: 800-394-2255; Toll-Free TTY: 800-211-7996
Website: http://www.ncvc.org

Rape, Abuse, and Incest National Network
2000 L Street NW, Suite 406
Washington, DC 20036
Toll-Free: 800-656-4673 ext. 3
Phone: 202-544-1034; Fax: 202-544-3556
Website: http://www.rainn.org
E-mail: info@rainn.org

Chapter 55

Hazing: Violent Teen Initiations

A group of seniors at Glenbrook North High School outside Chicago were caught on tape by a fellow classmate allegedly beating junior girls and covering them with mud, feces, pig entrails, garbage, and paint. Part of an annual powder puff touch football game held between girls in the senior and junior classes as a rite of passage for incoming seniors, the incident caused a firestorm of controversy, bringing the topic of high school hazing into the limelight.

An initiation rite most often associated with fraternities and sororities, hazing isn't a new phenomenon in older kids and young adults. And it could be a problem that's existed, without much media attention, for quite some time in high schools. Older, often popular kids—or those already accepted in a certain group—pass along traditions they likely succumbed to in years past. Those doing the hazing might contend that it's all just a long-lived facet of becoming a part of something—an upper class at school, a sports team, a club, a social group or clique, or even a gang.

Meanwhile, younger kids desiring acceptance just chalk it up to part of going through the ranks of their social crowd, class, or athletic team. Many figure that they have to endure the hazing this year, but that they'll be able to unleash the tradition on others next year.

This information was provided by KidsHealth, one of the largest resources online for medically reviewed health information written for parents, kids, and teens. For more articles like this one, visit www.KidsHealth.org, or www.TeensHealth.org. © 2003 The Nemours Center for Children's Health Media, a division of The Nemours Foundation.

The annual powder puff football hazing at Glenbrook North High had reportedly been occurring off-campus for years. The latest incident sent five girls to the hospital (one for a broken ankle, another for gashes in her scalp). Twelve girls and three boys allegedly involved were charged with battery, 33 seniors were expelled, and 20 juniors were suspended by the school. Although the powder puff football game was held off-campus at a local park and the students apparently kept the date and location hush-hush, many are wondering if something could have been done to prevent the annual event from happening again.

What Is Hazing?

Much attention has been paid to the often over-the-top rituals at institutions of higher learning, but little has been reported about why younger kids are putting their peers through these emotional and physical rites of passage. The end result of hazing is usually embarrassment and demoralization, but that's not always the intention, says child and adolescent psychologist D'Arcy Lyness, Ph.D. "I don't think that's on anyone's mind as hazing begins," Lyness explains. "Hazing has to do with earning entry—and making it hard to earn entry—into whatever group it is."

Hazing is a way to have people demonstrate their commitment to a group and to show how much they want to be in that club. However, many who go through hazing endure not only embarrassment, but harassment, ridicule, and even injuries that can be severe or life-threatening.

Hazing can include a number of types of mental and physical insults of varying degrees that may not be perceived as abuse or victimization, even by those perpetuating and enduring it. Although some forms of subtle hazing—being called demeaning names or having to refer to peers as Ms. or Mr.—are seemingly benign, they can still cause feelings of degradation. Emotional distress can come from more serious types of hazing—verbal abuse, public displays in which participants have to wear ridiculous apparel or perform embarrassing stunts, and being required to perform certain duties or menial tasks for others.

But there's a difference between forcing someone to dress up in an embarrassing outfit and being beaten and covered in feces, as in the incident at Glenbrook North High. The effects can be increasingly dangerous when hazing involves risk-taking, being forced to drink excess amounts of alcohol, or physical abuse.

"Perhaps the biggest problem is that the line can get crossed very quickly," Lyness says. "People are relaxing their individual responsibility and judgment and getting peer validation for their actions. The momentum can build quickly and a situation can get out of control."

Why Do Good Kids Participate In or Watch Hazing?

In the Illinois hazing incident, a crowd of students reportedly stood by, cheering on the activities as they drank beer. Meanwhile, many of the accused students' parents attested that their daughters are good girls and wouldn't do something like this. But why would otherwise nice kids willingly participate in or observe such abusive acts?

"When people are in a group, they often relax individual responsibility, assuming that someone else will act when it's appropriate," Lyness says. "This explains why a group of bystanders often does nothing, but the same individuals might take action if they were the only bystander."

In social situations in which there's uncertainty, people—especially kids—often look to leaders (in the Illinois case, the accused seniors) for cues and social proof about what is and isn't acceptable behavior, says Lyness. Being told what to do and how to participate reduces the discomfort of social uncertainty. The most easily influenced will do what leaders tell them, then others may follow, too. Watching others, kids may think, "It must be okay. Everyone else is doing it. They must know what they're doing."

"Everyone is looking to others and getting peer validation that the correct action is just what everyone else is doing. This might also help explain why no one takes the initiative to stop what's going on, speak up, or take themselves out of the situation," Lyness says.

Although it might seem like kids who haze are the same ones who bully, that's not necessarily the case. Bullying is often an attempt to exclude someone from a group or activity, whereas hazing is an attempt to include someone through an initiation process. "Bullying is about using uneven power to make yourself feel more powerful at someone else's expense, and many bullies are the kids who lack social conscience," Lyness explains. "But hazing is the difficult rite of passage to earn membership."

Both bullies and hazers can feel a sense of higher power or status. However, bullies exhibit a pattern of intentionally hurting others on repeated occasions; hazers are often simply caught up in a role within a group or team on one occasion or limited occasions, says Lyness. Though some kids who haze may have some of the same characteristics as those who bully, bullying doesn't explain hazing.

What Are Some Alternatives to Hazing?

It might seem contradictory that those who endure hazing would feel allegiance toward a group of people inflicting discomfort—even pain—on them, but Lyness says hazing does, in fact, build commitment, even if it is often an emotionally unhealthy sense of commitment.

"There is a psychological principle that's sometimes referred to as 'commitment and consistency' at work. When a person has put themselves through a difficult rite of passage to become a member, he or she does feel more committed to the group," she says. Going through hazing can make a person believe their actions are consistent with their commitment.

But there are other ways for organized groups or teams to foster unity, commitment, and communication:

* Plan events in which the whole group, team, or organization attends (such as field trips, retreats, dances, movies, and plays).

* Participate in team-building activities (for example, visit a ropes course).

* Plan a social event with another group.

* Develop a peer mentor program within the group, teaming seasoned members with new members.

* Work together on a community service project or plan fundraisers for local charitable organizations.

What Can You Do about Hazing?

Anti-hazing laws and policies do exist in most states, as well in many individual schools. And you'd be hard-pressed to find a college or university without a very clear anti-hazing policy in place. But just because there are policies and laws doesn't mean students know about or abide by them. The students involved in the powder puff football incident in Illinois clearly violated Glenbrook North High School's hazing policy, even though the activities occurred off-campus.

Students—and even parents—may dismiss annual hazing-oriented rites as good old tradition, silly fun, or harmless high jinks. But this mentality could only perpetuate a problem that, Lyness says, shouldn't be overlooked. "No one intends the harm that sometimes happens at hazing rituals, but the same is true for bullying—often adults minimize it as a normal childhood behavior, and it can have harmful consequences."

Even the most benign types of hazing can easily go awry, turning ugly, and sometimes dangerous, says Lyness. But there are steps you, as a parent, can take to help prevent your child from ever having to endure this type of hazing:

- Educate yourself about your state's anti-hazing laws (all but seven states have some sort of law applying to schools, colleges, universities, and other educational institutions). Some schools—and states—may group hazing and bullying together in policies and laws.

- Make sure your child's school and/or district has clearly defined policies that prohibit hazing, is taking measures to proactively prevent hazing from occurring, and is acting immediately with repercussions when hazing does occur.

- Ask your parent-teacher association and/or school administrators to invite a local law-enforcement official to speak to parents and/or the student body about hazing and the state's anti-hazing law.

- Work with school personnel and student leaders to create powerful—and safe—experiences to promote positive alternatives to hazing that would foster cohesion in group, club, and team membership.

- Talk to other parents—especially those of upperclassmen and your child's sports teammates—about what their children may have seen or experienced. If you know that the problem exists at your child's school, you'll be better prepared to discuss it with your child, fellow parents, and school officials.

- Clichéd as it is, have the "if everyone else was jumping off the bridge, would you do it, too?" conversation with your child, Lyness advises. Talk about why your child shouldn't feel pressured to participate in anything, even if "everyone else is doing it" or "it's always been done this way."

  - Talk specifically about hazing and what your child would do in a hypothetical hazing situation. Discuss how the group mentality can sometimes cause people to wait for someone else to do the right thing, stop something dangerous, speak out, etc.

- "Discuss the topic in a way that doesn't lecture or tell your child what to think or do. It's better to ask kids to tell you what they would do, or what they think about it," Lyness encourages. "Kids are more committed to the ideas they state themselves, so get them to actively state their own values and ideas to you. Let your child know that often it just takes one person to speak out or take different action to change a situation. Others will follow if someone has the courage to be first to do something different, or to be first to refuse to go along with the group. Allow kids to consider themselves leaders, and to know that they have the potential to make a difference."

- Explain to your child that physical and mental abuse, no matter how harmless it may seem, isn't part of becoming a member of the in crowd or a specific group, and that it may even be against the law. Emphasize the importance of telling you and an adult at school whenever another kid or group of kids causes your child or anyone else physical harm.

- If your child has experienced hazing, talk to school officials immediately. If physical abuse was involved, talk to your local law-enforcement agency. Though he or she may be unwilling or may feel uneasy about telling on peers, get precise details from your child about the incident—who, what, when, where, and how.

Above all, maintain open communication with your child. Always ask what's going on at school, what peers are doing, and what pressures are present—physically, academically, and socially. Encourage your child to come to you in any uncomfortable situation, big or small.

Part Eight

Adolescent Mental Health

Chapter 56

Managing Stress during Adolescence

What is stress?

Stress is what you feel when you react to pressure, either from the outside world (school, work, after-school activities, family, friends) or from inside yourself (wanting to do well in school, wanting to fit in). Stress is a normal reaction for people of all ages. It is caused by your body's instinct to protect itself from emotional or physical pressure or, in extreme situations, from danger.

Is stress always bad?

No. In fact, a little bit of stress is good. Most of us could not push ourselves to do well at things—sports, music, dance, work, school—without feeling the pressure of competition. Without the stress of deadlines, most of us also would not be able to finish projects or get to work or school on time.

If stress is so normal, why do I feel so bad?

With all the things that happen during the teen years, it is easy to feel overwhelmed. Things that you cannot control are often the most frustrating. Maybe your parents are fighting, or your social life is a mess. You can also feel bad when you put pressure on yourself—like pressure to get good grades or to get promoted at your part-time job. A common reaction to stress is to criticize yourself. You may even get so upset that things do not seem fun anymore and life looks pretty grim. When this happens, it is easy to think there is nothing you can do to change things. But you can. See the following tips.

Signs you are stressed out:

- feeling depressed, edgy, guilty, tired

- having headaches, stomachaches, trouble sleeping

- laughing or crying for no reason

- blaming other people for bad things that happen to you

- only seeing the down side of a situation

- feeling like things that you used to enjoy are not fun or are a burden

- resenting other people or your responsibilities

Managing Stress

Things that help fight stress:

- eating well-balanced meals on a regular basis

- drinking less caffeine

- getting enough sleep

- exercising on a regular basis

How can I deal with stress?

Although you cannot always control the things that are stressing you, you can control how you react to them. The way you feel about things results from the way you think about things. If you change how you think, you can change the way you feel. Try some of these tips to cope with your stress:

Make a list of the things that are causing your stress. Think about your friends, family, school and other activities. Accept that you cannot control everything on your list.

Take control of what you can. For example, if you are working too many hours and you do not have time to study enough, ask your boss if you can cut back.

Give yourself a break. Remember that you cannot make everyone in your life happy all the time, and it is okay to make mistakes now and then.

Do not commit yourself to things you cannot do or do not want to do. If you are already too busy, do not promise to decorate for the school dance. If you are tired and do not want to go out, tell your friends you will go another night.

Find someone to talk to. Talking to your friends or family can help because it gives you a chance to express your feelings. However, problems in your social life or family can be the hardest to talk about. If you feel like you cannot talk to your family or a friend, talk to someone outside the situation. This could be your priest or minister, a school counselor, or your family doctor.

Things That Do Not Help You Deal with Stress

There are safe and unsafe ways to deal with stress. It is dangerous to try to escape your problems by using drugs and alcohol. Both can be very tempting, and your friends may offer them to you. Drugs and alcohol may seem like easy answers, but they are not. Using drugs and alcohol to deal with stress just adds new problems, like addiction, or family and health problems.

Danger Sign

I have tried dealing with my stress, but I just feel like giving up.

This is a danger sign. Stress can become too much to deal with. It can lead to such awful feelings that you may think about hurting— or even killing—yourself. When you feel like giving up, it may seem like things will never get better. Talk to someone right away. Talking about your feelings is the first step in learning to deal with them and starting to feel better.

Additional Help

National Youth Crisis Hotline
Toll-Free: 800-448-4663

National Adolescent Suicide Hotline
(also called the National Runaway Switchboard)
Toll-Free: 800-621-4000

Chapter 57

Warning Signs of Teen Mental Health Problems

Child and Adolescent Mental Health

Mental Health Is Important

Mental health is how people think, feel, and act as they face life's situations. It affects how people handle stress, relate to one another, and make decisions. Mental health influences the ways individuals look at themselves, their lives, and others in their lives. Like physical health, mental health is important at every stage of life.

All aspects of our lives are affected by our mental health. Caring for and protecting our children is an obligation and is critical to their daily lives and their independence.

Children and Adolescents Can Have Serious Mental Health Problems

Like adults, children and adolescents can have mental health disorders that interfere with the way they think, feel, and act. When untreated, mental health disorders can lead to school failure, family conflicts, drug abuse, violence, and even suicide. Untreated mental health disorders can be very costly to families, communities, and the health care system.

This chapter includes: Excerpts from "Child and Adolescent Mental Health," Substance Abuse and Mental Health Services Administration (SAMHSA), November 2003; and "America's Children: Parents Report Estimated 2.7 Million Children with Emotional and Behavioral Problems," National Institute of Child Health and Human Development (NICHD), July 20, 2005.

In this chapter, mental health problems for children and adolescents refers to the range of all diagnosable emotional, behavioral, and mental disorders. They include depression, attention-deficit/hyperactivity disorder (ADHD), and anxiety, conduct, and eating disorders. Mental health problems affect one in every five young people at any given time. Serious emotional disturbances for children and adolescents refers to the above disorders when they severely disrupt daily functioning in home, school, or community. Serious emotional disturbances affect one in every ten young people at any given time.

The Causes Are Complicated

Mental health disorders in children and adolescents are caused mostly by biology and environment. Examples of biological causes are genetics, chemical imbalances in the body, or damage to the central nervous system, such as a head injury. Many environmental factors also put young people at risk for developing mental health disorders. Examples include:

- exposure to environmental toxins, such as high levels of lead;

- exposure to violence, such as witnessing or being the victim of physical or sexual abuse, drive-by shootings, muggings, or other disasters;

- stress related to chronic poverty, discrimination, or other serious hardships; and

- the loss of important people through death, divorce, or broken relationships.

Signs of Mental Health Disorders Can Signal a Need for Help

Children and adolescents with mental health issues need to get help as soon as possible. A variety of signs may point to mental health disorders or serious emotional disturbances in children or adolescents. Pay attention if a child or adolescent you know has any of the following warning signs.

A child or adolescent is troubled by feeling:

- sad and hopeless for no reason, and these feelings do not go away

- very angry most of the time and crying a lot or overreacting to things
- worthless or guilty often
- anxious or worried often
- unable to get over a loss or death of someone important
- extremely fearful or having unexplained fears
- constantly concerned about physical problems or physical appearance
- frightened that his or her mind either is controlled or is out of control

A child or adolescent experiences big changes, such as:

- showing declining performance in school
- losing interest in things once enjoyed
- experiencing unexplained changes in sleeping or eating patterns
- avoiding friends or family and wanting to be alone all the time
- daydreaming too much and not completing tasks
- feeling life is too hard to handle
- hearing voices that cannot be explained
- experiencing suicidal thoughts

A child or adolescent experiences:

- poor concentration and is unable to think straight or make up his or her mind
- inability to sit still or focus attention
- worry about being harmed, hurting others, or doing something bad
- a need to wash, clean things, or perform certain routines hundreds of times a day, in order to avoid an unsubstantiated danger
- racing thoughts that are almost too fast to follow
- persistent nightmares

A child or adolescent behaves in ways that cause problems, such as:

- using alcohol or other drugs

- eating large amounts of food and then purging, or abusing laxatives, to avoid weight gain

- dieting and/or exercising obsessively

- violating the rights of others or constantly breaking the law without regard for other people

- setting fires

- doing things that can be life threatening

- killing animals

Finding the Right Services Is Critical

To find the right services for their children, families can do the following:

- Get accurate information from hotlines, libraries, or other sources.

- Seek referrals from professionals.

- Ask questions about treatments and services.

- Talk to other families in their communities.

- Find family network organizations.

It is critical that people who are not satisfied with the mental health care they receive discuss their concerns with providers, ask for information, and seek help from other sources.

Important Messages about Child and Adolescent Mental Health

- Every child's mental health is important.

- Many children have mental health problems.

- These problems are real, painful, and can be severe.

- Mental health problems can be recognized and treated.

- Caring families and communities working together can help.

- Information is available from the Substance Abuse and Mental Health Services Administration (SAMHSA); call 800-789-2647.

Parents Report Estimated 2.7 Million Children with Emotional and Behavioral Problems

A special feature in the report, *America's Children: Key National Indicators of Well-Being 2005* shows that nearly 5 percent—or an estimated 2.7 million children—are reported by their parents to suffer from definite or severe emotional or behavioral difficulties, problems that may interfere with their family life, their ability to learn, and their formation of friendships. These difficulties may persist throughout a child's development and lead to lifelong disability, including more serious illness, more difficult to treat illness, and co-occurring mental illnesses.

This special child mental health indicator is based on responses from a sample of parents of children ages 4–17. They were asked to rate their child's difficulty with emotions, concentration, behavior, and ability to get along with other people.

"Parents are usually the first to notice emotional and behavioral difficulties in their children," said Thomas R. Insel, M.D., Director of the National Institute of Mental Health of the National Institutes of Health. "We encourage them to talk to a health care or mental health professional if they are concerned about their child's mental, behavioral or emotional health."

This indicator reports that 65 percent of parents of children with definite or severe difficulties had contacted a mental health professional or general doctor, or that their child had received special education services, for emotional or behavioral problems. Nine percent of parents of these children said that they wanted mental health services for their child but were unable to afford them.

Parents also reported:

- Boys were more likely than girls to have definite or severe emotional and behavioral difficulties.

- Children ages eight and over were more likely than younger children to have emotional or behavioral difficulties.

- Children from poor families were more likely to have emotional or behavioral difficulties than other children.

Additional Information

National Mental Health Information Center
P.O. Box 42557
Washington DC 20015
Toll-Free: 800-789-2647
Toll-Free TDD: 866-889-2647
Fax: 240-747-5470
Website: http://www.mentalhealth.samhsa.gov

Chapter 58

Anxiety Disorders

Most people experience feelings of anxiety before an important event such as a big exam, business presentation, or first date. Anxiety disorders, however, are illnesses that fill people's lives with overwhelming anxiety and fears that are chronic, unremitting, and can grow progressively worse. Tormented by panic attacks, obsessive thoughts, flashbacks of traumatic events, nightmares, or countless frightening physical symptoms, some people with anxiety disorders even become housebound. Fortunately, through research supported by the National Institute of Mental Health (NIMH), there are effective treatments that can help.

How common are anxiety disorders?

Anxiety disorders, as a group, are the most common mental illness in America. More than 19 million American adults are affected by these debilitating illnesses each year. Children and adolescents can also develop anxiety disorders.

What are the different kinds of anxiety disorders?

Panic disorder—Repeated episodes of intense fear that strike often and without warning. Physical symptoms include chest pain, heart palpitations, shortness of breath, dizziness, abdominal distress, feelings of unreality, and fear of dying.

Excerpted from "Facts about Anxiety Disorders," National Institute of Mental Health (NIMH), February 2006.

Obsessive-compulsive disorder—Repeated, unwanted thoughts or compulsive behaviors that seem impossible to stop or control.

Posttraumatic stress disorder—Persistent symptoms that occur after experiencing or witnessing a traumatic event such as rape or other criminal assault, war, child abuse, natural or human-caused disasters, or crashes. Nightmares, flashbacks, numbing of emotions, depression, and feeling angry, irritable or distracted and being easily startled are common. Family members of victims can also develop this disorder.

Phobias—Two major types of phobias are social phobia and specific phobia. People with social phobia have an overwhelming and disabling fear of scrutiny, embarrassment, or humiliation in social situations, which leads to avoidance of many potentially pleasurable and meaningful activities. People with specific phobia experience extreme, disabling, and irrational fear of something that poses little or no actual danger; the fear leads to avoidance of objects or situations and can cause people to limit their lives unnecessarily.

Generalized anxiety disorder—Constant, exaggerated worrisome thoughts and tension about everyday routine life events and activities, lasting at least six months. Almost always anticipating the worst even though there is little reason to expect it; accompanied by physical symptoms, such as fatigue, trembling, muscle tension, headache, or nausea.

What are effective treatments for anxiety disorders?

Treatments have been largely developed through research conducted by NIMH and other research institutions. They help many people with anxiety disorders and often combine medication and specific types of psychotherapy.

A number of medications that were originally approved for treating depression have been found to be effective for anxiety disorders as well. Some of the newest of these antidepressants are called selective serotonin reuptake inhibitors (SSRIs). Other antianxiety medications include groups of drugs called benzodiazepines and beta-blockers. If one medication is not effective, others can be tried. New medications are currently under development to treat anxiety symptoms.

Two clinically-proven effective forms of psychotherapy used to treat anxiety disorders are behavioral therapy and cognitive-behavioral therapy. Behavioral therapy focuses on changing specific actions and uses several techniques to stop unwanted behaviors. In addition to the behavioral therapy techniques, cognitive-behavioral therapy teaches patients to understand and change their thinking patterns so they can react differently to the situations that cause them anxiety.

Do anxiety disorders coexist with other physical or mental disorders?

It is common for an anxiety disorder to accompany depression, eating disorders, substance abuse, or another anxiety disorder. Anxiety disorders can also coexist with illnesses such as cancer or heart disease. In such instances, the accompanying disorders will also need to be treated. Before beginning any treatment, however, it is important to have a thorough medical examination to rule out other possible causes of symptoms.

Additional Information

Crisis Hotlines
Toll-Free for Anxiety Disorders: 888-269-4389
Toll-Free for Depression: 800-421-4211

National Institute of Mental Health
Public Information and Communications Branch
6001 Executive Blvd.
Room 8184, MSC 9663
Bethesda, MD 20892-9663
Toll-Free: 866-615-6464
Toll-Free TTY: 866-415-8051
Phone: 301-443-8431
Fax: 301-443-4279
Website: http://www.nimh.nih.gov
E-mail: nimhinfo@nih.gov

Anxiety Disorders Association of America
8730 Georgia Ave., Suite 600
Silver Spring, MD 20910
Phone: 240-485-1001
Fax: 240-485-1035
Website: http://www.adaa.org

Obsessive-Compulsive Foundation (OCF)
676 State St.
New Haven, CT 06511
Phone: 203-401-2070
Website: http://www.ocfoundation.org

OCF offers a webzine, *Organized Chaos*, for teens and young adults.
It is available at http://www.ocfoundation.org/1000/oc100a.htm

National Mental Health Association
2000 N. Beauregard St., 6th Floor
Alexandria, VA 22311
Toll-Free: 800-969-6642
Toll-Free Crisis Helpline: 800-784-2433
Toll-Free TTY: 800-433-5959
Phone: 703-684-7722
Fax: 703-684-5968
Website: http://www.nmha.org

Chapter 59

Attention Deficit Hyperactivity Disorder (ADHD)

In recent years, attention deficit hyperactivity disorder (ADHD) has been a subject of great public attention and concern. Children with ADHD—one of the most common of the psychiatric disorders that appear in childhood—cannot stay focused on a task, cannot sit still, act without thinking, and rarely finish anything. If untreated, the disorder can have long-term effects on a child's ability to make friends or do well at school or work. Over time, children with ADHD may develop depression, poor self-esteem, and other emotional problems.

- ADHD affects an estimated 4.1 percent of youth ages 9–17 in a six month period.

- About two to three times more boys than girls have ADHD.

- Children with untreated ADHD have higher than normal rates of injury.

- ADHD often co-occurs with other problems, such as depressive and anxiety disorders, conduct disorder, drug abuse, or antisocial behavior.

- Symptoms of ADHD usually become evident in preschool or early elementary years. The disorder frequently persists into adolescence and occasionally into adulthood.

This chapter includes: Excerpts from "Attention Deficit Hyperactivity Disorder (Overview)," National Institute of Mental Health (NIMH), NIH Publication No. 01-4589, February 2006; and excerpts from "Attention Deficit Hyperactivity Disorder," NIMH, NIH Publication No. 3572, 2003.

Your Teenager with ADHD

Your child with ADHD has successfully navigated the early school years and is beginning his or her journey through middle school and high school. Although your child has been periodically evaluated through the years, this is a good time to have a complete re-evaluation of your child's health.

The teen years are challenging for most children; for the child with ADHD these years are doubly hard. All the adolescent problems—peer pressure, the fear of failure in both school and socially, low self-esteem—are harder for the ADHD child to handle. The desire to be independent, to try new and forbidden things—alcohol, drugs, and sexual activity—can lead to unforeseen consequences. The rules that once were, for the most part, followed, are often now flaunted. Parents may not agree with each other on how the teenager's behavior should be handled.

Now, more than ever, rules should be straightforward and easy to understand. Communication between the adolescent and parents can help the teenager to know the reasons for each rule. When a rule is set, it should be clear why the rule is set. Sometimes it helps to have a chart, posted in a central location such as the kitchen, which lists all household rules and all rules for outside the home (social and school). Another chart could list household chores with space to check off a chore once it is done.

When rules are broken—and they will be—respond to this inappropriate behavior as calmly and matter-of-factly as possible. Use punishment sparingly. Even with teens, a time-out can work. Impulsivity and hot temper often accompany ADHD. A short time alone can help.

As the teenager spends more time away from home, there will be demands for a later curfew and the use of the car. Listen to your child's request, give reasons for your opinion, listen to his or her opinion, and negotiate. Communication, negotiation, and compromise will prove helpful.

Your Teenager and the Car

Teenagers, especially boys, begin talking about driving by the time they are 15. In some states, a learner's permit is available at 15 and a driver's license at 16. Statistics show that 16-year-old drivers have more accidents per driving mile than any other age. In the year 2000, 18 percent of those who died in speed-related crashes were youth ages

15 to 19. Sixty-six percent of these youth were not wearing safety belts. Youth with ADHD, in their first two to five years of driving, have nearly four times as many automobile accidents, are more likely to cause bodily injury in accidents, and have three times as many citations for speeding as the young drivers without ADHD.

Most states, after looking at the statistics for automobile accidents involving teenage drivers, have begun to use a graduated driver licensing system. This system eases young drivers onto the roads by a slow progression of exposure to more difficult driving experiences. The program, as developed by the National Highway Traffic Safety Administration and the American Association of Motor Vehicle Administrators, consists of three stages: learner's permit, intermediate (provisional) license, and full licensure. Drivers must demonstrate responsible driving behavior at each stage before advancing to the next level. During the learner's permit stage, a licensed adult must be in the car at all times. This period of time will give the learner a chance to practice, practice, and practice. The more your child drives, the more efficient he or she will become. The sense of accomplishment the teenager with ADHD will feel when the coveted license is finally in his or her hands will make all the time and effort involved worthwhile.

Chapter 60

Bipolar Disorder in Adolescents

Bipolar disorder (also known as manic-depression) is a serious but treatable medical illness. It is a disorder of the brain marked by extreme changes in mood, energy, thinking, and behavior. Symptoms may be present since infancy or early childhood, or may suddenly emerge in adolescence or adulthood. Until recently, a diagnosis of the disorder was rarely made in childhood. Doctors can now recognize and treat bipolar disorder in young children.

Early intervention and treatment offer the best chance for children with emerging bipolar disorder to achieve stability, gain the best possible level of wellness, and grow up to enjoy their gifts and build upon their strengths. Proper treatment can minimize the adverse effects of the illness on their lives and the lives of those who love them.

Families of affected children and adolescents are almost always baffled by early-onset bipolar disorder and are desperate for information and support.

How common is bipolar disorder in children?

It is not known, because epidemiological studies are lacking. However, bipolar disorder affects an estimated 1–2 percent of adults worldwide. The more we learn about this disorder, the more prevalent it appears to be among children.

Excerpts from "About Pediatric Bipolar Disorder," © 2002 Child and Adolescent Bipolar Foundation. All rights reserved. Reprinted with permission.

- It is suspected that a significant number of children diagnosed in the United States with attention-deficit disorder with hyperactivity (ADHD) have early-onset bipolar disorder instead of, or along with, ADHD.

- Depression in children and teens is usually chronic and relapsing. According to several studies, a significant proportion of the 3.4 million children and adolescents with depression in the United States may actually be experiencing the early onset of bipolar disorder, but have not yet experienced the manic phase of the illness.

What are the symptoms of bipolar disorder in adolescents?

In adolescents, bipolar disorder may resemble any of the following classical adult presentations of the illness.

Bipolar I. In this form of the disorder, the adolescent experiences alternating episodes of intense and sometimes psychotic mania and depression.
Symptoms of mania include:

- elevated, expansive, or irritable mood

- decreased need for sleep

- racing speech and pressure to keep talking

- grandiose delusions

- excessive involvement in pleasurable but risky activities

- increased physical and mental activity

- poor judgment

- in severe cases, hallucinations

Symptoms of depression include:

- pervasive sadness and crying spells

- sleeping too much or inability to sleep

- agitation and irritability

- withdrawal from activities formerly enjoyed

- drop in grades and inability to concentrate

- thoughts of death and suicide
- low energy
- significant change in appetite

Periods of relative or complete wellness occur between the episodes.

Bipolar II. In this form of the disorder, the adolescent experiences episodes of hypomania between recurrent periods of depression. Hypomania is a markedly elevated or irritable mood accompanied by increased physical and mental energy. Hypomania can be a time of great creativity.

Cyclothymia. Adolescents with this form of the disorder experience periods of less severe, but definite, mood swings.

Bipolar Disorder NOS (not otherwise specified). Doctors make this diagnosis when it is not clear which type of bipolar disorder is emerging.

For some adolescents, a loss or other traumatic event may trigger a first episode of depression or mania. Later episodes may occur independently of any obvious stresses, or may worsen with stress. Puberty is a time of risk. In girls, the onset of menses may trigger the illness, and symptoms often vary in severity with the monthly cycle.

Once the illness starts, episodes tend to recur and worsen without treatment. Studies show that after symptoms first appear, typically there is a ten year lag until treatment begins. The Child and Adolescent Bipolar Foundation (CABF) encourages parents to take their adolescent for an evaluation if four or more of the listed symptoms persist for more than two weeks. Early intervention and treatment can make all the difference in the world during this critical time of development.

Is substance abuse and addiction related to bipolar disorder?

A majority of teens with untreated bipolar disorder abuse alcohol and drugs. Any child or adolescent who abuses substances should be evaluated for a mood disorder.

Adolescents who seemed normal until puberty and experience a comparatively sudden onset of symptoms are thought to be especially vulnerable to developing addiction to drugs or alcohol. Substances may be readily available among their peers and teens may use them to attempt to control their mood swings and insomnia. If addiction develops, it is essential to treat both the bipolar disorder and the substance abuse at the same time.

Diagnosing Bipolar Disorder in Children

Healthy children often have moments when they have difficulty staying still, controlling their impulses, or dealing with frustration. The *Diagnostic and Statistical Manual IV* (*DSM-IV*) still requires that, for a diagnosis of bipolar disorder, adult criteria must be met. There are as yet no separate criteria for diagnosing children. Some behaviors by a child, however, should raise a red flag including:

- destructive rages that continue past the age of four
- talk of wanting to die or kill themselves
- trying to jump out of a moving car

How Does Bipolar Disorder Differ from Other Conditions?

Even when a child's behavior is unquestionably not normal, correct diagnosis remains challenging. Bipolar disorder is often accompanied by symptoms of other psychiatric disorders. In some children, proper treatment for the bipolar disorder clears up the troublesome symptoms thought to indicate another diagnosis. In other children, bipolar disorder may explain only part of a more complicated case that includes neurological, developmental, and other components.

Diagnoses that mask or sometimes occur along with bipolar disorder include:

- depression
- conduct disorder (CD)
- oppositional-defiant disorder (ODD)
- attention-deficit disorder with hyperactivity (ADHD)
- panic disorder
- generalized anxiety disorder (GAD)
- obsessive-compulsive disorder (OCD)
- Tourette syndrome (TS)
- intermittent explosive disorder
- reactive attachment disorder (RAD)

In adolescents, bipolar disorder is often misdiagnosed as:

- borderline personality disorder
- posttraumatic stress disorder (PTSD)
- schizophrenia

The Need for Prompt and Proper Diagnosis

Tragically, after symptoms first appear in children, years often pass before treatment begins, if ever. Meanwhile, the disorder worsens and the child's functioning at home, school, and in the community is progressively more impaired. The results of untreated or improperly treated bipolar disorder can include:

- an unnecessary increase in symptomatic behaviors leading to removal from school, placement in a residential treatment center, hospitalization in a psychiatric hospital, or incarceration in the juvenile justice system
- the development of personality disorders such as narcissistic, antisocial, and borderline personality
- a worsening of the disorder due to incorrect medications
- drug abuse, accidents, and suicide

It is important to remember that a diagnosis is not a scientific fact. It is a considered opinion based upon the behavior of the child over time, what is known of the child's family history, the child's response to medications, his or her developmental stage, the current state of scientific knowledge and the training and experience of the doctor making the diagnosis. These factors (and the diagnosis) can change as more information becomes available. Competent professionals can disagree on which diagnosis fits an individual best. Diagnosis is important, however, because it guides treatment decisions and allows the family to put a name to the condition that affects their child. Diagnosis can provide answers to some questions but raises others that are unanswerable given the current state of scientific knowledge.

How Can I Help My Child?

Parents concerned about their child's behavior, especially suicidal talk and gestures, should have the child immediately evaluated by a professional familiar with the symptoms and treatment of early-onset bipolar disorder. There is no a blood test or brain scan, as yet, that can establish a diagnosis of bipolar disorder.

Parents who suspect that their child has bipolar disorder (or any psychiatric illness) should take daily notes of their child's mood, behavior, sleep patterns, unusual events, and statements by the child of concern to the parents. Share these notes with the doctor making the evaluation and with the doctor who eventually treats your child. Some parents fax or e-mail a copy of their notes to the doctor before each appointment. A good evaluation takes at least two appointments and includes a detailed family history.

Treatment

Although there is no cure for bipolar disorder, in most cases treatment can stabilize mood and allow for management and control of symptoms. A good treatment plan includes medication, close monitoring of symptoms, education about the illness, counseling or psychotherapy for the individual and family, stress reduction, good nutrition, regular sleep and exercise, and participation in a network of support.

The response to medications and treatment varies. Factors that contribute to a better outcome are:

- access to competent medical care
- early diagnosis and treatment
- adherence to medication and treatment plan
- a flexible, low-stress home and school environment
- a supportive network of family and friends

Factors that complicate treatment are:

- lack of access to competent medical care
- time lag between onset of illness and treatment
- not taking prescribed medications
- stressful and inflexible home and school environment
- the co-occurrence of other diagnoses
- use of substances such as illegal drugs and alcohol

The good news is that with appropriate treatment and support at home and at school, many children with bipolar disorder achieve a marked reduction in the severity, frequency, and duration of episodes of illness. With education about their illness (as is provided to children with epilepsy, diabetes, and other chronic conditions), they learn how to manage and monitor their symptoms as they grow older.

The Parent's Role in Treatment

As with other chronic medical conditions such as diabetes, epilepsy, and asthma, children and adolescents with bipolar disorder and their families need to work closely with their doctor and other treatment professionals. Having the entire family involved in the child's treatment plan can usually reduce the frequency, duration, and severity of episodes. It can also help improve the child's ability to function successfully at home, in school, and in the community.

Parents need to learn all they can about bipolar disorder. Read, join support groups, and network with other parents. There are many questions still unanswered about early onset bipolar disorder, but early intervention and treatment can often stabilize mood and restore wellness. Relapses can best be managed by prompt intervention at the first re-occurrence of symptoms.

Medication

Few controlled studies have been done on the use of psychiatric medications in children. The U.S. Food and Drug Administration (FDA) has approved only a handful for pediatric use. Psychiatrists must adapt what they know about treating adults to children and adolescents.

Medications used to treat adults are often helpful in stabilizing mood in children. Most doctors start medication immediately upon diagnosis if both parents agree. If one parent disagrees, a short period of watchful waiting and charting of symptoms can be helpful. Treatment should not be postponed for long, however, because of the risk of suicide and school failure.

A symptomatic child should never be left unsupervised. If parental disagreement makes treatment impossible, as may happen in families undergoing divorce, a court order regarding treatment may be necessary.

Other treatments, such as psychotherapy, may not be effective until mood stabilization occurs. In fact, stimulants and antidepressants given without a mood stabilizer (often the result of misdiagnosis) can cause havoc in bipolar children, potentially inducing mania, more frequent cycling, and increases in aggressive outbursts.

No one medication works in all children. The family should expect a trial-and-error process lasting weeks, months, or longer as doctors try several medications alone and in combination before they find the best treatment for your child. It is important not to become discouraged during the initial treatment phase. Two or more mood stabilizers, plus additional medications for symptoms that remain, are often necessary to achieve and maintain stability.

Parents often find it hard to accept that their child has a chronic condition that may require treatment with several medications. It is important to remember that bipolar disorder has a high rate of suicide. Estimates vary, but mortality rates of 5–10% from suicide are reported by various studies, rates equal to or greater than the mortality rates for many serious physical illnesses. The untreated disorder carries the risk of drug and alcohol addiction, damaged relationships, school failure, and difficulty finding and holding jobs. The risks of not treating are substantial and must be measured against the unknown risks of using medications whose safety and efficacy have been established in adults, but not yet in children.

Therapeutic Parenting™

Parents of children with bipolar disorder have discovered numerous techniques that CABF refers to as therapeutic parenting. These techniques help calm their children when they are symptomatic and can help prevent and contain relapses.

Such techniques include:

- practicing and teaching their child relaxation techniques

- using firm restraint holds to contain rages

- prioritizing battles and letting go of less important matters

- reducing stress in the home, including learning and using good listening and communication skills

- using music and sound, lighting, water, and massage to assist the child with waking, falling asleep, and relaxation

- becoming an advocate for stress reduction and other accommodations at school

- helping the child anticipate and avoid, or prepare for stressful situations by developing coping strategies beforehand

- engaging the child's creativity through activities that express and channel their gifts and strengths

- providing routine structure and a great deal of freedom within limits

- removing objects from the home (or locking them in a safe place) that could be used to harm self or others during a rage, especially guns, and keeping medications in a locked cabinet or box.

What Are the Educational Needs of A Child with Bipolar Disorder?

A diagnosis of bipolar disorder means the child has a significant health impairment (such as diabetes, epilepsy, or leukemia) that requires ongoing medical management. The child needs and is entitled to accommodations in school to benefit from his or her education. Bipolar disorder and the medications used to treat it can affect a child's school attendance; alertness and concentration; sensitivity to light, noise, and stress; motivation; and energy available for learning. The child's functioning can vary greatly at different times throughout the day, season, and school year.

These factors and any others that affect the child's education must be identified. A plan, called an individual education plan (IEP), will be written to accommodate the child's needs. The IEP should include accommodations for periods when the child is relatively well (when a less intense level of services may suffice), and accommodations available to the child in the event of relapse. Specific accommodations should be backed up by a letter or phone call from the child's doctor to the director of special education in the school district. Some parents find it necessary to hire a lawyer to obtain the accommodations and services that federal law requires public schools to provide for children with similar health impairments.

A Turning Point

Learning that one's child has bipolar disorder can be traumatic. Diagnosis usually follows months or years of the child's mood instability, school difficulties, and damaged relationships with family and friends. However, diagnosis can and should be a turning point for everyone concerned. Once the illness is identified, energies can be directed towards treatment, education, and developing coping strategies.

Additional Information

Child and Adolescent Bipolar Foundation
1000 Skokie Blvd., Suite 425
Wilmette, IL 60091
Phone: 847-256-8525
Fax: 847-920-9498
Website: http://www.bpkids.org
E-mail: cabf@bpkids.org

Chapter 61

Borderline Personality Disorder

Raising Questions, Finding Answers

Borderline personality disorder (BPD) is a serious mental illness characterized by pervasive instability in moods, interpersonal relationships, self-image, and behavior. This instability often disrupts family and work life, long-term planning, and the individual's sense of self-identity. Originally thought to be at the borderline of psychosis, people with BPD suffer from a disorder of emotion regulation. While less well-known than schizophrenia or bipolar disorder (manic-depressive illness), BPD is more common, affecting two percent of adults, mostly young women.[1] There is a high rate of self-injury without suicide intent, as well as a significant rate of suicide attempts and completed suicide in severe cases.[2, 3] Patients often need extensive mental health services, and account for 20 percent of psychiatric hospitalizations.[4] Yet, with help, many improve over time and are eventually able to lead productive lives.

Symptoms

While a person with depression or bipolar disorder typically endures the same mood for weeks, a person with BPD may experience intense bouts of anger, depression, and anxiety that may last only hours, or at most a day.[5] These may be associated with episodes of

National Institute of Mental Health (NIMH), NIH Publication No. 01-4928, February 2006.

impulsive aggression, self-injury, and drug or alcohol abuse. Distortions in cognition and sense of self can lead to frequent changes in long-term goals, career plans, jobs, friendships, gender identity, and values. Sometimes people with BPD view themselves as fundamentally bad, or unworthy. They may feel unfairly misunderstood or mistreated, bored, empty, and have little idea who they are. Such symptoms are most acute when people with BPD feel isolated and lacking in social support, and may result in frantic efforts to avoid being alone.

People with BPD often have highly unstable patterns of social relationships. While they can develop intense but stormy attachments, their attitudes towards family, friends, and loved ones may suddenly shift from idealization (great admiration and love) to devaluation (intense anger and dislike). Thus, they may form an immediate attachment and idealize the other person, but when a slight separation or conflict occurs, they switch unexpectedly to the other extreme and angrily accuse the other person of not caring for them at all. Even with family members, individuals with BPD are highly sensitive to rejection, reacting with anger and distress to such mild separations as a vacation, a business trip, or a sudden change in plans. These fears of abandonment seem to be related to difficulties feeling emotionally connected to important persons when they are physically absent, leaving the individual with BPD feeling lost and perhaps worthless. Suicide threats and attempts may occur along with anger at perceived abandonment and disappointments.

People with BPD exhibit other impulsive behaviors, such as excessive spending, binge eating, and risky sex. BPD often occurs together with other psychiatric problems, particularly bipolar disorder, depression, anxiety disorders, substance abuse, and other personality disorders.

Treatment

Treatments for BPD have improved in recent years. Group and individual psychotherapy are at least partially effective for many patients. Within the past 15 years, a new psychosocial treatment termed dialectical behavior therapy (DBT) was developed specifically to treat BPD, and this technique has looked promising in treatment studies.[6] Pharmacological treatments are often prescribed based on specific target symptoms shown by the individual patient. Antidepressant drugs and mood stabilizers may be helpful for depressed and/or labile mood. Antipsychotic drugs may also be used when there are distortions in thinking.[7]

Recent Research Findings

Although the cause of BPD is unknown, both environmental and genetic factors are thought to play a role in predisposing patients to BPD symptoms and traits. Studies show that many, but not all, individuals with BPD report a history of abuse, neglect, or separation as young children.[8] Forty to 71 percent of BPD patients report having been sexually abused, usually by a non-caregiver.[9] Researchers believe that BPD results from a combination of individual vulnerability to environmental stress, neglect or abuse as young children, and a series of events that trigger the onset of the disorder as young adults. Adults with BPD are also considerably more likely to be the victim of violence, including rape and other crimes. This may result from harmful environments as well as impulsivity and poor judgement in choosing partners and lifestyles.

NIMH-funded neuroscience research is revealing brain mechanisms underlying the impulsivity, mood instability, aggression, anger, and negative emotion seen in BPD. Studies suggest that people predisposed to impulsive aggression have impaired regulation of the neural circuits that modulate emotion.[10] The amygdala, a small almond-shaped structure deep inside the brain, is an important component of the circuit that regulates negative emotion. In response to signals from other brain centers indicating a perceived threat, it marshals fear and arousal. This might be more pronounced under the influence of drugs like alcohol, or stress. Areas in the front of the brain (pre-frontal area) act to dampen the activity of this circuit. Recent brain imaging studies show that individual differences in the ability to activate regions of the prefrontal cerebral cortex thought to be involved in inhibitory activity predict the ability to suppress negative emotion.[11]

Serotonin, norepinephrine, and acetylcholine are among the chemical messengers in these circuits that play a role in the regulation of emotions, including sadness, anger, anxiety, and irritability. Drugs that enhance brain serotonin function may improve emotional symptoms in BPD. Likewise, mood-stabilizing drugs that are known to enhance the activity of the brain's major inhibitory neurotransmitter may help people who experience BPD-like mood swings. Such brain-based vulnerabilities can be managed with help from behavioral interventions and medications, much like people manage susceptibility to diabetes or high blood pressure.[7]

References

1. Swartz M, Blazer D, George L, Winfield I. Estimating the prevalence of borderline personality disorder in the community. *Journal of Personality Disorders*, 1990; 4(3): 257–72.

2. Soloff PH, Lis JA, Kelly T, Cornelius J, Ulrich R. Self-mutilation and suicidal behavior in borderline personality disorder. *Journal of Personality Disorders*, 1994; 8(4): 257–67.

3. Gardner DL, Cowdry RW. Suicidal and parasuicidal behavior in borderline personality disorder. *Psychiatric Clinics of North America*, 1985; 8(2): 389–403.

4. Zanarini MC, Frankenburg FR. Treatment histories of borderline inpatients. *Comprehensive Psychiatry*, in press.

5. Zanarini MC, Frankenburg FR, DeLuca CJ, Hennen J, Khera GS, Gunderson JG. The pain of being borderline: dysphoric states specific to borderline personality disorder. *Harvard Review of Psychiatry*, 1998; 6(4): 201–7.

6. Koerner K, Linehan MM. Research on dialectical behavior therapy for patients with borderline personality disorder. *Psychiatric Clinics of North America*, 2000; 23(1): 151–67.

7. Siever LJ, Koenigsberg HW. The frustrating no-mans-land of borderline personality disorder. *Cerebrum*, The Dana Forum on Brain Science, 2000; 2(4).

8. Zanarini MC, Frankenburg. Pathways to the development of borderline personality disorder. *Journal of Personality Disorders*, 1997; 11(1): 93–104.

9. Zanarini MC. Childhood experiences associated with the development of borderline personality disorder. *Psychiatric Clinics of North America*, 2000; 23(1): 89–101.

10. Davidson RJ, Jackson DC, Kalin NH. Emotion, plasticity, context and regulation: perspectives from affective neuroscience. *Psychological Bulletin*, 2000; 126(6): 873–89.

11. Davidson RJ, Putnam KM, Larson CL. Dysfunction in the neural circuitry of emotion regulation—a possible prelude to violence. *Science*, 2000; 289(5479): 591–4.

Chapter 62

Conduct Disorder in Adolescents

Children with conduct disorder repeatedly violate the personal or property rights of others and the basic expectations of society. A diagnosis of conduct disorder is likely when symptoms continue for six months or longer. Conduct disorder is known as a disruptive behavior disorder because of its impact on children and their families, neighbors, and schools.

Another disruptive behavior disorder, called oppositional defiant disorder, may be a precursor of conduct disorder. A child is diagnosed with oppositional defiant disorder when he or she shows signs of being hostile and defiant for at least six months. Oppositional defiant disorder may start as early as the preschool years, while conduct disorder generally appears when children are older. Oppositional defiant disorder and conduct disorder are not co-occurring conditions.

What are the signs of conduct disorder?

Symptoms of conduct disorder include:

- aggressive behavior that harms or threatens other people or animals

- destructive behavior that damages or destroys property

- lying or theft

"Conduct Disorder in Children and Adolescents," Substance Abuse and Mental Health Services Administration (SAMHSA), April 2003.

- truancy or other serious violations of rules

- early tobacco, alcohol, and substance use and abuse

- precocious sexual activity

Children with conduct disorder or oppositional defiant disorder also may experience:

- higher rates of depression, suicidal thoughts, suicide attempts, and suicide

- academic difficulties

- poor relationships with peers or adults

- sexually transmitted diseases

- difficulty staying in adoptive, foster, or group homes

- higher rates of injuries, school expulsions, and problems with the law

How common is conduct disorder?

Conduct disorder affects one to four percent of 9- to 17-year-olds, depending on exactly how the disorder is defined (U.S. Department of Health and Human Services, 1999). The disorder appears to be more common in boys than in girls and more common in cities than in rural areas.

Who is at risk for conduct disorder?

Research shows that some cases of conduct disorder begin in early childhood, often by the preschool years. In fact, some infants who are especially fussy appear to be at risk for developing conduct disorder. Other factors that may make a child more likely to develop conduct disorder include:

- early maternal rejection

- separation from parents, without an adequate alternative caregiver

- early institutionalization

- family neglect

- abuse or violence

- parental mental illness
- parental marital discord
- large family size
- crowding
- poverty

What help is available for families?

Although conduct disorder is one of the most difficult behavior disorders to treat, young people often benefit from a range of services that include:

- training for parents on how to handle child or adolescent behavior
- family therapy
- training in problem solving skills for children or adolescents
- community-based services that focus on the young person within the context of family and community influences

What can parents do?

Some child and adolescent behaviors are hard to change after they have become ingrained. Therefore, the earlier the conduct disorder is identified and treated, the better the chance for success. Most children or adolescents with conduct disorder are probably reacting to events and situations in their lives. Some recent studies have focused on promising ways to prevent conduct disorder among at-risk children and adolescents. In addition, more research is needed to determine if biology is a factor in conduct disorder.

Parents or other caregivers who notice signs of conduct disorder or oppositional defiant disorder in a child or adolescent should try the following tips.

- Pay careful attention to the signs, try to understand the underlying reasons, and then try to improve the situation.
- If necessary, talk with a mental health or social services professional, such as a teacher, counselor, psychiatrist, or psychologist specializing in childhood and adolescent disorders.
- Get accurate information from libraries, hotlines, or other sources.

- Talk to other families in their communities.

- Find family network organizations.

People who are not satisfied with the mental health services they receive should discuss their concerns with their provider, ask for more information, and/or seek help from other sources.

Endnote

U.S. Department of Health and Human Services. (1999). *Mental Health: A Report of the Surgeon General.* Rockville, MD: U.S. Department of Health and Human Services.

Additional Information

National Institute of Mental Health
Public Information and Communications Branch
6001 Executive Blvd.
Room 8184, MSC 9663
Bethesda, MD 20892-9663
Toll-Free: 866-615-6464
Toll-Free TTY: 866-415-8051
Phone: 301-443-8431
Fax: 301-443-4279
Website: http://www.nimh.nih.gov
E-mail: nimhinfo@nih.gov

National Mental Health Information Center
P.O. Box 42557
Washington DC 20015
Toll-Free: 800-789-2647
Toll-Free TDD: 866-889-2647
Fax: 240-747-5470
Website: http://www.mentalhealth.samhsa.gov

Chapter 63

Depression Affects Teens

Major Depression in Children and Adolescents

Major depression is one of the mental, emotional, and behavior disorders that can appear during childhood and adolescence. This type of depression affects a young person's thoughts, feelings, behavior, and body. Major depression in children and adolescents is serious; it is more than the blues. Depression can lead to school failure, alcohol or other drug use, and even suicide.

Signs of Depression

Young people with depression may have a hard time coping with everyday activities and responsibilities, have difficulty getting along with others, and suffer from low self-esteem. Signs of depression often include:

- sadness that will not go away
- hopelessness, boredom
- unexplained irritability or crying
- loss of interest in usual activities

This chapter includes: Excerpts from "Major Depression in Children and Adolescents," Substance Abuse and Mental Health Services Administration (SAMHSA), April 2003; excerpts from "Antidepressant Medications for Children and Adolescents: Information for Parents and Caregivers," National Institute of Mental Health (NIMH), February 2005; and excerpts from "Suicidal Thoughts among Youths Aged 12 to 17 with Major Depressive Episode," SAMHSA, September 2005.

- changes in eating or sleeping habits

- alcohol or substance abuse

- missed school or poor school performance

- threats or attempts to run away from home

- outbursts of shouting, complaining

- reckless behavior

- aches and pains that do not get better with treatment

- thoughts about death or suicide

Adolescents with major depression are likely to identify themselves as depressed before their parents suspect a problem. The same may be true for children.

How Common Is Depression?

Population studies show that at any point in time 10 to 15 percent of children and adolescents have some symptoms of depression. Having a family history of depression, particularly a parent who had depression at an early age, also increases the chances that a child or adolescent may develop depression. Once a young person has experienced a major depression, he or she is at risk of developing another depression within the next five years. This young person is also at risk for other mental health problems.

What Help Is Available for a Young Person with Depression?

While several types of antidepressant medications can be effective to treat adults with depression, these medications may not be as effective in treating children and adolescents. Care must be used in prescribing and monitoring all medication.

Many mental health care providers use talk treatments to help children and adolescents with depression. A child or adolescent in need of treatment or services and his or her family may need a plan of care based on the severity and duration of symptoms. Optimally, this plan is developed with the family, service providers, and a service coordinator, who is referred to as a case manager. Whenever possible, the child or adolescent is involved in decisions. This system of care is designed to improve the child's ability to function in all areas of life— at home, at school, and in the community.

What Can Parents Do?

- Make careful notes about the behaviors that concern them. Note how long the behaviors have been going on, how often they occur, and how severe they seem.

- Make an appointment with a mental health professional or the child's doctor for evaluation and diagnosis.

- Get accurate information from libraries, hotlines, or other sources.

- Ask questions about treatments and services.

- Talk to other families in their community.

- Find family network organizations.

Antidepressant Medications for Children and Adolescents: Information for Parents and Caregivers

Research has shown that, as in adults, depression in children and adolescents can be treated. In particular, antidepressant medications—called selective serotonin reuptake inhibitors (SSRIs) because they specifically target the neurotransmitter serotonin—have been shown to be of benefit to children and adolescents with major depressive disorder. Certain types of psychological therapies have also been shown to be beneficial. In those with moderate to severe depression they are especially useful when combined with medication. Our knowledge of antidepressant treatments in youth, though growing substantially, remains limited when compared with what we know about treatment of depression in adults.

Recently, concerns have been raised that the use of antidepressant medications themselves may induce suicidal behavior in youths. In fact, following a thorough and comprehensive review of all the available published and unpublished controlled clinical trials of antidepressants in children and adolescents, the U.S. Food and Drug Administration (FDA) has warned the public about an increased risk of suicidal thoughts or behavior (suicidality) in children and adolescents treated with SSRI antidepressant medications.

The SSRIs (serotonin reuptake inhibitors) include:

- fluoxetine (Prozac)

- sertraline (Zoloft)

531

- paroxetine (Paxil)

- citalopram (Celexa)

- escitalopram (Lexapro)

- fluvoxamine (Luvox)

- venlafaxine (Effexor)—another antidepressant closely related to the SSRIs

SSRI medications are considered an improvement over older antidepressant medications because they have fewer side effects and are safer if taken in an overdose (which is an issue for patients at risk for suicide). They have been extensively tested in adult populations and have been proven to be safe and effective for adults.

Use of SSRI medications has risen dramatically in the past several years in children and adolescents age 10–19. Some studies show that this increase has coincided with a significant decrease in suicide rates in this age group, but it is not known if SSRI medications are directly responsible for this improvement.

Fluoxetine (also known as Prozac) is the only medication approved by the FDA for use to treat depression in children age eight and older. The other SSRI medications, such as sertraline, citalopram, and paroxetine, and the SSRI-related antidepressant venlafaxine, have not been approved for treatment of depression in children or adolescents, though they have been prescribed to children by physicians in off-label use—a use other than the FDA approved use. In June 2003, the FDA recommended that paroxetine not be used in children and adolescents for the treatment of major depressive disorder.

Fluoxetine leads to significant improvement of depression overall. The drug, however, may increase the risk for suicidal behaviors in a small subset of adolescents. As with all medical decisions, doctors and families have to weigh risks and benefits of treatment for each individual patient.

What Remains Unknown

Currently, there is no way of telling who may be sensitive to an SSRI's positive or adverse effects. Results thus far are based on populations— some individuals may show marked improvement, some may see no change, and some may be vulnerable to adverse effects. The response to medication of an individual patient cannot be predicted with certainty from the kind of studies that have been done so far.

It is extremely difficult to determine whether SSRI medications do or do not increase the risk of completed suicide, especially since depression itself increases the risk for suicide and because completed suicide is a rare event.

What Should You Do for A Child with Depression?

Major depression in children and adolescents is a serious condition that should be adequately treated, which includes careful follow-up and monitoring.

Each child should be carefully and thoroughly evaluated by a physician to determine if medication is appropriate. Those who are prescribed an SSRI medication should receive ongoing medical monitoring, with particular care paid in the first four weeks of taking the drug.

Psychotherapy is often used as an initial treatment for milder forms of depression. Many times, psychotherapy accompanied by an early follow-up appointment may help to establish the persistence of depression before a decision is made to try antidepressant medications. Psychotherapies include "cognitive behavioral therapy" and "interpersonal therapy."

Should suicidal thinking or behavior, nervousness, agitation, irritability, mood instability, or sleeplessness emerge or worsen during treatment with SSRI medications, parents should obtain a prompt evaluation by a clinician with expertise in these medications.

Children already on any of the SSRI medications should remain on the drug if it has been helpful, but they should also be carefully monitored by a physician for evidence of side effects. Once started, treatment with these medications should not be abruptly stopped, because of potential side effects. Families should not discontinue treatment without consulting with their physician.

Suicidal Thoughts among Youths Aged 12 to 17 with Major Depressive Episode

In 2003, suicide was the 11th leading cause of death among persons of all ages in the United States. However, among young people aged 15 to 24, suicide, or intentional self-harm, was the third leading cause of death, with 3,921 deaths, following accidents/unintentional injuries (14,966 deaths) and assaults/homicides (5,148 deaths).

The 2004 National Survey on Drug Use and Health (NSDUH) asked youths aged 12 to 17 about symptoms of depression, including thoughts about death or suicide. Major depressive episode (MDE) is defined as a period of at least two weeks when a person experienced a depressed mood or loss of interest or pleasure in daily activities and had at least five of the nine symptoms of depression as described in the *Diagnostic and Statistical Manual of Mental Disorders* (*DSM-IV*).

Prevalence of Major Depressive Episode (MDE)

An estimated 14 percent of youths aged 12 to 17, approximately 3.5 million youths, had experienced at least one MDE in their lifetime (Table 63.1). Almost 20 percent of females aged 12 to 17 and 8.5 percent of males had at least one of these depressive episodes. Rates of lifetime MDE were similar among racial/ethnic groups and increased with age.

Table 63.1. Numbers (in Thousands) and Percentages of Youths Aged 12 to 17 Reporting a Major Depressive Episode (MDE) in Their Lifetime: 2004

	Lifetime Major Depressive Episode	
Characteristic	Estimated Number (in Thousands)	Percent
Total	3,477	14.0
Age		
12 to 13	725	8.8
14 to 15	1,252	14.6
16 to 17	1,499	18.5
Gender		
Male	1,074	8.5
Female	2,403	19.7
Race/Ethnicity		
White	2,135	13.9
Black	485	12.9
Hispanic or Latino	630	15.2
American Indian or Alaska Native	20	12.0
Native Hawaiian or Other Pacific Islander	*	*
Asian	128	13.0

*Low precision, estimate not reported

Source: SAMHSA, 2004 NSDUH

MDE and Suicidal Thoughts

Among youths aged 12 to 17, about 9 percent, an estimated 2.3 million youths, had experienced MDE in their lifetime and thought, during their worst or most recent MDE, that it would be better if they were dead. Over 7 percent, an estimated 1.8 million youths, thought about killing themselves at the time of their worst or most recent MDE.

Females aged 12 to 17 were significantly more likely than their male peers to have had MDE and to report thinking about suicide and believing it would be better if they were dead.

Both 14 or 15 year olds and 16 or 17 year olds were significantly more likely than those aged 12 or 13 to have had MDE accompanied by thoughts that it would be better if they were dead and thoughts about committing suicide.

MDE with suicidal thoughts did not vary by urbanicity. Youths in large metropolitan areas, small metropolitan areas, and non-metropolitan areas were equally likely to have MDE with suicidal thoughts.

MDE and Suicide Attempts

An estimated 900,000 youths, or 3.6 percent of 12 to 17 year olds, made a plan to kill themselves at the time they were having their worst or most recent MDE. An estimated 712,000 youths had tried to kill themselves during such an episode; this represents 2.9 percent of those aged 12 to 17.

Female youths were more likely than male youths to have had MDE and made a plan to kill themselves (5.6 percent of females and 1.7 percent of males) or to have attempted suicide (4.7 percent of females and 1.1 percent of males).

Chapter 64

Eating Disorders Impact Adolescents

Who Has Eating Disorders?

Research shows that more than 90 percent of those who have eating disorders are women between the ages of 12 and 25 (National Alliance for the Mentally Ill, 2003). However, increasing numbers of older women and men have these disorders. In addition, hundreds of thousands of boys are affected by these disorders (U.S. DHHS Office on Women's Health, 2000).

Eating Disorders Information

Eating Disorders Are a Serious Health Issue

Eating disorders can pose serious health risks to young people. Approximately one out of every 100 adolescent girls develops anorexia nervosa, and another two to five develop bulimia nervosa. Both can lead to serious health complications and even death. Binge eating disorder affects millions more and can result in complications

This chapter includes: An excerpt titled "Who Has Eating Disorders?" from "Eating Disorders," Substance Abuse and Mental Health Services Administration (SAMHSA), April 2003; excerpts from "Eating Disorders Information Sheet: Health Care Providers," National Women's Health Information Clearinghouse, October 2005; and an excerpt titled "Treatment Strategies," from "Eating Disorders: Facts about Eating Disorders and the Search for Solutions," National Institute of Mental Health (NIMH), September 2005.

associated with obesity. Anorexia, bulimia, and binge eating disorder are serious and chronic mental health problems associated with anxiety and depression.

Children and Adolescents Should Be Routinely Screened for Eating Disorders

Eating disorders are often preceded by troublesome eating behaviors known as disordered eating in children as young as eight years old. Primary care providers are in a unique position to detect eating disorders in the early or subclinical stages. Early detection through routine screening greatly increases the likelihood of successful treatment and recovery. The prevalence of eating disorders is increasing in boys as well as girls, and these disorders affect young people of most ethnic, cultural, and socioeconomic groups. Routine screening for eating disorders is an increasingly important aspect of young patients' care.

Adolescence Is a Time of Change

Pre- and early adolescence is a time of dramatic physical and psychological change. Along with physical changes such as height and weight gains and sexual maturation, pre-adolescents often experience mood swings and wavering self-esteem. Influenced by the media and susceptible to peer pressure, young people may become increasingly concerned about body image during these years and base their feelings of self-esteem and self-worth on their appearance. They may be teased about their developing bodies by family or friends or may use food as a way of coping with the pressures in their lives. Body dissatisfaction, fear of fat, being teased, dieting, and using food to deal with stress are major risk factors associated with disordered eating.

Anorexia Nervosa Symptoms

- Refusal to maintain body weight at or above a minimally normal weight for height and age, or failure to make expected weight gain during period of growth, leading to body weight 15% below that expected.

- Intense fear of gaining weight or becoming fat, even though underweight.

- Disturbance in the way one's body weight or shape is experienced, undue influence of body shape and weight on self-evaluation, or denial of the seriousness of current low body weight.

- In menarcheal females, amenorrhea—the absence of at least three consecutive menstrual cycles.

Restricting type of anorexia: The person does not regularly engage in binge eating or purging during the anorexia episode.

Binge eating/purging type of anorexia: The person regularly engages in binge eating or purging during the anorexia episode.

Bulimia Nervosa Symptoms

- Recurrent episodes of binge eating (eating an abnormally large amount of food in a discrete period of time, with a sense of lack of control over eating during the episode).

- Recurrent inappropriate compensatory behavior to prevent weight gain, such as self-induced vomiting; misuse of laxatives, diuretics, or other medications; fasting; or excessive exercise.

- Binge eating and inappropriate compensatory behaviors both occur, on average, at least twice a week for three months.

- Self-evaluation is unduly influenced by body shape and weight.

- The disturbance does not occur exclusively during episodes of anorexia nervosa.

Binge Eating Disorder Symptoms

- Recurrent episodes of food consumption substantially larger than most people would eat in a similar period of time under similar circumstances.

- A feeling of being unable to control what or how much is being eaten.

- Associated with three (or more) of the following:
  - eating very rapidly
  - eating until feeling uncomfortably full
  - eating large amounts of food when not feeling physically hungry
  - eating alone because of being embarrassed by how much one is eating
  - feeling disgust, guilt, or depression after overeating

539

- Marked distress or unpleasant feelings during and after the binge episode, as well as concerns about the long-term effect of binge eating on body weight and shape.

- Binge eating that occurs, on average, at least two days a week for six months.

- The binge eating is not associated with the regular use of inappropriate compensatory behaviors (for example, purging, fasting, excessive exercise) and does not occur exclusively during the course of anorexia nervosa or bulimia nervosa.

Symptoms of Other Types of Eating Disorders and Disordered Eating

- Eating disorder not otherwise specified (EDNOS) includes characteristics of one or more eating disorders but does not fit the diagnostic criteria for any one disorder.

- Disordered eating refers to troublesome eating behaviors that are less frequent or less severe than those that occur in an eating disorder.

- Over-exercising is exercising compulsively for long periods of time as a way to control weight. It is often viewed as a type of purging behavior, frequently associated with bulimia or anorexia.

Eating Disorders Can Cause Serious Complications

Anorexia has the highest rate of premature death of any psychiatric illness, with one in ten cases leading to death by cardiac arrest, starvation, other medical complications, or suicide. Complications of anorexia may include heart failure due to malnutrition, hypometabolism, and increased risk of osteoporosis. Young women with anorexia have an increased risk of bone fractures. In addition, anemia, reduced muscle mass, cessation of menstruation, and edema may accompany weight loss in anorexia.

Most complications of bulimia result from electrolyte imbalance or trauma from repeated purging behaviors. Loss of potassium damages heart muscle, increasing the risk for cardiac arrest. Repeated vomiting can cause esophagitis, enlargement of salivary glands, and erosion of tooth enamel.

Individuals with anorexia and bulimia have high rates of clinical depression, and often suffer from anxiety or personality disorders. Eating disorders may be related to other health risk behaviors, such as substance abuse and unprotected sexual activity.

Binge eating disorder affects up to four percent of the general population. Complications are similar to those found in obesity, including high blood pressure, diabetes, and increased risk of gallbladder disease, heart disease, and some types of cancer. Individuals with binge eating disorder also have high rates of depression.

Although large numbers of teenagers who have disordered eating do not meet the strict DSM-IV criteria for either anorexia nervosa or bulimia nervosa, many have similar levels of emotional distress. Up to 60 percent of adolescent girls consider themselves overweight and have attempted to diet. In one study, more than half of the adolescents evaluated for eating disorders had subclinical disease but suffered a similar degree of emotional distress as those who met strict diagnostic criteria.

Eating Disorders Should Be Diagnosed in the Context of Multiple Aspects of Normal Growth and Development

Severe nutritional deficits can occur even in the absence of weight loss in early adolescence. The use of strict criteria may also make it more difficult to recognize eating disorders in their early stages and subclinical form. It is essential to diagnose eating disorders in adolescents in the context of the multiple and varied aspects of normal adolescent growth and development. The rate of most rapid weight gain for girls is from age 9 to 14. Families and health care providers may notice this rapid weight gain but fail to provide adequate reassurance to the girls that their body sizes and weights are in the normal range. Adolescent depression may camouflage an underlying eating disorder that may go undetected but which requires a separate treatment plan.

Communicate with Patients and Parents

Patients with eating disorders often feel shame, guilt, and fear that their illness will be discovered. Their eating disorder is not simply a physical problem; it is a way of coping with emotional distress. They may distrust health care providers and resist pressure to give up the disorder. It is important that health care providers be sensitive to and validate the patient's feelings; provide a nonjudgmental, caring environment; and maintain confidentiality.

Treatment Strategies

Eating disorders can be treated and a healthy weight restored. The sooner these disorders are diagnosed and treated, the better the outcomes are likely to be. Because of their complexity, eating disorders require a comprehensive treatment plan involving medical care and monitoring, psychosocial interventions, nutritional counseling, and when appropriate, medication management. At the time of diagnosis, the clinician must determine whether the person is in immediate danger and requires hospitalization.

Treatment of anorexia calls for a specific program that involves three main phases: (1) restoring weight lost to severe dieting and purging; (2) treating psychological disturbances such as distortion of body image, low self-esteem, and interpersonal conflicts; and (3) achieving long-term remission and rehabilitation, or full recovery. Early diagnosis and treatment increases the treatment success rate. Use of psychotropic medication in people with anorexia should be considered only after weight gain has been established. Certain selective serotonin reuptake inhibitors (SSRIs) have been shown to be helpful for weight maintenance and for resolving mood and anxiety symptoms associated with anorexia.

The acute management of severe weight loss is usually provided in an inpatient hospital setting, where feeding plans address the person's medical and nutritional needs. In some cases, intravenous feeding is recommended. Once malnutrition has been corrected and weight gain has begun, psychotherapy (often cognitive-behavioral or interpersonal psychotherapy) can help people with anorexia overcome low self-esteem and address distorted thought and behavior patterns. Families are sometimes included in the therapeutic process.

The primary goal of treatment for bulimia is to reduce or eliminate binge eating and purging behavior. To this end, nutritional rehabilitation, psychosocial intervention, and medication management strategies are often employed. Establishment of a pattern of regular, non-binge meals, improvement of attitudes related to the eating disorder, encouragement of healthy but not excessive exercise, and resolution of co-occurring conditions such as mood or anxiety disorders are among the specific aims of these strategies. Individual psychotherapy (especially cognitive-behavioral or interpersonal psychotherapy), group psychotherapy that uses a cognitive-behavioral approach, and family or marital therapy have been reported to be effective. Psychotropic medications, primarily antidepressants such as the selective serotonin reuptake inhibitors (SSRIs), have been found helpful for people with bulimia, particularly those with significant symptoms of depression or anxiety, or those who have not responded adequately to psychosocial treatment alone. These medications also may help prevent relapse. The treatment goals and strategies for binge-eating disorder are similar to those for bulimia, and studies are currently evaluating the effectiveness of various interventions.

People with eating disorders often do not recognize or admit that they are ill. As a result, they may strongly resist getting and staying in treatment. Family members or other trusted individuals can be helpful in ensuring that the person with an eating disorder receives needed care and rehabilitation. For some people, treatment may be long-term.

Chapter 65

Schizophrenia in Young People

Childhood-Onset Schizophrenia

A child's stage of development must be taken into account when considering a diagnosis of mental illness. Behaviors that are normal at one age may not be at another. Rarely, a healthy young child may report strange experiences—such as hearing voices—that would be considered abnormal at a later age. Clinicians look for a more persistent pattern of such behaviors. Parents may have reason for concern if a child of seven years or older often hears voices saying derogatory things about him or her, or voices conversing with one another, talks to himself or herself, stares at scary things—snakes, spiders, shadows—that are not really there, and shows no interest in friendships. Such behaviors could be signs of schizophrenia, a chronic and disabling form of mental illness.

Fortunately, schizophrenia is rare in children, affecting only about one in 40,000, compared to one in 100 in adults. The average age of onset is 18 in men and 25 in women. Ranking among the top ten causes of disability worldwide, schizophrenia, at any age, exacts a heavy toll on patients and their families. Children with schizophrenia experience difficulty in managing everyday life. With their adult counterparts, they share psychotic symptoms (hallucinations, delusions), social withdrawal, flattened emotions, increased risk of suicide, and

This chapter includes: Excerpts from "Childhood-Onset Schizophrenia: An Update from the NIMH," National Institute of Mental Health (NIMH), February 17, 2006; and "Teens with Deletion Syndrome Confirm Gene's Role in Psychosis," NIMH, October, 23, 2005.

loss of social and personal care skills. They may also share some symptoms with—and be mistaken for—children who suffer from autism or other pervasive developmental disabilities, which affect about one in 500 children. Although they tend to be harder to treat and have a worse prognosis than adult-onset schizophrenia patients, researchers are finding that many children with schizophrenia can be helped by the new generation of antipsychotic medications.

Symptoms and Diagnosis

While schizophrenia sometimes begins as an acute psychotic episode in young adults, it emerges gradually in children, often preceded by developmental disturbances, such as lags in motor and speech/language development. Such problems tend to be associated with more pronounced brain abnormalities. The diagnostic criteria are the same as for adults, except that symptoms appear prior to age 12, instead of in the late teens or early 20s. Children with schizophrenia often see or hear things that do not really exist, and harbor paranoid and bizarre beliefs. For example, they may think people are plotting against them or can read their minds. Other symptoms of the disorder include problems paying attention, impaired memory and reasoning, speech impairments, inappropriate or flattened expression of emotion, poor social skills, and depressed mood. Such children may laugh at a sad event, make poor eye contact, and show little body language or facial expression.

Misdiagnosis of schizophrenia in children is all too common. It is distinguished from autism by the persistence of hallucinations and delusions for at least six months, and a later age of onset—seven years or older. Autism is usually diagnosed by age three. Schizophrenia is also distinguished from a type of brief psychosis sometimes seen in affective, personality, and dissociative disorders in children. Adolescents with bipolar disorder sometimes have acute onset of manic episodes that may be mistaken for schizophrenia. Children who have been victims of abuse may sometimes claim to hear voices of—or see visions of—the abuser. Symptoms of schizophrenia characteristically pervade the child's life, and are not limited to just certain situations, such as at school. If children show any interest in friendships, even if they fail at maintaining them, it is unlikely that they have schizophrenia.

Treatment

Treatments that help young patients manage their illness have improved significantly in recent decades. Antipsychotic medications are especially helpful in reducing hallucinations and delusions. The newer generation atypical antipsychotics, such as olanzapine and clozapine, may also help improve motivation and emotional expressiveness in some patients. They also have a lower likelihood of producing disorders of movement, including tardive dyskinesia, than the other antipsychotic drugs such as haloperidol. However, even with these newer medications, there are side effects, including excess weight gain that can increase risk of other health problems. Children with schizophrenia and their families can also benefit from supportive counseling, psychotherapies, and social skills training aimed at helping them cope with the illness. They most likely will require special education and/or other accommodations to succeed in the classroom.

Causes

Although it is unclear whether schizophrenia has a single or multiple underlying causes, evidence suggests that it is a neurodevelopmental disease likely involving a genetic predisposition, a prenatal insult to the developing brain, and stressful life events. The role of genetics has long been established; the risk of schizophrenia rises from one percent with no family history of the illness, to ten percent if a first degree relative has it, to 50 percent if an identical twin has it. Prenatal insults may include viral infections, such as maternal influenza in the second trimester, starvation, lack of oxygen at birth, and untreated blood type incompatibility. Studies find that children and adults share many of the same abnormal brain structural, physiological, and neuropsychological features associated with schizophrenia. The children seem to have more severe cases than adults, with more pronounced neurological abnormalities. This makes childhood-onset schizophrenia potentially one of the clearest windows available for research into a still obscure illness process.

Children who become psychotic prior to puberty show conspicuous evidence of progressively abnormal brain development. In the first longitudinal brain imaging study of adolescents, magnetic resonance imaging (MRI) scans revealed fluid-filled cavities in the middle of the brain enlarging abnormally between ages 14 and 18 in teens with early-onset schizophrenia, suggesting a shrinkage in brain tissue volume. These children lost four times as much gray matter, neurons, and their branch-like extensions, in their frontal lobes as normally occurs in teens. This gray matter loss engulfs the brain in a progressive wave from back to front over five years, beginning in rear structures involved in attention and perception, eventually spreading to frontal areas responsible for organizing, planning, and other executive functions impaired in schizophrenia. Since losses in the rear areas are influenced mostly by environmental factors, the researchers suggest that some non-genetic trigger contributes to the onset and initial progression of the illness. The final loss pattern is consistent with that seen in adult schizophrenia. Adult-onset patients' brains may have undergone similar changes when they were teens that went unnoticed because symptoms had not yet emerged, suggest the researchers.

Researchers are also examining a group of measures associated with genetic risk for schizophrenia. Early-onset cases of illness have recently proven crucial in the discovery of genes linked to other genetically complex disorders like breast cancer, and Alzheimer and Crohn diseases. Hence, children with schizophrenia and their families may play an important role in deciphering schizophrenia's molecular roots. Evidence suggests that the rate of genetically linked abnormalities is twice as high in children as in adults with the illness. Similarly, schizophrenia spectrum disorders, thought to be genetically related to schizophrenia, are about twice as prevalent among first-degree relatives of childhood-onset patients. In one recent study, a third of the families of individuals with childhood onset schizophrenia had at least one first-degree relative with a diagnosis of schizophrenia, or schizotypal or paranoid personality disorder. This profile of psychiatric illness is remarkably similar to that seen in parents of adult-onset patients, adding to the likelihood that both forms share common genetic roots. Other anomalies associated with adult schizophrenia, such as abnormal eye movements, are also more common in families of children with the illness.

Teens with Deletion Syndrome Confirm Gene's Role in Psychosis

A study in youth who are missing part of a chromosome is further implicating a suspect gene in schizophrenia. Youth with this genetic chromosomal deletion syndrome already had a nearly 30-fold higher-than-normal risk of schizophrenia, but those who also had one of two common versions of the suspect gene had worse symptoms. They were more prone to cognitive decline, psychosis, and frontal lobe tissue loss by late adolescence when schizophrenia symptoms begin to emerge.

The gene version appeared to worsen symptoms of the deletion syndrome by chronically boosting the chemical messenger dopamine to excessive levels in the brain's executive hub, the prefrontal cortex, during development. The study is the first to show the long-term effects of the dopamine-regulating gene in a disorder related to schizophrenia.

"It's not that there's a good or bad version of this gene," explained NIMH director Thomas Insel, M.D. "Either version can be an accomplice via interactions with other genes and environmental factors in creating a dopamine imbalance that disturbs information processing. In this case, one version conspired with a rare mutation to produce too much dopamine. In other cases, the other version may tip the balance in the opposite direction."

While most people inherit two copies of the gene for the enzyme that breaks down dopamine, one in 4000 children are born with just one copy of the catechol-O-methyltransferase (COMT) gene. The gene is located in the tiny part of chromosome 22 that is partly missing in the 22q11.2 deletion syndrome, also known as the velocardiofacial syndrome. A mutation causes a variable array of problems, including cleft palate, heart defects and cognitive deficits.

Since about 30 percent of people with the chromosomal deletion syndrome also develop schizophrenia or related psychotic disorders— compared to only one percent of the general population—Reiss and colleagues suspected that people with the syndrome may hold unique clues about how the COMT gene influences development of the mental disorder.

A variation in the COMT gene's sequence results in two common versions: Val and Met—one version produces an enzyme that has the amino acid valine in the same position as the other has a methionine. The Val version results in stronger COMT enzyme activity. For example, people who inherit two copies of Val have 40 percent higher prefrontal cortex enzyme activity, resulting in more rapid chemical breakdown and markedly lower dopamine levels than people with two copies of Met.

In some studies, Val has been associated with slightly increased risk for schizophrenia, but evidence now suggests that either version can potentially increase risk, depending on how prefrontal dopamine is affected by interactions with other genes and environmental events. Since people with the deletion syndrome carry only one copy of the COMT gene, their enzyme activity is already compromised. If that copy is a Met, its weak enzyme action would likely expose their developing brains to excessive, potentially damaging prefrontal dopamine levels, with attendant adverse consequences, hypothesized the researchers at Stanford's Center for Interdisciplinary Brain Sciences Research, Department of Psychiatry and Behavioral Sciences.

They followed 24 subjects with the deletion syndrome and 23 matched control subjects with developmental disabilities. When first tested in childhood, subjects with the syndrome and Met did not suffer from psychotic disorders and performed cognitive tasks as well or better than subjects with Val. Yet, when they were re-tested in late adolescence/early adulthood, seven (29.2 percent) subjects with the syndrome had developed schizophrenia or other psychotic disorders, compared to only one from the developmental disabilities group. The syndrome group showed significant declines in tests of verbal intelligence quotient (IQ), and expressive language. Subjects with Met showed more robust decreases on these measures, as well as more severe psychotic symptoms, and more loss of prefrontal cortical gray matter volume than subjects with Val.

The researchers propose that dopamine increases that normally occur during adolescence are further boosted in syndrome-affected teens with Met, leading to "reduced efficiency of cognitive processing" during adolescence.

Chapter 66

Self-Injury in Adolescents

What does hurting yourself or self-injury mean?

Hurting yourself, sometimes called self-injury, is when a person deliberately hurts his or her own body. Some self-injuries can leave scars that will not go away, while others leave marks or bruises that eventually will go away. These are some forms of self-injury:

- cutting yourself (such as using a razor blade, knife or other sharp object to cut the skin)

- punching yourself or other objects

- burning yourself with cigarettes, matches, or candles

- pulling out your hair

- poking objects through body openings

- breaking your bones or bruising yourself

- plucking hair for hours

Why do some teens want to hurt themselves?

Many people cut themselves because it gives them a sense of relief. Some people use cutting as a means to cope with any problem. Some teens say that when they hurt themselves, they are trying to stop feeling lonely,

"Hurting Yourself," National Women's Health Information Center, August 2005.

angry, or hopeless. Some teens who hurt themselves have low self-esteem, may feel unloved by their family and friends, may have an eating disorder, an alcohol or drug problem, or may have been victims of abuse.

Teens who hurt themselves often keep their feelings bottled up inside and have a hard time letting their feelings show. Some teens who hurt themselves say that feeling the pain provides a sense of relief from intense feelings. Cutting can relieve the tension from bottled up sadness or anxiety. Others hurt themselves in order to feel. Often people who hold back strong emotions can begin feeling numb, and cutting can be a way to cope with this because it causes them to feel something. Some teens also may hurt themselves because they want to fit in with others who do it.

If you are hurting yourself, please get help—it is possible to overcome the urge to cut. There are other ways to find relief and cope with your emotions. Please talk to your parents, your doctor, or an adult you trust, like a teacher or religious leader.

Who are the people who hurt themselves?

People who hurt themselves come from all walks of life, no matter their age, gender, race, or ethnicity. About one in 100 people hurts himself or herself on purpose. More females hurt themselves than males. Teens usually hurt themselves by cutting with sharp objects.

These are some signs of self-injury:

- cuts or scars on the arms or legs

- hiding cuts or scars by wearing long sleeved shirts or pants, even in hot weather

- making poor excuses about how the injuries happened

Self-injury can be dangerous—cutting can lead to infections, scars, numbness, and even hospitalization and death. People who share tools to cut themselves are at risk of getting and spreading diseases like human immunodeficiency virus (HIV) and hepatitis. Teens who continue to hurt themselves are less likely to learn how to cope with negative feelings.

Are you or a friend depressed, angry, or having a hard time coping with life?

If you are thinking about hurting yourself, please ask for help. Talk with an adult you trust, like a teacher or minister or doctor. There is nothing wrong with asking for help—everyone needs help sometimes. You have a right to be strong, safe, and happy.

Do you have a friend who hurts herself or himself?

Please try to get your friend to talk to a trusted adult. Your friend may need professional counseling and treatment. Help is available—counselors can teach positive ways to cope with problems without turning to self-injury.

Have you been pressured to cut yourself by others who do it?

If so, think about how much you value that friendship or relationship. Do you really want a friend who wants you to hurt yourself, cause you pain, and put you in danger? Try to hang out with other friends who do not pressure you in this way.

Additional Information

Self Abuse Finally Ends (SAFE)
Toll-Free: 800-366-8288
Website: http://www.selfinjury.com

If it is an emergency, please call 911.

Chapter 67

Teen Response to Disaster

Reaction of Children to a Disaster

How Do Children Typically React to Disasters?

Many feelings and reactions are shared by people of all ages in response to a disaster. However, special attention is required to meet the needs of children. Typical reactions for children of all ages include:

- fears of future disasters
- loss of interest in school
- regressive behavior
- sleep disturbances and night terrors
- fears of events associated with disaster

Pre-Adolescent (Ages 11–14) Response

Peer reactions are especially significant in this age group. The child needs to feel that his/her fears are both appropriate and shared by others. Responses should be aimed at lessening tensions and anxieties and possible guilt feelings.

This chapter includes: Excerpts from "Reaction of Children to a Disaster," Substance Abuse and Mental Health Services Administration (SAMHSA), April 2003; and excerpts from "Tips for Talking to Children in Trauma," SAMHSA, October 2002; also, "After Disaster: What Teens Can Do," SAMHSA, October 2002.

Typical responses include:

- sleep disturbance, appetite disturbance
- rebellion in the home
- refusal to do chores
- school problems (such as fighting, withdraw, loss of interest, attention seeking behavior)
- physical problems (such as headaches, vague aches and pains, skin eruptions, bowel problems, psychosomatic complaints)
- loss of interest in peer social activities

Some things that may be helpful are:

- group activities geared toward the resumption of routines
- involvement with same age group activity
- group discussions geared toward relieving the disaster and rehearsing appropriate behavior for future disasters
- structured but undemanding responsibilities
- temporary relaxed expectations of performance at school or at home
- additional individual attention and consideration

Adolescent (Ages 14–18) Response

Most of the activities and interest of the adolescent are focused in his/her own age group peers. They tend to be especially distressed by the disruption of their peer group activities and the lack of access to full adult responsibilities in community efforts.

Typical responses include:

- psychosomatic symptoms (such as rashes, bowel problems, asthma)
- headaches and tension
- appetite and sleep disturbance
- hypochondriasis
- amenorrhea or dysmenorrhea

- agitation or decrease in energy level

- apathy

- irresponsible and/or delinquent behavior

- decline in emancipatory struggles over parental control

- poor concentration

Some things that might be helpful include:

- participation in the community rehabilitation or reclamation work

- resumption of social activities, athletics, clubs, etc.

- discussion of disaster experiences with peers, extended family members, significant others

- temporary reduced expectations for level of school and general performance

- discussion of disaster fears within the family setting

(Source: Merrin County Community Mental Health Services and Santa Cruz County Mental Health Services, California)

Tips for Talking to Adolescents in Trauma

Children are just as affected as adults are by a disaster or traumatic event. Some may be affected even more, but no one realizes it. Without intending to, parents may send children a message that it is not all right to talk about the experience. This may cause confusion, self-doubt, and feelings of helplessness for a child. Children need to hear that it is normal to feel frightened during and after a disaster or traumatic event. When you acknowledge and normalize these feelings for your children, it will help them make peace with their experience and move on.

Following exposure to a disaster or traumatic event, children are likely to show signs of stress. Signs include sadness and anxiety, outbursts and tantrums, aggressive behavior, a return to earlier behavior that was outgrown, stomach aches and headaches, and an ongoing desire to stay home from school or away from friends. These reactions are normal and usually do not last long. You can help your pre-adolescent or adolescent child by following these suggestions.

- Provide extra attention and consideration.

- Be there to listen to your children, but do not force them to talk about feelings and emotions.

- Encourage discussion of trauma experiences among peers.

- Promote involvement with community recovery work.

- Urge participation in physical activities.

- Encourage resumption of regular social and recreational activities.

- Rehearse family safety measures for future incidents.

It is important to remember that you do not have to fix how your child feels. Instead, focus on helping your child understand and deal with his or her experiences. Healing is an evolving state for most children, but some may need professional help. If signs of stress do not subside after a few weeks, or if they get worse, consider consulting a mental health professional who has special training in working with children. In time and with help, your children will learn that life does go on.

After Disaster: What Teens Can Do

- Whether or not you were directly affected by a disaster or violent event, it is normal to feel anxious about your own safety, to picture the event in your own mind, and to wonder how you would react in an emergency.

- People react in different ways to trauma. Some become irritable or depressed, others lose sleep or have nightmares, others deny their feelings or simply blank out the troubling event.

- While it may feel better to pretend the event did not happen, in the long run it is best to be honest about your feelings and to allow yourself to acknowledge the sense of loss and uncertainty.

- It is important to realize that, while things may seem off balance for a while, your life will return to normal. It is important to talk with someone about your sorrow, anger, and other emotions, even though it may be difficult to get started.

- You may feel most comfortable talking about your feelings with a teacher, counselor, or church leader. The important thing is that you have someone you trust to confide in about your thoughts and feelings.

- It is common to want to strike back at people who have caused great pain. This desire comes from our outrage for the innocent victims. We must understand, though, that it is futile to respond with more violence. Nothing good is accomplished by hateful language or actions.

- While you will always remember the event, the painful feelings will decrease over time, and you will come to understand that, in learning to cope with tragedy, you have become stronger, more adaptable, and more self-reliant.

Source: This information was developed by Project Heartland—A Project of the Oklahoma Department of Mental Health and Substance Abuse Services in response to the 1995 bombing of the Murrah Federal Building in Oklahoma City. Project Heartland was developed with funds from the Federal Emergency Management Agency in consultation with the Federal Center for Mental Health Services.

Chapter 68

Finding Help for Mental Health Disorders

Where to Go for Help

If you or someone you know could benefit from seeing a mental health professional, these resources can help you find the right care:

- your family physician or health care provider
- mental health division of your local health department
- community mental health center
- family services agency, such as Catholic Charities, Family Services, or Jewish Social Services
- employee assistance program provided by your employer
- professional counselor who works in a mental health center, outpatient clinic, private or group practice, general or psychiatric hospital, or nursing home
- pastoral counselor/member of the clergy
- self-help or mutual support group
- mental health or crisis hotline, drug hotline, or suicide prevention center
- hospital emergency room

This chapter includes: "Finding Mental Health Services," Substance Abuse and Mental Health Services Administration (SAMHSA), July 2003, and "How to Pay for Mental Health Services," SAMHSA, April 2003. All contact information was verified as correct as of May 2006.

How to Pay for Mental Health Services

Why Are Payment Methods Important?

The high cost of health care makes treatment out of reach for many people. Those who do not have health insurance—more than 38 million Americans—often avoid treatment entirely, because costs can be staggering.

What Is Private Insurance?

The majority of working Americans are covered under employer-provided health insurance plans. One type of plan is a standard indemnity policy, which gives people freedom to visit a health care provider of their choice and pay out of pocket for their treatment. The insurance plan reimburses members for some portion of the cost. The other common plan is a managed care plan. Under this plan, medically necessary care is provided in the most cost-effective, or least expensive, way available. Plan members must visit health care providers chosen by the managed care plan. Generally, a co-payment is charged to the patient, but sometimes all care received from providers within the plan is covered. Managed care companies provide services in many States for low-income Medicare and Medicaid beneficiaries. Both types of private health coverage may offer some coverage for mental health treatment. However, this treatment often is not paid for at the same rate as other health care costs.

Resources for the Uninsured

Community-based resources: Many communities have community mental health centers (CMHC). These centers offer a range of mental health treatment and counseling services, usually at a reduced rate for low-income people. CMHC generally require you to have a private insurance plan or to be a recipient of public assistance.

Pastoral counseling: Your church or synagogue can put you in touch with a pastoral counseling program. Certified pastoral counselors, who are ministers in a recognized religious body, have advanced degrees in pastoral counseling, as well as professional counseling experience. Pastoral counseling is often provided on a sliding-scale fee basis.

Self-help groups: Another option is to join a self-help or support group. Such groups give people a chance to learn about, talk about, and work on their common problems, such as alcoholism, substance abuse, depression, family issues, and relationships. Self-help groups are generally free and can be found in virtually every community in America. Many people find them to be effective.

Public assistance: People with severe mental illness may be eligible for several forms of public assistance, both to meet the basic costs of living and to pay for health care. Examples of such programs are Social Security, Medicare, and Medicaid.

- Social Security has two types of programs to help individuals with disabilities. Social Security Disability Insurance provides benefits for those individuals who have worked for a required length of time and have paid Social Security taxes. Supplemental Security Income provides benefits to individuals based on their economic needs (Social Security Administration, 2002).

- Medicare is America's primary Federal health insurance program for people who are 65 or older and for some with disabilities who are under 65. It provides basic protection for the cost of health care. Two programs exist to help people with low incomes receive benefits: the Qualified Medicare Beneficiary (QMB) and the Specified Low-Income Medicare Beneficiary (SLMB) programs.

- Medicaid pays for some health care costs for America's poorest and most vulnerable people. More information about Medicaid and eligibility requirements is available at local welfare and medical assistance offices. Although there are certain Federal requirements, each State also has its own rules and regulations for Medicaid.

Additional Information

American Association of Pastoral Counselors
9504-A Lee Highway
Fairfax, VA 22031-2303
Telephone: 703-385-6967
Fax: 703-352-7725
Website: http://www.aapc.org
E-mail: info@aapc.org

American Psychiatric Association
1000 Wilson Blvd., Suite 1825
Arlington, VA 22209-3901
Toll-Free: 888-357-7924
Phone: 703-907-7300
Website: http://www.psych.org
E-mail: apa@psych.org

Centers for Medicare and Medicaid Services
Toll-Free: 800-633-4227
Toll-Free TTY: 877-486-2048
Website: http://www.cms.gov

Your local social service or welfare office will have further information about Medicaid services in your State.

Depression and Bipolar Support Alliance (DBSA)
730 N. Franklin St., Suite 501
Chicago, IL 60610-7224
Toll-Free: 800-826-3632
Fax: 312-642-7243
Website: http://www.dbsalliance.org
E-mail: questions@dbsalliance.org

National Alliance for the Mentally Ill
Colonial Place Three
2107 Wilson Blvd., Suite 300
Arlington, VA 22201-3042
Toll-Free: 800-950-6264
Fax: 703-524-9094
Website: http://www.nami.org

National Empowerment Center
599 Canal Street
Lawrence, MA 01840
Toll-Free: 800-769-3728
Phone: 978-685-1494
Fax: 978-681-6426
Website: http://www.power2u.org
E-mail: info4@power2u.org

National Institute of Mental Health
NIMH Public Inquiries
6001 Executive Blvd.
Room 8184, MSC 9663
Bethesda, MD 20892-9663
Toll-Free: 866-615-6464
Toll-Free TTY: 866-415-8051
Fax: 301-443-4279
Website: http://www.nimh.nih.gov
E-mail: nimhinfo@nih.gov

National Mental Health Association
2000 N. Beauregard St., 6th Floor
Alexandria, VA 22311
Toll-Free: 800-969-6642
Toll-Free Crisis Helpline: 800-784-2433
Toll-Free TTY: 800-433-5959
Phone: 703-684-7722
Fax: 703-684-5968
Website: http://www.nmha.org

National Mental Health Information Center
P.O. Box 42557
Washington DC 20015
Toll-Free: 800-789-2647
Toll-Free TDD: 866-889-2647
Fax: 240-747-5470
Website: http://www.mentalhealth.samhsa.gov
E-mail: info@mentalhealth.org

Social Security Administration
Office of Public Inquiries
Windsor Park Building
6401 Security Blvd.
Baltimore, MD 21235
Toll-Free: 800-772-1213
Toll-Free TTY: 800-325-0778
Website: http://www.ssa.gov

Part Nine

Teens and Substance Abuse

Chapter 69

Alcohol's Impact on Underage Drinkers

Understanding Underage Drinking

Alcohol is the drug of choice among youth. Many young people are experiencing the consequences of drinking too much, at too early an age. As a result, underage drinking is a leading public health problem in the United States.

Research shows that alcohol drinking is widespread among adolescents. For example, 2002 data from *Monitoring the Future*, an annual survey of U.S. youth, show that more than three-fourths of 12th graders, two-thirds of 10th graders, and nearly half of 8th graders have drunk alcohol at some point in their lives. And when youth drink, they tend to drink heavily. Underage drinkers between the ages of 12 and 17 consume on average four to five drinks per occasion, about five times a month. By comparison, adult drinkers aged 26 and older consume on average two to three drinks per occasion, about nine times a month.

Underage drinking can result in a range of adverse short- and long-term consequences, including academic and/or social problems; physical problems such as hangovers or illnesses; unwanted, unintended, and unprotected sexual activity; physical and sexual assault; memory

This chapter includes: Excerpts from "Understanding Underage Drinking," National Institute on Alcohol Abuse and Alcoholism (NIAAA), NIH Publication No. 04–5465, September 2004; and "Tips for Teens: The Truth about Alcohol," Substance Abuse and Mental Health Services Administration (SAMHSA), August 2004.

problems; increased risk of suicide and homicide; alcohol-related car crashes and other unintentional injuries such as burns, falls, and drowning; and death from alcohol poisoning.

Understanding the Problem

Research suggests that the kind of serious drinking problems previously associated with middle adulthood (including alcoholism) often emerge during adolescence and young adulthood. Analyses of data from the *National Longitudinal Alcohol Epidemiologic Survey* of persons 18 and older in the United States show that drinking early in life increases the likelihood of developing an alcohol use disorder later. For example, the survey showed that young people who began drinking before age 15 were four times more likely to develop alcoholism than those who began drinking at age 21.

The college drinking initiative, launched by the National Institute on Alcohol Abuse and Alcoholism (NIAAA) in 1998, has advanced our understanding of drinking by college students, particularly the heavy episodic consumption commonly called binge drinking. It has also underscored the fact that while some students begin drinking in college, most begin much earlier—in high school, middle school, and even elementary school.

These and other findings that have helped scientists develop a better understanding of alcohol consumption during adolescence have led to a fundamental change in the way researchers think about alcohol abuse and dependence. Scientists now believe that alcohol problems are probably best characterized as developmental disorders, with consequences that play out over the life span.

Significant changes occur in the body during adolescence, including rapid hormonal alterations and the formation of new neural networks in the brain. Adolescence is also a time for trying new experiences and activities that emphasize socializing with peers and conforming to peer-group standards. These new activities may place young people at particular risk for initiating and continuing alcohol consumption. Exposing the brain to alcohol during this period may interfere with important developmental processes and possibly result in short- and/or long-term cognitive impairment. It may also increase the risk for alcohol dependence.

A recent brain imaging study has shown structural differences in the brains of 17-year-olds being treated for alcohol dependence as compared with the brains of those who are not alcohol dependent. Specifically, the hippocampus—a part of the brain important for learning and memory—was smaller in alcohol-dependent research participants than it was in nondependent participants.

It is not clear whether starting to drink at an early age actually causes alcoholism or whether it simply indicates an existing vulnerability to alcohol use disorders. Some evidence indicates that genetic, physiologic, and psychiatric factors may contribute to the relationship between early drinking and subsequent alcoholism. Environmental factors may also be involved, especially in alcoholic families, where children may start drinking earlier because of easier access to alcohol at home, family acceptance of drinking, and lack of parental monitoring.

Future Directions

A variety of prevention and intervention tools directed at the individual, family, school, and community have brought about some positive behavioral change with regard to underage drinking. To determine whether these interventions are enduring and broadly applicable or whether other strategies are needed will require further studies to follow cohorts of young people from childhood through college. Finding lasting solutions to such an entrenched problem will not be easy, but we are confident that diligent research efforts will meet this urgent challenge.

To fully understand the risk and protective factors for, and consequences of, alcohol consumption during the first decades of life, alcohol consumption must be studied as a developmental phenomenon that begins in childhood and continues through adolescence and into young adulthood. A single approach for preventing or treating underage drinking will likely be less effective than multiple, developmentally appropriate approaches.

Tips for Teens: The Truth about Alcohol

The Facts

Alcohol affects your brain. Drinking alcohol leads to a loss of coordination, poor judgment, slowed reflexes, distorted vision, memory lapses, and even blackouts.

Alcohol affects your body. Alcohol can damage every organ in your body. It is absorbed directly into your bloodstream and can increase your risk for a variety of life-threatening diseases, including cancer.

Alcohol affects your self-control. Alcohol depresses your central nervous system, lowers your inhibitions, and impairs your judgment. Drinking can lead to risky behaviors, such as driving when you shouldn't, or having unprotected sex.

Alcohol can kill you. Drinking large amounts of alcohol at one time or very rapidly can cause alcohol poisoning, which can lead to coma or even death. Driving and drinking also can be deadly. In 2003, 31 percent of drivers age 15 to 20 who died in traffic accidents had been drinking alcohol.[1]

Alcohol can hurt you—even if you are not the one drinking. If you are around people who are drinking, you have an increased risk of being seriously injured, involved in car crashes, or affected by violence. At the very least, you may have to deal with people who are sick, out of control, or unable to take care of themselves.

Before You Risk It

Know the law. It is illegal to buy or possess alcohol if you are under age 21.

Get the facts. One drink can make you fail a breath test. In some States, people under age 21 can lose their driver's license, be subject to a heavy fine, or have their car permanently taken away.

Stay informed. Binge drinking means having five or more drinks on one occasion. Studies show that more than 35 percent of adults with an alcohol problem developed symptoms—such as binge drinking—by age 19.[2]

Know the risks. Alcohol is a drug. Mixing it with any other drug can be extremely dangerous. Alcohol and acetaminophen—a common ingredient in over-the-counter (OTC) pain and fever reducers—can damage your liver. Alcohol mixed with other drugs can cause nausea, vomiting, fainting, heart problems, and difficulty breathing.[3] Mixing alcohol and drugs also can lead to coma and death.

Keep your edge. Alcohol is a depressant, or downer, because it reduces brain activity. If you are depressed before you start drinking, alcohol can make you feel worse.

Look around you. Most teens are not drinking alcohol. Research shows that 71 percent of people ages 12–20 have not had a drink in the past month.[4]

Know the Signs

How can you tell if a friend has a drinking problem? Sometimes it is tough to tell. But there are signs you can look for. If your friend has one or more of the following warning signs, he or she may have a problem with alcohol:

- getting drunk on a regular basis

- lying about how much alcohol he or she is using

- believing that alcohol is necessary to have fun

- having frequent hangovers

- feeling rundown, depressed, or even suicidal

- having blackouts—forgetting what he or she did while drinking

Are beer and wine safer than liquor?

No. One 12-ounce bottle of beer or a 5-ounce glass of wine (about a half-cup) has as much alcohol as a 1.5-ounce shot of liquor. Alcohol can make you drunk and cause you problems no matter how you consume it.

Why can't teens drink if their parents can?

Teens' brains and bodies are still developing; alcohol use can cause learning problems or lead to adult alcoholism.[5] People who begin drinking by age 15 are five times more likely to abuse or become dependent on alcohol than those who begin drinking after age 20.[6]

References

1. *Traffic Safety Facts 2003 Data: Young Drivers*, National Highway Traffic Safety Administration. U.S. Department of Transportation, 2004.

2. *Prevention Alert: The Binge Drinking Epidemic.* Substance Abuse and Mental Health Services Administration, 2002.

3. *Harmful Interactions: Mixing Alcohol with Medicines.* National Institute on Alcohol Abuse and Alcoholism, 2003.

4. *2004 National Survey on Drug Use and Health.* Substance Abuse and Mental Health Services Administration, 2005.

5. *Underage Drinking: A Major Public Health Challenge.* National Institute on Alcohol Abuse and Alcoholism, 2003.

6. *The NSDUH Report: Alcohol Dependence or Abuse and Age at First Use.* Substance Abuse and Mental Health Services Administration, 2004.

Additional Information

National Clearinghouse for Alcohol and Drug Information (NCADI)
Toll-Free: 800-729-6686
Toll-Free TDD: 800-487-4889
Website: http://ncadi.samhsa.gov

National Institute on Alcohol Abuse and Alcoholism (NIAAA)
5635 Fishers Lane, MSC 9304
Bethesda, MD 20892-9304
Website: http://www.niaaa.nih.gov
E-mail: niaaaweb-r@exchange.nih.gov

National Youth Anti-Drug Media Campaign
Drug Policy Information Clearinghouse
P.O. Box 6000
Rockville, MD 20849-6000
Toll-Free: 800-666-3332
Phone: 301-519-5212
Website: http://www.mediacampaign.org

Chapter 70

Teen Abuse of Anabolic Steroids

Anabolic Steroids

Have you ever wondered how those bulky weight lifters got so big? While some may have gotten their muscles through a strict regimen of weight-lifting and diet, others may have gotten that way through the illegal use of steroids.

Steroids are synthetic substances similar to the male sex hormone testosterone. They do have legitimate medical uses. Sometimes doctors prescribe anabolic steroids to help people with certain kinds of anemia and men who do not produce enough testosterone on their own. Doctors also prescribe a different kind of steroid, called corticosteroids, to reduce swelling. Corticosteroids are not anabolic steroids and do not have the same harmful effects.

But doctors never prescribe anabolic steroids to young, healthy people to help them build muscles. Without a prescription from a doctor, steroids are illegal.

There are many different kinds of steroids. Here's a list of some of the most common anabolic steroids taken today: Anadrol, Oxandrin, Dianabol, Winstrol, Deca Durabolin, and Equipoise.[1, 5]

Common Street Names

Slang words for steroids are hard to find. Most people just say steroids. On the street, steroids may be called roids or juice.[2] The

"NIDA for Teens: Facts on Drugs: Anabolic Steroids," National Institute on Drug Abuse (NIDA), June 10, 2005.

scientific name for this class of drugs is anabolic androgenic steroids. Anabolic refers to muscle-building. Androgenic refers to increased male characteristics. But even scientists shorten it to anabolic steroids.[3]

How Are They Used?

Some steroid users pop pills. Others use hypodermic needles to inject steroids directly into muscles. When users take more and more of a drug over and over again, they are called abusers. Abusers have been known to take doses 10 to 100 times higher than the amount prescribed for medical reasons by a doctor.

Many steroid users take two or more kinds of steroids at once. Called stacking, this way of taking steroids is supposed to get users bigger faster. Some abusers pyramid their doses in 6–12 week cycles. At the beginning of the cycle, the steroid user starts with low doses and slowly increases to higher doses. In the second half of the cycle, they gradually decrease the amount of steroids. Neither of these methods has been proven to work.[1]

Teens Using Steroids

Most teens are smart and stay away from steroids. As part of a 2002 NIDA-funded study, teens were asked if they ever tried steroids—even once. Only 2.5% of 8th graders ever tried steroids; only 3.5% of 10th graders; and 4% of 12th graders.[4]

Steroids Cause Hormone Imbalances

For teens, hormone balance is important. Hormones are involved in the development of a girl's feminine traits and a boy's masculine traits. When someone abuses steroids, gender mix-ups happen.

Using steroids, guys can experience shrunken testicles and reduced sperm count. They can also end up with breasts, a condition called gynecomastia.

Using steroids, girls can become more masculine. Their voices deepen. They grow excessive body hair. Their breast size decreases.[1]

Teens at Risk for Stunted Growth

Teens who abuse steroids before the typical adolescent growth spurt risk staying short and never reaching their full adult height.

Why? Because the body is programmed to stop growing after puberty. When hormone levels reach a certain point, the body thinks it has already gone through puberty. So, bones get the message to stop growing way too soon.[1]

Steroid Abuse Can Be Fatal

When steroids get into the body, they go to different organs and muscles. Steroids affect individual cells and make them create proteins. These proteins spell trouble.[6]

The liver, for example, can grow tumors and develop cancer. Steroid abusers may also develop a rare condition called peliosis hepatis in which blood-filled cysts crop up on the liver. Both the tumors and cysts can rupture and cause internal bleeding.

Steroids are no friend of the heart, either. Abusing steroids can cause heart attacks and strokes, even in young athletes. Steroid use can lead to a condition called atherosclerosis, which causes fat deposits inside arteries to disrupt blood flow. When blood flow to the heart is blocked, a heart attack can occur. If blood flow to the brain is blocked, a stroke can result.[1]

To bulk up the artificial way—using steroids—puts teens at risk for more than liver disease and cardiovascular disease. Steroids can weaken the immune system, which is what helps the body fight against germs and disease. That means that illnesses and diseases have an easy target in a steroid abuser.[5]

By injecting steroids by needle, teens can add human immunodeficiency virus (HIV, the virus that causes acquired immune deficiency syndrome, or AIDS) and hepatitis B and C to their list of health hazards. Many abusers share non-sterile works or drug injection equipment that can spread life-threatening viral infections.[1]

Steroids Can Cause Extreme Mood Changes

Steroids can also mess with your head. Research shows that high doses of steroids can cause extreme fluctuations in emotions, from euphoria to rage. That's right. Rage can come from how steroids act on your brain.[7]

Your moods and emotions are balanced by the limbic system of your brain. Steroids act on the limbic system and may cause irritability and mild depression. Eventually, steroids can cause mania, delusions, and violent aggression or roid rage.[5]

Steroids' Disfiguring Effects

Last, but not least, steroids have disfiguring effects—severe acne, greasy hair, and baldness (in both guys and girls).[1] The bottom line is: Science proves the serious risks of steroid use.

References

1. National Institute on Drug Abuse. *NIDA Research Report— Steroid Abuse and Addiction* (http://www.drugabuse.gov/ ResearchReports/Steroids/ AnabolicSteroids.html). NIH Pub. No. 00-3721. Bethesda, MD: NIDA, NIH, DHHS. Printed 1991. Reprinted 1994, 1996. Revised April, 2000.

2. National Institute on Drug Abuse. *Commonly Abused Drugs Chart* (http://www.drugabuse.gov/DrugPages/DrugsofAbuse .html). Bethesda, MD: NIDA, NIH, DHHS, 2000.

3. National Institute on Drug Abuse. *NIDA InfoFacts: Steroids* (Anabolic-Androgenic) (http://www.drugabuse.gov/Infofax/ steroids.html). Bethesda, MD: NIDA, NIH, DHHS. Retrieved June 2000.

4. National Institute on Drug Abuse. *NIDA InfoFacts: High School and Youth Trends* (http://www.drugabuse.gov/Infofax/ HSYouthtrends.html). Bethesda, MD: NIDA, NIH, DHHS. Retrieved June 2003.

5. National Institute on Drug Abuse. *Mind Over Matter: The Brain's Response to Steroids* (http://teens.drugabuse.gov/mom/ mom_ster1.asp). NIH Pub. No. 00—3858. Bethesda, MD: NIDA, NIH, DHHS. Printed 1997. Reprinted 1998, 2000.

6. National Institute on Drug Abuse. *Mind Over Matter: The Brain's Response to Drugs Teacher's Guide* (http://teens.drug abuse.gov/mom/tg_intro.asp). NIH Pub. No. 020—3592. Bethesda, MD: NIDA, NIH, DHHS. Printed 1997. Reprinted 1998, 2002. Revised 2000.

7. Pope, H.G., Jr.; Kouri, E.M.; and Hudson, J.I. Effects of supra-physiologic doses of testosterone on mood and aggression in normal men: A randomized controlled trial. *Archives of General Psychiatry* 57(2):133-140, 2000.

Chapter 71

Tobacco and Teens

Chapter Contents

Section 71.1

What Youth Should Know about Tobacco

This section includes: Excerpts from "Youth and Tobacco Use: Current Estimates," Centers for Disease Control and Prevention (CDC), November 2005; "Tips 4 Youth: Teens and Tobacco," CDC, January 2005; excerpts from "You(th) and Tobacco," CDC, June 2005; and "Parents: Nicotine Is a Real Threat to Your Kids," by Alan I. Leshner, Ph.D., Director, National Institute on Drug Abuse (NIDA), February 2005.

Youth and Tobacco Use: Current Estimates

Cigarette Smoking

*   Twenty-two percent of high school students in the United States are current cigarette smokers—21.9 percent of females and 21.8 percent of males.

*   Twenty–five percent of whites, 18 percent of Hispanics, and 15 percent of African Americans in high school are current cigarette smokers.

*   Eight percent of middle school students in this country are current cigarette smokers, with estimates slightly higher for females (nine percent) than males (eight percent).

*   Nine percent of whites, ten percent of Hispanics, eight percent of African Americans, and three percent of Asian Americans in middle school are current cigarette smokers.

*   Each day, approximately 3,900 young people between the ages of 12 and 17 years initiate cigarette smoking in the United States. In this age group, each day an estimated 1,500 young people become daily cigarette smokers in this country.

Other Tobacco Use

*   Thirteen percent of high school students are current cigar smokers, with estimates higher for males (18 percent) than for females (eight percent). Nationally, an estimated five percent of

all middle school students are current cigar smokers, with estimates of seven percent for males and four percent for females.

- An estimated ten percent of males in high school are current smokeless tobacco users, as are an estimated four percent of males in middle school.

- An estimated three percent of high school students are current users of bidis; bidi use is more common among males (four percent) than females (two percent). An estimated two percent of middle school students are bidi users, with estimates of three percent for males and two percent for females.

Factors Associated with Tobacco Use among Youth

- Factors associated with youth tobacco use include low socioeconomic status, use and approval of tobacco use by peers or siblings, smoking by parents or guardians, accessibility, availability and price of tobacco products, a perception that tobacco use is normative, lack of parental support or involvement, low levels of academic achievement, lack of skills to resist influences to tobacco use, lower self-image or self-esteem, belief in functional benefits of tobacco use, and lack of self-efficacy to refuse offers of tobacco.

- Tobacco use in adolescence is associated with many other health risk behaviors, including higher risk sexual behavior and use of alcohol or other drugs.

Tips for Youth

You are educated, you are smart, and you are aware. You know what is in and you know what is out. But do you know the whole story about what is really in cigarettes?

- Did you know that cigarettes contain formaldehyde—the same stuff used to preserve dead frogs?

- Did you know that the same cyanide found in rat poison is available in the cigarette smoke nearest you—whether you are a smoker or just hanging around people who smoke?

- How about the nicotine in cigarettes? You probably already know that it is addictive, but did you know that it is also a potent insecticide found in bug spray?

Youth and Tobacco

Tobacco and Athletic Performance

- Do not get trapped. Nicotine in cigarettes, cigars, and spit tobacco is addictive.

- Nicotine narrows your blood vessels and puts added strain on your heart.

- Smoking can wreck lungs and reduce oxygen available for muscles used during sports.

- Smokers suffer shortness of breath almost three times more often than nonsmokers.

- Smokers run slower and cannot run as far, affecting overall athletic performance.

- Cigars and spit tobacco are not safe alternatives.

Tobacco and Personal Appearance

- Tobacco smoke can make hair and clothes stink.

- Tobacco stains teeth and causes bad breath.

- Short-term use of spit tobacco can cause cracked lips, white spots, sores, and bleeding in the mouth.

- Surgery to remove oral cancers caused by tobacco use can lead to serious changes in the face. Sean Marcee, a high school star athlete who used spit tobacco, died of oral cancer when he was 19 years old.

Know the Truth

Despite all the tobacco use on television and in movies, music videos, billboards, and magazines—most teens, adults, and athletes do not use tobacco. Make friends, develop athletic skills, control weight, be independent, be cool, play sports. Do not waste (burn) money on tobacco. Spend it on music, clothes, computer games, and movies. Get involved: make your team, school, and home tobacco-free; teach others; join community efforts to prevent tobacco use.

Parents—Help Keep Your Kids Tobacco-Free

Kids who use tobacco may:

- cough and have asthma attacks more often and develop respiratory problems leading to more sick days, more doctor bills, and poorer athletic performance

- be more likely to use alcohol and other drugs such as cocaine and marijuana

- become addicted to tobacco and find it extremely hard to quit

Spit tobacco and cigars are not safe alternatives to cigarettes; low-tar and additive-free cigarettes are not safe either. Tobacco use is the single most preventable cause of death in the United States causing heart disease, cancers, and strokes.

Take a Stand at Home—Early and Often

- Despite the impact of movies, music, and television, parents can be the greatest influence in their kids' lives.

- Talk directly to children about the risks of tobacco use; if friends or relatives died from tobacco-related illness, let your kids know.

- If you use tobacco, you can still make a difference. Your best move, of course, is to try to quit. Meanwhile, do not use tobacco in your children's presence, do not offer it to them, and do not leave it where they can easily get it.

- Start the dialog about tobacco use at age five or six and continue through their high school years. Many kids start using tobacco by age 11, and many are addicted by age 14.

- Know if your kids' friends use tobacco. Talk about ways to refuse tobacco.

- Discuss with kids the false glamorization of tobacco on billboards, and other media, such as movies, television, and magazines.

Parents: Nicotine Is a Real Threat to Your Kids

Parents naturally worry about the health and safety of their children. Many parents teach their kids to avoid getting involved with drugs, although sometimes adults forget about the drug most abused by adolescents—nicotine.

Every year, teens continue to light up even though there is strong public awareness about the health hazards of smoking. When you are young, it is hard to think about the consequences of your actions. Kids do not project that smoking today can lead to negative effects in their futures—increased risk of cancer, heart attack, and stroke in adulthood.

Many kids think they will just try one cigarette or two or three. These young smokers believe that they will be able to control their habit over time. Young people may experiment with cigars and chewing tobacco, which are also dangerous. Others try bidis, thinking they are a safe alternative to cigarettes.

Colorfully packaged with a variety of flavors like cinnamon, orange, and chocolate, these unfiltered cigarettes from India have 28 percent higher nicotine concentration than regular cigarettes.

There is good news—the number of teens who currently smoke has gradually declined since 1996. But there is also bad news—over four million youth between the ages of 12 and 17 are smokers. In fact, by the time they leave high school, more than one-third of graduates are active smokers.

Nicotine is a powerfully addictive drug. Once your teen is addicted, it will be very difficult to quit. The cause of addiction is simple. Nicotine goes straight to the brain. The human brain has circuits that control feelings of pleasure. Dopamine—a brain chemical—contributes to the desire to consume drugs. Nicotine spikes an increase in dopamine.

When your teen smokes, he or she inhales the nicotine. It goes quickly to the brain. In just ten seconds, the pleasurable effects of smoking reach peak levels. Within a few minutes, the pleasure is gone, and the craving for a cigarette begins a new cycle. A teen can easily get hooked on nicotine, although it takes much more effort to quit. Many smokers find it hard to stay away from the drug's effects.

The National Institute on Drug Abuse (NIDA) is concerned about teen nicotine addiction and is working to determine the best methods for helping adolescents quit. NIDA has opened a Teen Tobacco Addiction Treatment Research Center in Baltimore, Maryland, to find the best treatments for young smokers. Currently, the Center is assessing the nicotine patch and nicotine gum to see how safe, tolerable, and effective they are for adolescents. The Center is also determining whether teens use these quitting aids properly. At the same time, researchers are trying to find out whether these therapies work better alone or in combination with counseling and group support.

Nicotine addiction is a disease. But it is preventable. Not starting to smoke is the best form of prevention. Talk to your kids about the threat of smoking. With your guidance, maybe they will not light up.

Section 71.2

Bidis, Kreteks, and Hookah Pipes Deliver Nicotine to Teens

This section includes: Excerpts from "Bidis and Kreteks Fact Sheet," Centers for Disease Control and Prevention (CDC), November 2005; and "Hookah Pipes—More or Less Harmful Than Cigarettes?" reprinted with permission from Go Ask Alice!, Columbia University's Health Q&A Internet Service, at www.goaskalice.columbia.edu. Copyright © 2006 by The Trustees of Columbia University.

Bidis and Kreteks

Bidis (pronounced bee-dees) are small, thin hand-rolled cigarettes imported to the United States primarily from India and other Southeast Asian countries. They consist of tobacco wrapped in a tendu or temburni leaf (plants native to Asia), and may be secured with a colorful string at one or both ends. Bidis can be flavored (chocolate, cherry, and mango) or unflavored. They have higher concentrations of nicotine, tar, and carbon monoxide than conventional cigarettes sold in the United States.

Kreteks (pronounced cree-techs) are sometimes referred to as clove cigarettes. Imported from Indonesia, kreteks typically contain a mixture consisting of tobacco, cloves, and other additives. As with bidis, standardized machine-smoking analyses indicate that kreteks deliver more nicotine, carbon monoxide, and tar than conventional cigarettes. There is no evidence to indicate that bidis or kreteks are safe alternatives to conventional cigarettes.

Health Effects

* No research studies on the health effects of bidis have been conducted in the United States. Research studies from India indicate that bidi smoking is associated with an increased risk for oral cancer, as well as an increased risk for cancer of the lung, stomach, and esophagus.

- Research studies in India have shown that bidi smoking is associated with a more than three-fold increased risk for coronary heart disease and acute myocardial infarction (heart attack), and a nearly four-fold increased risk for chronic bronchitis.

- Kretek smoking is associated with an increased risk for acute lung injury, especially among susceptible individuals with asthma or respiratory infections.

- No research studies on the long-term health effects of kreteks have been conducted in the United States. Research in Indonesia has shown that regular kretek smokers have 13–20 times the risk for abnormal lung function compared with nonsmokers.

Current Estimates

- There are no national adult estimates for bidi or kretek smoking in the United States.

- An estimated three percent of high school students are current bidi smokers. Bidi smoking is more than twice as common among male (four percent) compared with female (two percent) high school students.

- An estimated two percent of middle school students are current bidi smokers. Bidi smoking is more common among male (three percent) compared with female (two percent) middle school students.

- An estimated three percent of high school students are current kretek smokers. Kretek smoking is more common among male (three percent) than female (two percent) high school students.

- An estimated two percent of middle school students are current kretek smokers. Kretek use is more common among male (two percent) compared with female (one percent) middle school students.

Hookah Pipes—More or Less Harmful Than Cigarettes?

Hookah pipes (also known as water pipes, sheesha, nargile, and argileh) originated in what is today Turkey and are now popular throughout the Middle East as a leisurely, social, after-meal activity. Across the United States, bars and cafes that offer hookah pipes are popping up. In a hookah pipe, the tobacco (often fruit flavored) is heated by coals, and the resulting smoke passes through tubes and water so that it cools down by the time the person inhales. The tobacco mixture used in the pipes is usually 30 percent tobacco and 70 percent fruit flavorings, molasses, and/or honey—though the amounts can vary by manufacturer.

Some people feel that smoking a hookah is safer than other methods of tobacco smoking since the water is thought to filter out the harmful compounds before the smoke is inhaled. But, compared to cigarettes, little research exists on the health risks of hookah smoking. To date, there have been no studies looking specifically at the consequences of smoking the non-tobacco substances that are used for flavoring. The little research that does exist, though, shows preliminary evidence that suggest hookahs are not any safer than cigarettes, and as with cigarettes, effects may include a higher chance of developing heart disease and/or lung cancer. On the other hand, because hookah smoking is usually a social activity, those who use hookah pipes might not be smoking as often or as much as cigarette, cigar, and pipe smokers.

To risk stating the obvious, the tobacco used in a hookah is still tobacco, so its smokers are still exposed to:

- Nicotine: The addictive chemical in tobacco products. Research suggests that hookah smoke delivers equal or greater amounts of nicotine compared to cigarettes, meaning hookah smoking has the potential to be addictive.

- Tar: The brown, sticky material that leads to cancer, emphysema, and other health problems in smokers, as well as causes stains on teeth and fingers.

- Carbon monoxide: A colorless, odorless gas that is toxic to humans. The amount produced by a hookah pipe depends on several factors, including the kind of tobacco, the type of charcoal, and the size of the pipe being used. In general, using commercial (quick-lighting) charcoal makes for higher levels of carbon monoxide. Also, smaller hookah pipes appear to deliver the most carbon monoxide, followed by cigarettes, with larger hookahs producing relatively less.

Source: Reprinted with permission from Go Ask Alice!, Columbia University's Health Q&A Internet Service, at www.goaskalice. columbia.edu. Copyright © 2006 by The Trustees of Columbia University.

Section 71.3

Myths about Smokeless Tobacco

"Smokeless Tobacco: Especially for Kids!" National Cancer Institute (NCI), and excerpts from "Smokeless Tobacco Fact Sheet," Centers for Disease Control and Prevention (CDC), November 2005.

Smokeless Tobacco

The makers of smokeless tobacco spend a lot of money to advertise and promote their products because the more people who use smokeless tobacco and the more smokeless tobacco each person uses, the more money they make. Promotional strategies, including free sampling, sponsorships, and coupons, are a large part of advertising. In 2001, $219 million was spent to advertise moist and dry snuff and about $18 million was spent to advertise chewing tobacco. (It is the tobacco companies' job to get you to use smokeless tobacco and keep on using it.) A Federal Trade Commission Report released in 2003, shows that in 2001 smokeless tobacco advertising in magazines increased to a record high of $21.96 million. The spending for distribution of free samples of smokeless tobacco products also reached a record high of $17.89 million in 2001.

Smokeless tobacco companies have used many methods to get people to use their products. Here are some of the ways they advertise:

- give away free samples and gifts

- show how smokeless tobacco users are independent, macho men who take risks, are cool, and enjoy life—making your think that if you use their products, you will be like the people in the ads

- show you how to use starter packs of dip in order to make it easy for you to use it

- make starter packs with less nicotine and add flavorings such as mint and cherry, so that it is not as strong or as bad tasting as full-strength smokeless tobacco to get you used to it

- offer pouches that are packets of smokeless tobacco so you will not get a lot of loose tobacco or float in your mouth, making it appear cleaner than loose smokeless tobacco

- offer clothing and other stuff for sale

- say it is an alternative to smoking—implying that it is safe—even by naming it smokeless implies safety

- sponsor events such as rodeos and car races implying that smokeless tobacco can make you a better athlete or you can be like the rodeo or car racing star if you use smokeless tobacco

- sponsor music concerts

Once you know what the smokeless tobacco advertisers do to try to get you to start using smokeless tobacco, you can resist them. Advertisers want you to believe what they are saying so you will buy and use their products.

Myths and Truths about Smokeless Tobacco

Myth: Smokeless tobacco is a safe alternative to cigarettes.

Truth: Just because there is no smoke, does not mean that smokeless tobacco is safe. Smokeless tobacco can cause cancer and a whole bunch of other bad health effects.

Myth: Smokeless tobacco makes you a better athlete.

Truth: No way. You may feel like you can perform better in sports, but you do not because you cannot. Studies have shown that athletes who use smokeless tobacco do not play better or move faster.

Myth: You can use a little smokeless tobacco and not get hooked.

Truth: Even a little smokeless tobacco has enough nicotine in it to get you addicted if you keep using it. Do not be fooled by thinking you can use just a little and not get addicted.

Myth: Because baseball players and other sports figures use smokeless tobacco, it is okay for you to use it, too.

Truth: The baseball players who use smokeless tobacco say they want to quit, but they are hooked. They did not know when they started using smokeless tobacco that they would not be able to quit or that using smokeless tobacco is bad for your health.

Myth: Since most people use smokeless tobacco and other tobacco, you might as well too.

Truth: Actually, most people do not use tobacco, but kids tend to think more people use tobacco than actually do. When you see so much advertising, smokeless tobacco for sale on the store counters, or people who use smokeless tobacco, you may think most people use it, but they do not.

Myth: Since smokeless tobacco is sold in stores in the United States where kids shop and in areas where kids go, kids can buy smokeless tobacco.

Truth: It is illegal to sell smokeless tobacco or any other kind of tobacco, including cigarettes and cigars to anyone under the age of 18. The Food and Drug Administration requires that sellers of tobacco ask for identification that includes the birth date and picture of the person trying to buy tobacco to make sure they are not selling to people who are under 18 years of age.

Myth: Even if you use smokeless tobacco, you can quit any time you want.

Truth: Kids overrate their ability to be able to quit. The truth is that if you are hooked, it is not easy to quit. But you can do it.

Do Not Start—You Have the Power!

By being aware of the myths and truths about smokeless tobacco, and the truth about smokeless tobacco advertising, you have the power to not start using smokeless tobacco.

When you become addicted to smokeless tobacco, you can feel like you have lost your power over the choice of whether or not to use it. Smokeless tobacco contains the same addictive chemical as cigarettes—nicotine. When you are addicted to a drug, like the nicotine in tobacco, you continue to use it even though you know it is causing you harm. This means that you may plan to only use smokeless tobacco occasionally or for a short while, but when you become addicted you may not be able to stop when you want to. The best thing to do is to never start using smokeless tobacco. You may see your friends, relatives, and other kids using smokeless tobacco or they may ask you to try it with them. Kids do not think anything bad will happen to them because they are young and feel like nothing can hurt them. It is hard to imagine that you may some day get cancer from using smokeless tobacco today.

Sports and Other Events

Baseball—It is true that about 35 to 40% of major league baseball players use smokeless tobacco. But most of them want to kick the habit. For most players, health concerns are the main reason they want to quit. Others want to quit for their families. And some have made quitting a personal challenge.

Baseball players have been using smokeless tobacco since the mid-1800s. At first they used smokeless tobacco to help keep their mouths wet on the dry, dusty fields. Eventually using smokeless tobacco was the thing to do. Although more baseball players smoked cigarettes than used smokeless tobacco in the 1950s, they started going back to smokeless tobacco in the 1970s when people learned about the dangers of smoking cigarettes. In 1990, Major League Baseball® issued a report on the hazards of smokeless tobacco and started efforts to help players stay off smokeless tobacco or quit using smokeless tobacco. Since then, efforts have continued with many baseball players helping educate young baseball players about the dangers of smokeless tobacco.

It is estimated that 40–50% or minor league baseball players use smokeless tobacco. In 1991, minor league baseball banned the use of smokeless tobacco at the rookie level and in 1993 extended the ban throughout all of minor leagues.

College sports—In 1994, the National Collegiate Athletic Association (NCAA) banned the use of all tobacco products, including smokeless tobacco, for coaches, game officials, and student athletes in all sports during practice and competition. A student athlete who uses tobacco products during practice or competition is automatically disqualified for the remainder of that practice or game.

Rodeos, car racing, and music concerts—Some smokeless tobacco manufacturers sponsor events as a way to tie smokeless tobacco with images such as rodeos, car racing, and music concerts. It is another type of promotion to get you to use smokeless tobacco.

Smokeless Tobacco Health Effects

The two main types of smokeless tobacco in the United States are chewing tobacco and snuff. Chewing tobacco comes in the form of loose leaf, plug, or twist. Snuff is finely ground tobacco that can be dry, moist, or in sachets (tea bag-like pouches). Although some forms of snuff can be used by sniffing or inhaling into the nose, most smokeless tobacco users place the product in their cheek or between their gum and cheek. Users then suck on the tobacco and spit out the tobacco juices, which is why smokeless tobacco is often referred to as spit or spitting tobacco. Smokeless tobacco is a significant health risk and is not a safe substitute for smoking cigarettes.

Health Effects

- Smokeless tobacco contains 28 cancer-causing agents (carcinogens). It is a known cause of human cancer, as it increases the risk of developing cancer of the oral cavity. Oral health problems strongly associated with smokeless tobacco use are leukoplakia (a lesion of the soft tissue that consists of a white patch or plaque that cannot be scraped off) and recession of the gums.

- Smokeless tobacco use can lead to nicotine addiction and dependence.

- Adolescents who use smokeless tobacco are more likely to become cigarette smokers.

High-Risk Populations and Current Estimates

- Smokeless tobacco use in the United States is higher among young white males; American Indians/Alaska Natives; people living in southern and north central states; and people who are employed in blue collar occupations, service/laborer jobs, or who are unemployed.

- Nationally, an estimated three percent of adults are current smokeless tobacco users. Smokeless tobacco use is much higher among men (six percent) than women (0.3 percent).

- In the United States, four percent of American Indian/Alaska Natives, four percent of whites, one percent of African Americans, one percent of Hispanics, and 0.6 percent of Asian-American adults are current smokeless tobacco users.

- An estimated seven percent of high school students are current smokeless tobacco users. Smokeless tobacco is more common among males (11 percent) than female high school students (two percent). Estimates by race/ethnicity are eight percent for white, five percent for Hispanic, and three percent for African American high school students.

- An estimated three percent of middle school students are current smokeless tobacco users. Smokeless tobacco is more common among male (four percent) than female (two percent) middle school students. Estimates by race/ethnicity are three percent for white, one percent for Asian, two percent for African American, and four percent for Hispanic middle school students.

Other Information

- During 2001, the five largest tobacco manufacturers spent $236.7 million on smokeless tobacco advertising and promotion.

- The two leading smokeless tobacco brands for users aged 12 years or older are Skoal (30 percent) and Copenhagen (22 percent).

Additional Information

CDC Office on Smoking and Health
Mailstop K-50
4770 Buford Hwy. NE
Atlanta, GA 30341-3717
Toll-Free: 800-232-4636
Phone: 770-488-5705
Website: http://www.cdc.gov/tobacco
E-mail: tobaccoinfo@cdc.gov

Chapter 72

Teen Abuse of Prescription and Over-the-Counter Medications

Prescription Medicine Misuse and Abuse: A Growing Problem

Prescription medication misuse by teens and young adults is a growing problem in the United States. As reported in the Partnership for a Drug Free America's annual tracking study:

- One in six teens has abused a prescription pain medication.
- One in ten report abusing prescription stimulants and tranquilizers.
- One in eleven has abused cough medication.

Many teens think these drugs are safe because they have legitimate uses, but taking them without a prescription to get high or self-medicate can be as dangerous—and addictive—as using street narcotics and other illicit drugs.

What Age Teens Are Abusing Prescription Medications?

Kids as young as 12 are trying or using prescription medications non-medically—to get high or for self-medicating.

This chapter includes: "Prescription Medicine Misuse and Abuse: A Growing Problem," © Partnership for a Drug-Free America, 2005. Used with permission. And, "Legal but Lethal: The Danger of Abusing Over-the-Counter Drugs," Substance Abuse and Mental Health Services Administration (SAMHSA), May 2005.

Pharmaceuticals are often more available to 12 year olds than illicit drugs because they can be taken from the medicine cabinet at home, rather than marijuana which necessitates knowing someone who uses or sells the drug. Also, pills may have a perception of safety because they are easier to take than smoking pot or drinking alcohol and are professionally manufactured in a lab.

What Types of Prescription Medications Are Teens Abusing?

The National Survey on Drug Use and Health identifies four types of prescription medications that are commonly abused—pain relievers, stimulants, sedatives, and tranquilizers. Eleven percent of teens (aged 12–17) reported lifetime non-medical use of pain relievers and four percent reported lifetime non-medical use of stimulants.

Do Different Groups Abuse Different Types of Medications?

Yes. Painkillers are the most common pharmaceutical abused by teens, especially by younger teens. Stimulant abuse is more common among older teens and college students than younger teens. Girls are more likely to be current (past month) abusers of prescription medications than boys (4.3 vs. 3.6 percent). (Source: 2002 National Survey on Drug Use and Health.)

What Can I Do to Help to Prevent My Child from Misusing Prescription Medications?

One easy way to prevent it is to keep all prescription medication hidden: Parents and family members whose homes teens visit should keep prescription medications out of teens' reach, rather than in the medicine cabinet. You should also talk to your teen and warn them that taking prescription medications without a doctor's supervision can be just as dangerous and as potentially lethal as taking illicit drugs. For example, pain killers are made from opioids, the same substance as in heroin.

How Can I Talk to My Kids about Pharmaceutical Medication Abuse?

Starting a conversation about drugs with your kids is never easy—but it also is not as difficult as you may think. Take advantage of everyday teachable moments and, in no time at all, you will have developed an ongoing dialogue with your child. Teachable moments refer to using everyday events in your life to point out things you would like your child to know about. When you talk to your kids about drugs, make a special point to tell kids how dangerous prescription medication abuse is.

What to Tell Your Child about Prescription Medications

- Pharmaceuticals taken without a prescription or a doctor's supervision can be just as dangerous as taking illicit drugs or alcohol.

- Abusing painkillers is like abusing heroin because their ingredients (both are opioids) are very similar.

- Prescription medications are powerful substances. While sick people taking medication under a doctor's care can benefit enormously, prescription medication can have a very different impact on a well person.

- Many pills look pretty much the same, but depending on the drug and the dosage the effects can vary greatly from mild to lethal.

- Prescription medications, as all drugs, can cause dangerous interactions with other drugs or chemicals in the body.

Legal but Lethal: The Danger of Abusing Over-the-Counter Drugs

Parents worry about their child being offered drugs from a stranger on a street corner or a friend at a party. But a child can get deadly drugs from a person you might never suspect—you. The over-the-counter (OTC) drugs you use to soothe a cough or clear a stuffy nose can be abused by kids looking for an easy and cheap way to get high.

OTC drugs are legal and mostly safe when used as directed, which may lead kids to believe that these drugs are always safe to take. The truth is, medication abuse can lead to addiction, overdose, and death. It is up to you to keep track of your child's use of OTC drugs and to stay alert for signs of abuse.

A Dangerous Dose

Nearly half of OTC drugs, more than 125 products, contain an ingredient called dextromethorphan (or DXM). It is in cough suppressants that can be found in stores in caplet or liquid form. It also can be ordered on the Internet.

Street names for DXM include:

- candy
- C-C-C
- dex
- DM
- drex
- red devils
- robo
- rojo
- skittles
- tussin
- velvet
- vitamin D

Street names for DXM abuse include:

- dexing
- robotripping
- robodosing

When taken in very large doses, DXM can produce a high. It also can pose a real danger to the user, including:

- impaired judgment and mental functioning
- loss of coordination
- dizziness
- nausea
- hot flashes
- hallucinations
- brain damage
- seizure
- death

Watch for Signs

Watch for signs that your child may be abusing DXM or other OTC drugs:

- Your child takes large amounts of cold or cough remedies or takes a medication even when not ill.
- OTC drugs seem to vanish from your medicine cabinet.
- You find OTC drugs stashed in your child's room or backpack.

Falling grades, mood swings, and changes in normal habits or appearance also can signal a possible drug abuse problem. One in 11 teens abused OTC medications, such as cough medicine. The problem is more common than you might think.

Keep Your Child Safe

Because OTC drugs are easy to get and legal to purchase, young people may not realize how harmful they can be. As parents, you need to know the facts about OTC drugs and warn your children. Let them know that OTC products are not safer to misuse simply because they are legal, have a legitimate purpose, and are easy to buy. Other ways you can protect your children include:

- Monitor the OTC drugs in your home. Keep track of how much medicine is in each bottle.
- Avoid overstocking OTC drugs in your home.
- Do not allow your child to keep OTC drugs in his bedroom, backpack, or school locker.
- Monitor your child's Internet use. Watch out for Web sites your child may be visiting that promote OTC or other drug abuse.
- Role model responsible use of OTC and prescription medications.

Talking with your child about the responsible use of OTC drugs is one of the best ways to keep your child safe. Teach your child how to read and follow directions on the labels of all OTC drugs, and always monitor your child's use of these medications. OTC drugs are meant to help people, not hurt them, so make sure your child knows the health risks of abusing medicines.

Chapter 73

Teen Use of Illicit Drugs

How significant is teen drug use?

Drug use among teenagers in the United States is a serious concern. In 2003 more than 7.5 million individuals aged 12 to 17 reported having used an illicit drug at least once in their lifetime. In the same year students in grades nine through twelve indicated that 40.2 percent of respondents had used marijuana, 12.1 percent had used inhalants, 11.1 percent had used MDMA (also known as ecstasy), 8.7 percent had used cocaine, 7.6 percent had used methamphetamine, 6.1 percent had illegally used steroids, 3.3 percent had used heroin, and 3.2 percent had injected an illegal drug one or more times during their lifetime. Furthermore, 9.9 percent of student respondents nationwide tried marijuana for the first time before the age of 13, 28.7 percent had been offered, sold, or given an illegal drug on school property during the year preceding the survey, and 5.8 percent had used marijuana on school property one or more times during the 30 days preceding the survey.

What is the correlation between age of first drug use and dependence?

Adults who first used drugs at a younger age were more likely to be classified with illicit drug dependence or abuse than adults who

"Teens and Drugs: Fast Facts," National Drug Intelligence Center of the U.S. Department of Justice, Product No. 2004-L0559-011, November 2004.

initiated use at an older age. For example, among adults aged 18 or older who first tried marijuana at age 14 or younger, 13.0 percent were classified with illicit drug dependence or abuse compared with only 2.8 percent of adults who had first used marijuana at age 18 or older.

Teens who first used marijuana before age 17 were shown to have smaller brains and to be physically smaller in height and weight than teens who first used marijuana after age 17. Exposure to marijuana and other drugs at certain critical periods, such as early adolescence, may alter normal patterns of development.

What are some of the risks specific to marijuana use?

Marijuana use, which is prevalent among youth, has been shown to interfere with short-term memory, learning, and psychomotor skills. Motivation and psychosexual/emotional development also may be affected.

Early adolescent marijuana use increases the risk in late adolescence of not graduating from high school, delinquency, having multiple sexual partners, and not always using condoms. Such marijuana use can result in perceiving drugs as not harmful, having long-term problems with cigarettes, alcohol, and marijuana, and having friends who exhibit deviant behavior.

In addition, early adolescent marijuana use is related to later adolescent problems that limit the acquisition of skills necessary for employment and heighten the risks of contracting human immunodeficiency virus (HIV) and abusing legal and illegal substances.

What are some risks associated with the use of other illicit drugs?

Any illicit drug use by adolescents can have immediate and long-term health and social consequences. Overall, mental health problems including depression, developmental lags, apathy, withdrawal, conduct problems, personality disorders, suicidal thoughts, attempted suicide, suicide, and other psychosocial dysfunctions are frequently linked to substance abuse among adolescents. Drug abuse has been shown to increase the likelihood of psychiatric disorders.

Abuse of specific drugs exposes users to a range of serious consequences. Cocaine use is linked with health problems including eating disorders, disabilities, and death from heart attacks and strokes. Hallucinogens can affect brain chemistry and result in problems with learning new information and memory. Methamphetamine can cause rapid heart rate, increased blood pressure, and damage to the small blood vessels in the brain that can lead to stroke. Heroin use can result in slow and shallow breathing, convulsions, coma, and even death.

Young people who inject drugs expose themselves to additional risks, including contracting HIV, hepatitis B and C, and other blood-borne viruses. Chronic injection drug users also risk scarred or collapsed veins, infection of the heart lining and valves, abscesses, pneumonia, tuberculosis, and liver and kidney disease.

Substance abuse among youth has also been strongly linked to delinquency. Arrest, adjudication, and intervention by the juvenile justice system are eventual consequences for many youths engaged in alcohol and other drug use.

What are some common signs of teen drug abuse?

Sudden and extreme changes in personality, physical appearance, social activity, or school performance may signal teen drug use. Personality changes may include becoming disrespectful and verbally or physically abusive, extreme mood swings, paranoia, confusion, anger, depression, and secretive behavior. Teens who abuse drugs may lie about what they are doing and where they are going. They may also steal, claim to lose possessions they once valued, have a lot of money, ask for money, and withdraw from family and family activities. With regard to physical effects, teens using drugs may exhibit a lack of hygiene and grooming, weight loss or gain, hyperactivity or lethargy, and insomnia or excessive sleeping. These teens may also drop old friends and activities, skip school, lose interest in school, receive low grades, sleep in class, lose concentration, and have trouble with memory.

Chapter 74

Adolescent Use of Inhalants

Inhalant Abuse Statistics

- In 2002, the nation's hospital emergency departments reported almost 1,500 mentions of inhalant abuse by patients.

- Most inhalant abusers are younger than 25. Data suggest that inhalant abuse reaches its peak during the seventh through ninth grades.

- A NIDA survey of drug use by 8th–12th graders shows that lifetime inhalant use for 8th graders has increased significantly in the past year.

When most people think of drug abuse, they think of illegal substances like heroin, cocaine and lysergic acid diethylamide (LSD). Would it surprise you to know that some of the most toxic substances abused by children and teens can be found in the home? Certain household and office products, including glue, shoe polish, gasoline, and cleaning fluids can cause intoxication when their vapors are inhaled. Called inhalants, these vapors can have devastating side effects. They pose a particularly significant problem because they are readily accessible, legal, and inexpensive. In a 2003 study, 12.7% of

---

"Sniffing Out Drugs," *News in Health*, September 2005, National Institutes of Health (NIH).

10th graders and 11.2% of 12th graders said they had abused inhalants at least once.

When the chemical vapors released by inhalants are breathed in by nose or mouth, they are absorbed by the lungs and travel rapidly through the blood to the brain and other organs. In minutes, the user feels alcohol-like effects such as slurred speech, clumsy movements, dizziness, and euphoria. These effects usually last only a few minutes, but the user can extend them for hours by inhaling the vapors repeatedly. Successive inhalations can also break down inhibitions and self-control. Inhalants also have serious side effects, from headaches, nausea, and vomiting to unconsciousness or even death.

How inhalants cause their effects is a topic currently being investigated by the National Institutes of Health (NIH)'s National Institute on Drug Abuse (NIDA). The vapors in inhalants contain chemicals that change the way the brain works, causing the user to feel happy for a short time. But these vapors often contain more than one chemical. Some may leave the body quickly, but others are absorbed into fatty substances in the brain and nervous system, where they can stay for a long time.

One of these fatty substances is myelin—a protective cover that surrounds many of the body's nerve cells. Nerve cells in your brain and spinal cord are sort of like command central for your body. They send and receive messages that control just about everything you think and do. If nerve cells are your body's electrical wiring, then myelin is the rubber insulation that protects the electrical cords. The chemicals in inhalants can break down myelin. If myelin breaks down, nerve cells may not be able to transmit messages as effectively.

As a result, people taking inhalants may have trouble solving complex problems and planning ahead. They might start losing control over their movement and coordination, making them slow or clumsy. They also may lose the ability to learn new things or have a hard time keeping track of simple conversations.

Regular abuse of inhalants can also cause serious damage to major organs, including the brain, liver, heart, kidneys, and lungs. A single session of repeated inhalations can lead to cardiac arrest and death by altering normal heart rhythms or by preventing oxygen from entering the lungs, causing suffocation.

There are three general types of inhalants.

- Solvents include paint thinners or removers, degreasers, dry-cleaning fluids, gasoline, glue, correction fluids, and felt tip marker fluid.

- Gas inhalants which can be found in butane lighters and pro-pane tanks, whipped cream aerosols or dispensers (whippets), spray paints, hair or deodorant sprays, and fabric protector sprays.

- Nitrites, commonly known as poppers, generally contain the chemicals isobutyl nitrite or butyl nitrite. They are available il-legally and come in small brown bottles, sometimes labeled as video head cleaner or liquid aroma.

It is difficult to know how many emergency room visits and deaths are caused by inhalants. There are probably many more emergency room admissions due to inhalants than we know about. Inhalant use is easily hidden, and they leave the body quickly so they are long gone by the time someone gets to the emergency room. NIDA continues to support new research on the prevention and treatment of inhalant abuse, but early identification and intervention remain the best ways to stop inhalant abuse, before it causes serious health consequences. Parents should store household products carefully to prevent acciden-tal inhalation by very young children. They should also remain aware of the temptations that these dangerous substances pose to children and teens in their homes.

Wise Choices: How to Recognize Inhalant Abuse

Parents, educators, family physicians, and other health care prac-titioners should be alert to the following signs of a serious inhalant abuse problem:

- chemical odors in breath or clothing

- paint or other stains on face, hands or clothes

- hidden empty spray paint or solvent containers and chemical-soaked rags or clothing

- drunk or disoriented appearance

- slurred speech

- nausea or loss of appetite

- inattentiveness, lack of coordination, irritability, and depres-sion

Additional Information

National Institute on Drug Abuse (NIDA)

6001 Executive Blvd., Room 5213
Bethesda, MD 20892-9561
Phone: 301-443-1124
Website: http://www.nida.nih.gov
NIDA Inhalants Website: http://www.inhalants.drugabuse.gov
NIDA for Teens Website: http://www.teens.drugabuse.gov
E-mail: information@nida.nih.gov

Chapter 75

Talk to Your Child about Alcohol and Drugs

Plan now to discuss alcohol and drugs with your family. There are many resources available, including community planning kits, booklets about alcohol use, studies with facts, and frequently asked questions that can help you get ready to talk to your child about alcohol. Think seriously about the example you set for your children. Perhaps the most important thing you can do to get ready for this talk is to seriously think about your own thoughts and feelings about alcohol and the way your children see you use alcohol.

Answer the following questions[1] to help you understand alcohol's place in your life or the life of someone you know. It is an easy, risk-free way to find out if alcohol may be affecting the way you, your friends, or your family members work and live. People with an alcohol problem often answer yes to one or more of the questions.

1. Have you ever felt you should cut down on your drinking?

2. Have people annoyed you by criticizing your drinking?

3. Have you ever felt bad or guilty about your drinking?

4. Have you ever had a drink first thing in the morning to steady your nerves or get rid of a hangover (eye opener)?

This chapter includes: Excerpts from "Talk to Your Child about Alcohol," Substance Abuse and Mental Health Services Administration (SAMHSA), April 2004; and, "Teach Your Child Refusal Skills," SAMHSA, December 2005.

Think about Factors That Put Your Child at Risk

Some children are more likely than others to drink alcohol and develop alcohol-related problems, including health, school, legal, family, and emotional problems. Risk factors include:[2]

- alcohol or other drug use before the age of 15

- a parent who is a problem drinker or an alcoholic

- close friends who use alcohol and/or other drugs

- aggressive, antisocial, or hard-to-control behavior from an early age

- childhood abuse and/or other major traumas

- current behavioral problems and/or problems with school work

- parents who do not support, talk to, or keep track of their child's whereabouts

- ongoing anger or rejection from parents and/or harsh, inconsistent discipline

Know the Facts about Alcohol

Remind yourself and other adults in your family, or in your child's life, about the dangers of alcohol. Know the facts when you talk with your child.[2]

- Alcohol is a strong drug that slows down the body and mind. It impairs coordination; slows reaction time; and impairs vision, clear thinking, and judgment.

- Beer and wine are not safer than hard liquor. A 12-ounce can of beer, a 5-ounce glass of wine, and 1.5 ounces of hard liquor all have the same amount of alcohol and have the same effects on the body and mind.

- On average, it takes two to three hours for a single drink to leave the body's system. Nothing can speed up the process, including drinking coffee, taking a cold shower, or walking it off.

- People tend to be very bad at judging how seriously alcohol has affected them. That means many people who drive after drinking think they can control a car but actually cannot.

- Anyone can develop a serious alcohol problem, including a teenager.

Be Clear in Your Own Mind about Your Expectations

Think about the rules and expectations you already have made in your family or those you want to make. Here are some ideas:[2]

- People under 21 will not drink or be served alcohol.

- Older siblings, family members, or friends will not give alcohol to people under 21 or encourage them to drink.

- Your child should leave parties or activities where alcohol is being served.

- Do not ride in a car when the driver has been drinking, if you can avoid it. It is not safe. Walk or try to get a ride with an adult friend who has not been drinking. If you must get in a car with a drinking driver, sit in the back seat in the middle, lock your door, and put on your safety belt.[3]

Let Your Child Know Why You Are Having This Talk

Even if this is not a topic you have talked about openly before, get started and let your child know that:[3]

- You want your child to avoid alcohol.

- You want your child to have self-respect.

- You want him to know that drinking is illegal.

- You want him to know that drinking at his age can be dangerous.

- You may have a family history of alcoholism, or there may be other things that put your child at risk for alcohol abuse.

Let Your Child Know That Breaking the Rules Will Have Consequences

Plan to discuss ways your child can fit in and have fun without drinking and how to turn down alcohol when it is offered. Discuss the consequences of using alcohol with your children. Include the health, school, emotional, legal, and social problems as well as punishment. Make sure your child is an active part of the talk and of the decision-making process.

- Ask open-ended questions—ones that do not have a yes or no answer.

- Let your child share his/her thoughts and feelings without being stopped.

- Control your emotions. If your child says something that you do not agree with, take a deep breath and try to find a constructive answer.

- Let him/her know you respect his/her views. Your child will be more likely to respect yours.

Questions to Get Started

1. What do you think about the dangers of people under 21 using alcohol?

2. What do you think about people your age who use alcohol?

3. How many ways can you think of to say no when you are offered alcohol?

4. How can I help you avoid other children, pressures, and situations that may lead to you using alcohol?

5. If we were hosting a teen party, what kinds of snacks and nonalcoholic drinks could we serve? What fun activities can we plan, and what do you think we should do if someone brings alcohol?

6. What do you think is a fair punishment for breaking our family rules about alcohol?

Keep the Dialog Going

Tell your child that you love him/her and want him/her to have a healthy and happy life. Let your child know, by your actions and your words, that you respect and care about him/her. In numerous surveys, teens say that they pay attention to parents who are interested and involved in their children's lives. Emphasizing the family's expectation to not drink alcohol before the age of 21 is one of the most important talks you will have with your child. During these discussions, both the conversation's tone and content can help build a trusting relationship and encourage future dialog about alcohol and other tough issues.

References

1. U.S. Department of Health and Human Services Substance Abuse and Mental Health Services Administration, Center for

Substance Abuse Prevention. *The Quick Quiz Questionnaire*, last referenced March 8, 2004.

2. National Institute on Alcohol Abuse and Alcoholism. *Make A Difference—Talk to Your Child About Alcohol*, last referenced March 8, 2004.

3. National Association for Children of Alcoholics. *What Can Kids Do?*, last referenced March 8 2004.

Teach Your Child Refusal Skills

Your child faces a number of tough decisions in life. Since making friends and fitting in are important to many children, peer pressure has a big impact on decisions, especially on those about drug, alcohol, and tobacco use. Children may be afraid that if they say no to something harmful, they won't be accepted. It is important that you teach your child about the dangers of drugs, alcohol, and tobacco. Other important skills your child needs are refusal skills. If you teach how to say no to dangerous situations, your child will feel more confident in his/her decisions. There are a number of ways your child can refuse drugs, alcohol, and tobacco.

Ways to Say No

- Say, "No, thanks." It could be just as easy as that. However, if the person offering the cigarette, beer, or joint persists, your child will have to back up "No thanks" with other tactics.

- Be a broken record. Tell your child to keep saying no as many times as needed, either to cause the person pressuring them to stop, or to stall until he/she can think of something else to say.

- Give a reason. This reason could be simply, "I'm not allowed to do that," or, "That's bad for you." It could state the consequences, such as, "I don't want to do that; it will make me sick," or, "You can die from doing that." The important thing is that your child state a reason for saying no with confidence. It is important for your child not to get into an argument; the goal is to refuse what is being offered.

- Walk away or ignore the offer. This does not work in all situations. Sometimes your child will be alone or where he/she cannot walk away.

- Change the subject or suggest doing something else. By saying, "Let's do ____ instead," your child has the potential to not only refuse an offer of drugs, alcohol, or tobacco, but to prevent a friend from using them too.

- Assert yourself. This is an important part of all the above tactics. Being able to state your position assertively is a trait that is valued in adults, so if your child learns it now, he/she will be better off in the future.

Remember, the best way to refuse drugs, alcohol, and tobacco is to spend time with people who do not use these substances. Help your children establish positive friendships, and monitor your child's activities.

Put It Into Practice

Once you teach your child refusal skills, it is important that you practice them together. Different aged children may face different situations, and it is important to make sure you practice with situations that may actually happen. Start by asking your child what he/she does when someone tries to get him/her to do something he/she does not want to do. Do a number of role-play situations in which you pose as the person offering drugs, alcohol, or tobacco, and have your child practice different ways to say no. When you are finished, your child should feel confident that he/she has the power to make the right choice.

Additional Information

Substance Abuse and Mental Health Services Administration
1 Choke Cherry Rd.
Rockville, MD 20857
Toll-Free: 800-729-6686
Toll-Free TDD: 800-487-4889
Website: http://www.samhsa.gov

Part Ten

Additional Help and Information

Chapter 76

Glossary of Terms Related to Adolescent Health

Adolescence: The period of life beginning with puberty and ending with completed growth and physical maturity.

Addiction: A chronic, relapsing disease characterized by compulsive drug-seeking and abuse and by long-lasting chemical changes in the brain.

Amenorrhea: Absence or abnormal cessation of the menses.[1]

Amphetamine: Stimulant drugs whose effects are very similar to cocaine.

Anabolic effects: Drug-induced growth or thickening of the body's non-reproductive tract tissues—including skeletal muscle, bones, the larynx, and vocal cords—and decrease in body fat.

Androgenic effects: A drug's effects upon the growth of the male reproductive tract and the development of male secondary sexual characteristics.

Aplastic anemia: A disorder that occurs when the bone marrow produces too few of all three types of blood cells: red blood cells, white blood cells, and platelets.

Unmarked definitions in this chapter are from "NIDA for Teens Glossary," National Institute on Drug Abuse (NIDA), November 2005; Terms marked [1] are from *Stedman's Medical Dictionary 27th Edition.* © 2000, Lippincott Williams & Wilkins. All rights reserved.

Asthma: An inflammatory disease of the lungs characterized by re-versible (in most cases) airway obstruction.[1]

Behavior disorder: General term used to denote mental illness or psychological dysfunction, specifically those mental, emotional, or behavioral subclasses for which organic correlates do not exist.[1]

Brainstem: The major route by which the forebrain sends informa-tion to, and receives information from, the spinal cord and peripheral nerves.

Carcinogen: Any substance that causes cancer.

Cardiovascular system: The heart and blood vessels.

Central nervous system: The brain and spinal cord.

Cerebellum: A portion of the brain that helps regulate posture, bal-ance, and coordination.

Cerebral cortex: Region of the brain responsible for cognitive func-tions including reasoning, mood, and perception of stimuli.

Cerebral hemispheres: The two specialized halves of the brain. The left hemisphere is specialized for speech, writing, language, and cal-culation; the right hemisphere is specialized for spatial abilities, face recognition in vision, and some aspects of music perception and pro-duction.

Cerebrum: The upper part of the brain consisting of the left and right hemispheres.

Chronic: Refers to a disease or condition that persists over a long period of time.

Depressants: Drugs that relieve anxiety and produce sleep. Depres-sants include barbiturates, benzodiazepines, and alcohol.

Dopamine: A brain chemical, classified as a neurotransmitter, found in regions of the brain that regulate movement, emotion, motivation, and pleasure.

Drug: A chemical compound or substance that can alter the struc-ture and function of the body. Psychoactive drugs affect the function of the brain, and some of these may be illegal to use and possess.

Drug abuse: The use of illegal drugs or the inappropriate use of legal drugs. The repeated use of drugs to produce pleasure, to alleviate stress, or to alter or avoid reality (or all three).

Eating disorders: A group of mental disorders including anorexia nervosa, bulimia nervosa, pica, and rumination disorder of infancy.[1]

Forebrain: The largest division of the brain, which includes the cerebral cortex and basal ganglia. It is credited with the highest intellectual functions.

Frontal lobe: One of the four divisions of each cerebral hemisphere. The frontal lobe is important for controlling movement and associating the functions of other cortical areas.

Genital system: The complex system consisting of the male or female gonads (testis, ovaries), associated ducts, and external genitalia dedicated to the function of reproducing the species.[1]

Hepatitis: Inflammation of the liver.

Hereditary: Transmissible from parent to offspring by information encoded in the parental germ cell.[1]

Hippocampus: An area of the brain crucial for learning and memory.

Hormone: A chemical substance formed in glands in the body and carried in the blood to organs and tissues, where it influences function, structure, and behavior.

Hypothalamus: The part of the brain that controls many bodily functions, including feeding, drinking, and the release of many hormones.

Ingestion: The act of taking in food or other material into the body through the mouth.

Inhalation: The act of administering a drug or combination of drugs by nasal or oral respiration. Also, the act of drawing air or other substances into the lungs. Nicotine in tobacco smoke enters the body by inhalation.

Injection: A method of administering a substance such as a drug into the skin, subcutaneous tissue, muscle, blood vessels, or body cavities, usually by means of a needle.

Limbic system: A set of brain structures that generates our feelings, emotions, and motivations. It is also important in learning and memory.

Medication: A drug that is used to treat an illness or disease according to established medical guidelines.

Menstruation: Cyclic endometrial shedding and discharge of a bloody fluid from the uterus during the menstrual cycle.[1]

Mental illness: a broadly inclusive term, generally denoting one or all of the following: 1) a disease of the brain, with predominant behavioral symptoms, as in paresis or acute alcoholism; 2) a disease of the mind or personality, evidenced by abnormal behavior, as in hysteria or schizophrenia; also called mental or emotional disease, disturbance, or disorder, or behavior disorder.[1]

Metabolism: The processes by which the body breaks things down or alters them so they can be eliminated.

Musculoskeletal system: The muscles, bones, tendons, and ligaments.

Nicotine: The addictive drug in tobacco. Nicotine activates a specific type of acetylcholine receptor.

Nitrites: A special class of inhalants that act primarily to dilate blood vessels and relax the muscles. Whereas other inhalants are used to alter mood, nitrites are used primarily as sexual enhancers.

Parietal lobe: One of the four subdivisions of the cerebral cortex; it is involved in sensory processes, attention, and language.

Psychoactive drug: A drug that changes the way the brain works.

Puberty: Sequence of events by which a child becomes a young adult, characterized by the beginning of gametogenesis, secretion of gonadal hormones, development of secondary sexual characteristics and reproductive functions; sexual dimorphism is accentuated.[1]

Relapse: In drug abuse, relapse is the resumption of drug use after trying to stop taking drugs. Relapse is a common occurrence in many chronic disorders, including addiction, that require behavioral adjustments to treat effectively.

Reward: The process that reinforces behavior. It is mediated at least in part by the release of dopamine into the nucleus accumbens. Human subjects report that reward is associated with feelings of pleasure.

Serotonin: A neurotransmitter that regulates many functions, including mood, appetite, and sensory perception.

Sex hormones: Hormones that are found in higher quantities in one sex than in the other. Male sex hormones are the androgens, which include testosterone; and the female sex hormones are the estrogens and progesterone.

Stimulants: A class of drugs that elevates mood, increases feelings of well-being, and increases energy and alertness. These drugs produce euphoria and are powerfully rewarding. Stimulants include cocaine, methamphetamine, and methylphenidate (Ritalin).

Temporal lobe: The lobe of the cerebral cortex at the side of the head that hears and interprets music and language.

Tobacco: A plant widely cultivated for its leaves, which are used primarily for smoking; the tabacum species is the major source of tobacco products.

Tolerance: A condition in which higher doses of a drug are required to produce the same effect as during initial use; often leads to physical dependence.

Withdrawal: Symptoms that occur after chronic use of a drug is reduced or stopped.

Chapter 77

Additional Resources for Information about Adolescence

Government Agencies and Organizations That Provide Information about Adolescence

Centers for Disease Control and Prevention (CDC)
Office of Public Inquiries
1600 Clifton Rd.
Atlanta, GA 30333
Toll-Free: 800-311-3435
Phone: 404-639-3534
Website: http://www.cdc.gov
E-mail: cdcinfo@cdc.gov

CDC Healthy Youth
P.O. Box 8817
Silver Spring, MD 20907
Toll-Free: 888-231-6405
Toll-Free TTY: 888-232-6348
Website: http://www.cdc.gov/
healthyYouth
E-mail: CDC-INFO@cdc.gov

CDC National Prevention Information Network
P.O. Box 6003
Rockville, MD 20849-6003
Toll-Free: 800-458-5231
Toll-Free TTY: 800-243-7012
Fax/Fax-on-demand: 888-282-7681
Website: http://www.cdcnpin.org
E-mail: info@cdcnpin.org

CDC Office on Smoking and Health
Mailstop K-50
4770 Buford Hwy. NE
Atlanta, GA 30341-3717
Toll-Free: 800-232-4636
Phone: 770-488-5705
Website: http://www.cdc.gov/
tobacco
E-mail: tobaccoinfo@cdc.gov

Resources in this chapter were compiled from several sources deemed reliable. All contact information was verified and updated in May 2006.

National Cancer Institute (NCI)
Cancer Information Service
Toll-Free: 800-4-CANCER
(800-422-6237)
Toll-Free TTY: 800-332-8615
Website: http://www.cancer.gov
Live online assistance: https://cissecure.nci.nih.gov/livehelp/welcome.asp
E-mail: cancergovstaff@mail.nih.gov

National Clearinghouse for Alcohol and Drug Information (NCADI)
Toll-Free: 800-729-6686
Toll-Free TDD: 800-487-4889
Website: http://ncadi.samhsa.gov

National Clearinghouse on Child Abuse and Neglect Information
Children's Bureau/ACYF
1250 Maryland Ave. SW, 8th Floor
Washington, DC 20024
Toll-Free: 800-394-3366
Phone: 703-385-7565
Fax: 703-385-3206
Website: http://nccanch.acf.hhs.gov
E-mail: nccanch@caliber.com

National Diabetes Education Program (NDEP)
One Diabetes Way
Bethesda, MD 20814-9692
Toll-Free: 800-438-5383
Phone: 301-496-3583
Website: http://www.ndep.nih.gov
E-mail: ndep@mail.nih.gov

National Diabetes Information Clearinghouse
1 Information Way
Bethesda, MD 20892-3560
Toll-Free: 800-860-8747
Fax: 703-738-4929
Website: http://diabetes.niddk.nih.gov
E-mail: ndic@info.niddk.nih.gov

National Institute of Arthritis and Musculo-skeletal and Skin Diseases (NIAMS) Information Clearinghouse
1 AMS Circle
Bethesda, MD 20892-3675
Toll-Free: 877-22-NIAMS (64267)
Phone: 301-495-4484
TTY: 301-565-2966
Fax: 301-718-6366
Website: http://www.niams.nih.gov
E-mail: niamsinfo@mail.nih.gov

National Institute of Child Health and Human Development (NICHD)
Information Resource Center
P.O. Box 3006
Rockville, MD 20847
Toll-Free: 800-370-2943
Toll-Free TTY: 888-320-6942
Fax: 301-984-1473
Website: http://www.nichd.nih.gov/milk
E-mail: NICHDInformationResourceCenter@mail.nih.gov

National Institute of Mental Health
Public Information and
Communications Branch
6001 Executive Blvd.
Room 8184, MSC 9663
Bethesda, MD 20892-9663
Toll-Free: 866-615-6464
Toll-Free TTY: 866-415-8051
Phone: 301-443-8431
Fax: 301-443-4279
Website: http://
www.nimh.nih.gov
E-mail: nimhinfo@nih.gov

National Institute on Alcohol Abuse and Alcoholism (NIAAA)
5635 Fishers Lane, MSC 9304
Bethesda, MD 20892-9304
Website: http://
www.niaaa.nih.gov
E-mail: niaaaweb-r@exchange.nih.gov

National Institute on Drug Abuse (NIDA)
6001 Executive Blvd., Room 5213
Bethesda, MD 20892-9561
Phone: 301-443-1124
Website: http://
www.nida.nih.gov
NIDA Inhalants Website: http://
www.inhalants.drugabuse.gov
NIDA for Teens Website: http://
www.teens.drugabuse.gov
E-mail:
information@nida.nih.gov

National Kidney and Urologic Diseases Information Clearinghouse
3 Information Way
Bethesda, MD 20892-3580
Toll-Free: 800-891-5390
Fax: 703-738-4929
Website: http://
kidney.niddk.nih.gov
E-mail:
nkudic@info.niddk.nih.gov

National Mental Health Information Center
P.O. Box 42557
Washington DC 20015
Toll-Free: 800-789-2647
Toll-Free TDD: 866-889-2647
Fax: 240-747-5470
Website: http://
www.mentalhealth.samhsa.gov
E-mail: info@mentalhealth.org

National Women's Health Information Center (NWHIC)
Office on Women's Health,
DHHS
200 Independence Ave. SW,
Room 712E
Washington, DC 20201
Toll-Free: 800-994-9662
Toll-Free TDD: 888-220-5446
Website: http://
womenshealth.gov

*National Youth Anti-Drug
Media Campaign*
Drug Policy Information
Clearinghouse
P.O. Box 6000
Rockville, MD 20849-6000
Toll-Free: 800-666-3332
Phone: 301-519-5212
Website: http://
www.mediacampaign.org

*National Youth Violence
Prevention Resource Center*
P.O. Box 10809
Rockville, MD 20849-0809
Toll-Free: 866-723-3968
Toll-Free TTY: 888-503-3952
Fax: 301-562-1001
Website: http://
www.safeyouth.org
E-mail: NYVPRC@safeyouth.org

*Substance Abuse and
Mental Health Services
Administration (SAMHSA)*
1 Choke Cherry Rd.
Rockville, MD 20857
Toll-Free: 800-729-6686
Toll-Free TDD: 800-487-4889
Website: http://www.samhsa.gov

*U.S. Department of Labor
(DOL)*
Information Referral Service
Frances Perkins Building
200 Constitution Ave. NW
Washington DC 20210
Toll-Free: 866-487-2365
Toll-Free TTY: 877-889-5627
Website: http://www.dol.gov

Private and Nonprofit Organizations That Provide Information about Adolescence

*American Academy of
Dermatology*
P.O. Box 4014
Schaumburg, IL 60618-4014
Toll-Free: 866-503-7546
Fax: 847-240-1859
Website: http://www.aad.org
E-mail: MCR@aad.org

*American Association of
Diabetes Educators*
100 W. Monroe, Suite 400
Chicago, IL 60603
Toll-Free: 800-338-3633
Fax: 312-424-2427
Website: http://www.aadenet.org

American Association of Pastoral Counselors
9504-A Lee Highway
Fairfax, VA 22031-2303
Telephone: 703-385-6967
Fax: 703-352-7725
Website:
http://www.aapc.org
E-mail: info@aapc.org

American College of Obstetricians and Gynecologists (ACOG)
409 12th St. SW
P.O. Box 96920
Washington, DC 20024-2188
Phone: 202-863-2518
Website:
http://www.acog.org

American College of Sports Medicine
P.O. Box 1440
Indianapolis, IN 46206-1440
Phone: 317-637-9200
Fax: 317-634-7817
Website: http://www.acsm.org

American Diabetes Association
1701 N. Beauregard St.
Alexandria, VA 22311
Toll-Free: 800-DIABETES
(800-342-2383)
Website:
http://www.diabetes.org
E-mail: AskADA@diabetes.org

American Juvenile Arthritis Organization
1330 W. Peachtree St., Suite 100
Atlanta, GA 30309
Toll-Free: 800-568-4045
Phone: 404-965-7538
Website: http://www.arthritis.org
E-mail: help@arthritis.org

American Psychiatric Association
1000 Wilson Blvd., Suite 1825
Arlington, VA 22209-3901
Toll-Free: 888-357-7924
Phone: 703-907-7300
Website: http://www.psych.org
E-mail: apa@psych.org

American Physical Therapy Association
1111 N. Fairfax St.
Alexandria, VA 22314-1488
Toll-Free: 800-999-2782
Phone: 703-684-2782
TDD: 703-683-6748
Fax: 703-684-7343
Website: http://www.apta.org

Association of Cancer Online Resources (ACOR)
173 Duane St., Suite 3A
New York, NY 10013-3334
Phone: 212-226-5525
Website: http://www.acor.org

Anxiety Disorders Association of America
8730 Georgia Ave., Suite 600
Silver Spring, MD 20910
Phone: 240-485-1001
Fax: 240-485-1035
Website: http://www.adaa.org

Candlelighters Childhood Cancer Foundation
National Office
P.O. Box 498
Kensington, MD 20895-0498
Toll-Free: 800-366-CCCF
(800-366-2223)
Phone: 301-962-3520
Fax: 301-962-3521
Website: http://
www.candlelighters.org
E-mail: staff@candlelighters.org

Child and Adolescent Bipolar Foundation
1000 Skokie Blvd., Suite 425
Wilmette, IL 60091
Phone: 847-256-8525
Fax: 847-920-9498
Website: http://www.bpkids.org
E-mail: cabf@bpkids.org

Children with Diabetes/ Diabetes123
5689 Chancery Place
Hamilton, OH 45011
Website: http://www.children
withdiabetes.com/kids
E-mail: info@childrenwith
diabetes.com

Depression and Bipolar Support Alliance (DBSA)
730 N. Franklin St., Suite 501
Chicago, IL 60610-7224
Toll-Free: 800-826-3632
Fax: 312-642-7243
Website: http://www.dbs
alliance.org
E-mail: questions@
dbsalliance.org

Hormone Foundation
8401 Connecticut Ave.
Suite 900
Chevy Chase, MD 20815-5817
Toll-Free: 800-467-6663
Website: http://
www.hormone.org

Juvenile Diabetes Research Foundation International
120 Wall Street
New York, NY 10005-4001
Toll-Free: 800-223-1138 or
800-533-2873
Fax: 212-785-9595
Website: http://kids.jdrf.org
E-mail: info@idrf.org

National Adolescent Health Information Center
School of Medicine
University of California,
San Francisco
UCSF Box 0503
San Francisco, CA 94143-0503
Phone: 415-502-4856
Fax: 415-502-4858
Website: http://nahic.ucsf.edu
E-mail: nahic@ucsf.edu

National Alliance for the Mentally Ill
Colonial Place Three
2107 Wilson Blvd.
Suite 300
Arlington, VA 22201-3042
Toll-Free: 800-950-6264
Fax: 703-524-9094
Website: http://www.nami.org

National Athletic Trainers Association
2952 Stemmons Freeway
Dallas, TX 75247-6916
Toll-Free: 800-TRY-NATA
(800-879-6282)
Phone: 214-637-6282
Fax: 214-637-2206
Website: http://www.nata.org

National Campaign to Prevent Teen Pregnancy
1776 Massachusetts Ave. NW,
Suite 200
Washington, DC 20036
Phone: 202-478-8500
Fax: 202-478-8588
Website: http://
www.teenpregnancy.org
E-mail:
campaign@teenpregnancy.org

National Center for Victims of Crime
2000 M St. NW, Suite 480
Washington, DC 20036
Toll-Free: 800-394-2255
Toll-Free TTY: 800-211-7996
Website: http://www.ncvc.org

National Children's Cancer Society
1015 Locust St., Suite 600
St. Louis, MO 63101
Toll-Free: 800-5-FAMILY
(800-532-6459)
Phone: 314-241-1600 (Program
Services)
Fax: 314-241-1996
Website: http://www
.children-cancer.com

National Mental Health Association
2000 N. Beauregard St.
6th Floor
Alexandria, VA 22311
Toll-Free: 800-969-6642
Toll-Free Crisis Helpline:
800-784-2433
Toll-Free TTY: 800-433-5959
Phone: 703-684-7722
Fax: 703-684-5968
Website: http://www.nmha.org

National Scoliosis Foundation
5 Cabot Place
Stoughton, MA 02072
Toll-Free: 800-NSF-MYBACK
(673-6922)
Phone: 617-341-6333
Fax: 617-341-8333
Website: http://www.scoliosis.org
E-mail: nsf@scoliosis.org

Obsessive-Compulsive Foundation (OCF)
676 State St.
New Haven, CT 06511
Phone: 203-401-2070
Website: http://
www.ocfoundation.org

Rape, Abuse, and Incest National Network
2000 L St. NW, Suite 406
Washington, DC 20036
Toll-Free: 800-656-4673 ext. 3
Phone: 202-544-1034
Fax: 202-544-3556
Website: http://www.rainn.org
E-mail: info@rainn.org

Scoliosis Association, Inc.
P.O. Box 811705
Boca Raton, FL 33481-1705
Toll-Free: 800-800-0669
Phone: 561-994-4435
Fax: 561-994-2455
Website:
http://www.scoliosis-assoc.org

Scoliosis Research Society
555 E. Wells St.
Suite 1100
Milwaukee, WI 53202-3823
Phone: 414-289-9107
Fax: 414-276-3349
Website:
http://www.srs.org
E-mail: info@srs.org

Technical Assistance Alliance for Parent Centers
8161 Normandale Blvd.
Minneapolis, MN 55437
Toll-Free: 888-248-0822
Phone: 952-838-9000
Website: http://www.taalliance.org
E-mail: alliance@taalliance.org

ThinkFirst National Injury Prevention Foundation
26 S. La Grange Rd., Suite 103
La Grange, IL 60525
Toll-Free: 800-844-6556
Phone: 708-588-2000
Fax: 708-588-2002
Website:
http://www.thinkfirst.org
E-mail:
thinkfirst@thinkfirst.org

Index

Index

Page numbers followed by 'n' indicate a footnote. Page numbers in *italics* indicate a table or illustration.

adolescents
  bipolar disorder 511–20
  brain development overview
    29–34
  cancer 354–76
  conduct disorder 525–28
  depression 529–35
  diet and nutrition 69–75
  disaster response 556–59
  medical care 39–41
  medication abuse 595–99
  mental health problems
    497–502
  scoliosis 421–28
  self-injury 551–53
  sports injuries 291–92, 293–94
  underage drinking 569–74
  well-being indicators 19–27
  see also boys; girls
adoptions, overview 267–74
adult-onset diabetes *see* type 2
  diabetes
advertising *see* marketing
"After Disaster: What Teens
  Can Do" (SAMHSA) 555n
age factor
  calorie requirements *72, 73*
  depression *534*
  disability legislation 62
  milk requirements 77–84, *78*
  pregnancy statistics 213–16, *216*
  suicide statistics *55*
  testicular cancer 313
  toxic shock syndrome 181
agricultural work injuries 321–22
AIDS *see* acquired immune
  deficiency syndrome
"Aim for a Healthy Weight:
  Assess Your Risk" (NHLBI) 95n
albuterol 348
alcohol abuse, described 610
alcohol use
  diet pills 107
  motor vehicle accidents 302–3,
    333, *333*
  pregnancy 263
  sexual activity statistics *222*
  underage drinking 569–74
Alexander, Duane 20

allergies
  asthma 345
  body piercings 143
  tattoos 148
alopecia, permanent makeup 148
aluminum chloride hexahydrate 159
Alving, Barbara 99
amenorrhea
  defined 617
  described 188–89
American Academy of Adoption
  Attorneys, contact information 273
American Academy of Dermatology,
  contact information 160, 626
American Academy of Family
  Physicians (AAFP), publications
  pregnancy termination 275n
  tinea infections 161n
American Academy of Orthopaedic
  Surgeons (AAOS), contact
  information 415
American Adoption Congress,
  contact information 274
American Association of Diabetes
  Educators, contact information
  389, 395, 626
American Association of Pastoral
  Counselors, contact information
  563, 627
American College of Obstetricians
  and Gynecologists (ACOG),
  contact information 186, 627
American College of Rheumatology,
  contact information 415
American College of Sports Medicine,
  contact information 295, 627
American Diabetes Association,
  contact information 389, 395, 627
American Heart Association,
  physical activity publication 112n
American Juvenile Arthritis
  Organization, contact information
  415, 627
American Obesity Association
  contact information 103
  obesity publication 90n
American Osteopathic College of
  Dermatology (AOCD), warts
  publication 165n

National Campaign to Prevent
  Teen Pregnancy
  contact information 282, 629
  publications
    advice 244n
    pregnancy avoidance 247n
    pregnancy prevention 277n
    sex myths 245n
National Cancer Institute (NCI)
  contact information 375–76,
    624
  publications
    diet and nutrition 69n
    pediatric cancer 354n, 363n,
      367n
    smokeless tobacco 588n
National Center for Victims
  of Crime, contact information
  484, 629
National Children's Cancer
  Society, contact information
  376, 629
*National Children's Study Dietary
  Assessment Literature Review*
  (NCI) 69n
National Clearinghouse for
  Alcohol and Drug Information
  (NCADI), contact information
  574, 624
National Clearinghouse on Child
  Abuse and Neglect Information
  contact information 448, 624
  definitions publication, 443n
National Diabetes Education
  Program (NDEP)
  contact information 388, 396,
    624
  publications
    type 1 diabetes 377n
    type 2 diabetes 391n
National Diabetes Information
  Clearinghouse, contact
  information 389, 396, 624
National Dissemination Center
  for Children with Disabilities
  (NICHCY), disability information
  publication 61n
National Domestic Violence Hotline,
  contact information 478

National Empowerment Center,
  contact information 564
National Heart, Lung, and Blood
  Institute (NHLBI), publications
  chronic illnesses 429n
  obesity 95n
  screen time limitations 118n
National Highway Traffic Safety
  Administration (NHTSA), contact
  information 207
National Institute of Arthritis
  and Musculoskeletal and Skin
  Diseases (NIAMS)
  contact information 295, 299, 415,
    427, 624
  publications
    acne 125n
    growth plate injuries 297n
    juvenile rheumatoid arthritis
      407n
    scoliosis 421n
    sports injuries 285n
National Institute of Child
  Health and Human
  Development (NICHD)
  contact information 624
  publications
    adolescent birth rates 19n
    juvenile mental health 497n
    milk 77n
National Institute of Diabetes and
  Digestive and Kidney Diseases
  (NIDDK)
  contact information 211, 625
  publications
    obesity prevention 100n
    prostatitis 210n
National Institute of
  Environment Health Sciences
  (NIEHS), reproductive health
  publication 9n
National Institute of Mental Health
  (NIMH)
  contact information 185, 505,
    565, 625
  publications
    adolescent brain
      development 29n
    antidepressant medications 529n

Y

"You(th) and Tobacco" (CDC) 580n
"You Can't Get Pregnant if
  You Do It Standing Up and
  Other Myths" (National
  Campaign to Prevent Teen
  Pregnancy) 245n
"Young People with Cancer: A
  Handbook for Parents" (NCI) 354n
"Youth and Tobacco Use: Current
  Estimates" (CDC) 580n
"Youth Internet Safety" (DOJ) 458n
youth violence, overview 435–41

"Youth Violence: A National
  Problem" (CDC) 435n
"Youth Violence: Fact Sheet"
  (CDC) 435n
"Youth Violence Warning Signs"
  (CDC) 435n
Yurgelun-Todd, Deborah 31

Z

zirconium 132
Zoloft (sertraline) 185, 531
Zwerling, Charles 149
zygotes, described 204

Health Reference Series

COMPLETE CATALOG

List price $87 per volume. **School and library price $78 per volume.**

Adolescent Health Sourcebook, 2nd Edition

Basic Consumer Health Information about the Physical, Mental, and Emotional Growth and Development of Adolescents, Including Medical Care, Nutritional and Physical Activity Requirements, Puberty, Sexual Activity, Acne, Tanning, Body Piercing, Common Physical Illnesses and Disorders, Eating Disorders, Attention Deficit Hyperactivity Disorder, Depression, Bullying, Hazing, and Adolescent Injuries Related to Sports, Driving, and Work

Along with Substance Abuse Information about Nicotine, Alcohol, and Drug Use, a Glossary, and Directory of Additional Resources

Edited by Joyce Brennfleck Shannon. 683 pages. 2006. 0-7808-0943-2.

"It is written in clear, nontechnical language aimed at general readers. . . . Recommended for public libraries, community colleges, and other agencies serving health care consumers."
— *American Reference Books Annual, 2003*

"Recommended for school and public libraries. Parents and professionals dealing with teens will appreciate the easy-to-follow format and the clearly written text. This could become a 'must have' for every high school teacher." — *E-Streams, Jan '03*

"A good starting point for information related to common medical, mental, and emotional concerns of adolescents." — *School Library Journal, Nov '02*

"This book provides accurate information in an easy to access format. It addresses topics that parents and caregivers might not be aware of and provides practical, useable information."
— *Doody's Health Sciences Book Review Journal, Sep-Oct '02*

"Recommended reference source."
— *Booklist, American Library Association, Sep '02*

■

AIDS Sourcebook, 3rd Edition

Basic Consumer Health Information about Acquired Immune Deficiency Syndrome (AIDS) and Human Immunodeficiency Virus (HIV) Infection, Including Facts about Transmission, Prevention, Diagnosis, Treatment, Opportunistic Infections, and Other Complications, with a Section for Women and Children, Including Details about Associated Gynecological Concerns, Pregnancy, and Pediatric Care

Along with Updated Statistical Information, Reports on Current Research Initiatives, a Glossary, and Directories of Internet, Hotline, and Other Resources

Edited by Dawn D. Matthews. 664 pages. 2003. 0-7808-0631-X.

"The 3rd edition of the *AIDS Sourcebook*, part of Omnigraphics' *Health Reference Series*, is a welcome update. . . . This resource is highly recommended for academic and public libraries."
— *American Reference Books Annual, 2004*

"Excellent sourcebook. This continues to be a highly recommended book. There is no other book that provides as much information as this book provides."
— *AIDS Book Review Journal, Dec-Jan '00*

"Recommended reference source."
— *Booklist, American Library Association, Dec '99*

■

Alcoholism Sourcebook, 2nd Edition

Basic Consumer Health Information about Alcohol Use, Abuse, and Dependence, Featuring Facts about the Physical, Mental, and Social Health Effects of Alcohol Addiction, Including Alcoholic Liver Disease, Pancreatic Disease, Cardiovascular Disease, Neurological Disorders, and the Effects of Drinking during Pregnancy

Along with Information about Alcohol Treatment, Medications, and Recovery Programs, in Addition to Tips for Reducing the Prevalence of Underage Drinking, Statistics about Alcohol Use, a Glossary of Related Terms, and Directories of Resources for More Help and Information

Edited by Amy L. Sutton. 653 pages. 2006. 0-7808-0942-4.

"This title is one of the few reference works on alcoholism for general readers. For some readers this will be a welcome complement to the many self-help books on the market. Recommended for collections serving general readers and consumer health collections."
— *E-Streams, Mar '01*

"This book is an excellent choice for public and academic libraries."
— *American Reference Books Annual, 2001*

"Recommended reference source."
— *Booklist, American Library Association, Dec '00*

"Presents a wealth of information on alcohol use and abuse and its effects on the body and mind, treatment, and prevention." — *SciTech Book News, Dec '00*

"Important new health guide which packs in the latest consumer information about the problems of alcoholism." — *Reviewer's Bookwatch, Nov '00*

SEE ALSO Drug Abuse Sourcebook, Substance Abuse Sourcebook

Allergies Sourcebook, 2nd Edition

Basic Consumer Health Information about Allergic Disorders, Triggers, Reactions, and Related Symptoms, Including Anaphylaxis, Rhinitis, Sinusitis, Asthma, Dermatitis, Conjunctivitis, and Multiple Chemical Sensitivity

Along with Tips on Diagnosis, Prevention, and Treatment, Statistical Data, a Glossary, and a Directory of Sources for Further Help and Information

Edited by Annemarie S. Muth. 598 pages. 2002. 0-7808-0376-0.

"This book brings a great deal of useful material together. . . . This is an excellent addition to public and consumer health library collections."
— *American Reference Books Annual, 2003*

"This second edition would be useful to laypersons with little or advanced knowledge of the subject matter. This book would also serve as a resource for nursing and other health care professions students. It would be useful in public, academic, and hospital libraries with consumer health collections." — *E-Streams, Jul '02*

■

Alternative Medicine Sourcebook

SEE *Complementary & Alternative Medicine Sourcebook, 3rd Edition*

■

Alzheimer's Disease Sourcebook, 3rd Edition

Basic Consumer Health Information about Alzheimer's Disease, Other Dementias, and Related Disorders, Including Multi-Infarct Dementia, AIDS Dementia Complex, Dementia with Lewy Bodies, Huntington's Disease, Wernicke-Korsakoff Syndrome (Alcohol-Reated Dementia), Delirium, and Confusional States

Along with Information for People Newly Diagnosed with Alzheimer's Disease and Caregivers, Reports Detailing Current Research Efforts in Prevention, Diagnosis, and Treatment, Facts about Long-Term Care Issues, and Listings of Sources for Additional Information

Edited by Karen Bellenir. 645 pages. 2003. 0-7808-0666-2.

"This very informative and valuable tool will be a great addition to any library serving consumers, students and health care workers."
— *American Reference Books Annual, 2004*

"This is a valuable resource for people affected by dementias such as Alzheimer's. It is easy to navigate and includes important information and resources."
— *Doody's Review Service, Feb '04*

"Recommended reference source."
— *Booklist, American Library Association, Oct '99*

SEE ALSO *Brain Disorders Sourcebook*

Arthritis Sourcebook, 2nd Edition

Basic Consumer Health Information about Osteoarthritis, Rheumatoid Arthritis, Other Rheumatic Disorders, Infectious Forms of Arthritis, and Diseases with Symptoms Linked to Arthritis, Featuring Facts about Diagnosis, Pain Management, and Surgical Therapies

Along with Coping Strategies, Research Updates, a Glossary, and Resources for Additional Help and Information

Edited by Amy L. Sutton. 593 pages. 2004. 0-7808-0667-0.

"This easy-to-read volume is recommended for consumer health collections within public or academic libraries." — *E-Streams, May '05*

"As expected, this updated edition continues the excellent reputation of this series in providing sound, usable health information. . . . Highly recommended."
— *American Reference Books Annual, 2005*

"Excellent reference." — *The Bookwatch, Jan '05*

■

Asthma Sourcebook, 2nd Edition

Basic Consumer Health Information about the Causes, Symptoms, Diagnosis, and Treatment of Asthma in Infants, Children, Teenagers, and Adults, Including Facts about Different Types of Asthma, Common Co-Occurring Conditions, Asthma Management Plans, Triggers, Medications, and Medication Delivery Devices

Along with Asthma Statistics, Research Updates, a Glossary, a Directory of Asthma-Related Resources, and More

Edited by Karen Bellenir. 609 pages. 2006. 0-7808-0866-5.

"A worthwhile reference acquisition for public libraries and academic medical libraries whose readers desire a quick introduction to the wide range of asthma information." — *Choice, Association of College & Research Libraries, Jun '01*

"Recommended reference source."
— *Booklist, American Library Association, Feb '01*

"Highly recommended." — *The Bookwatch, Jan '01*

"There is much good information for patients and their families who deal with asthma daily."
— *American Medical Writers Association Journal, Winter '01*

"This informative text is recommended for consumer health collections in public, secondary school, and community college libraries and the libraries of universities with a large undergraduate population."
— *American Reference Books Annual, 2001*

■

Attention Deficit Disorder Sourcebook

Basic Consumer Health Information about Attention Deficit/Hyperactivity Disorder in Children and Adults, Including Facts about Causes, Symptoms, Diagnostic Criteria, and Treatment Options Such as Medications, Behavior Therapy, Coaching, and Homeopathy

Along with Reports on Current Research Initiatives, Legal Issues, and Government Regulations, and Featuring a Glossary of Related Terms, Internet Resources, and a List of Additional Reading Material

Edited by Dawn D. Matthews. 470 pages. 2002. 0-7808-0624-7.

"Recommended reference source."
— Booklist, American Library Association, Jan '03

"This book is recommended for all school libraries and the reference or consumer health sections of public libraries." *— American Reference Books Annual, 2003*

■

Back & Neck Sourcebook, 2nd Edition

Basic Consumer Health Information about Spinal Pain, Spinal Cord Injuries, and Related Disorders, Such as Degenerative Disk Disease, Osteoarthritis, Scoliosis, Sciatica, Spina Bifida, and Spinal Stenosis, and Featuring Facts about Maintaining Spinal Health, Self-Care, Pain Management, Rehabilitative Care, Chiropractic Care, Spinal Surgeries, and Complementary Therapies

Along with Suggestions for Preventing Back and Neck Pain, a Glossary of Related Terms, and a Directory of Resources

Edited by Amy L. Sutton. 633 pages. 2004. 0-7808-0738-3.

"Recommended . . . an easy to use, comprehensive medical reference book." *— E-Streams, Sep '05*

"The strength of this work is its basic, easy-to-read format. Recommended." *— Reference and User Services Quarterly, American Library Association, Winter '97*

■

Blood & Circulatory Disorders Sourcebook, 2nd Edition

Basic Consumer Health Information about the Blood and Circulatory System and Related Disorders, Such as Anemia and Other Hemoglobin Diseases, Cancer of the Blood and Associated Bone Marrow Disorders, Clotting and Bleeding Problems, and Conditions That Affect the Veins, Blood Vessels, and Arteries, Including Facts about the Donation and Transplantation of Bone Marrow, Stem Cells, and Blood and Tips for Keeping the Blood and Circulatory System Healthy

Along with a Glossary of Related Terms and Resources for Additional Help and Information

Edited by Amy L. Sutton. 659 pages. 2005. 0-7808-0746-4.

"Highly recommended pick for basic consumer health reference holdings at all levels."
— The Bookwatch, Aug '05

"Recommended reference source."
—Booklist, American Library Association, Feb '99

"An important reference sourcebook written in simple language for everyday, non-technical users. "
— Reviewer's Bookwatch, Jan '99

Brain Disorders Sourcebook, 2nd Edition

Basic Consumer Health Information about Acquired and Traumatic Brain Injuries, Infections of the Brain, Epilepsy and Seizure Disorders, Cerebral Palsy, and Degenerative Neurological Disorders, Including Amyotrophic Lateral Sclerosis (ALS), Dementias, Multiple Sclerosis, and More

Along with Information on the Brain's Structure and Function, Treatment and Rehabilitation Options, Reports on Current Research Initiatives, a Glossary of Terms Related to Brain Disorders and Injuries, and a Directory of Sources for Further Help and Information

Edited by Sandra J. Judd. 625 pages. 2005. 0-7808-0744-8.

"Highly recommended pick for basic consumer health reference holdings at all levels."
—The Bookwatch, Aug '05

"Belongs on the shelves of any library with a consumer health collection." *— E-Streams, Mar '00*

"Recommended reference source."
— Booklist, American Library Association, Oct '99

SEE ALSO *Alzheimer's Disease Sourcebook*

■

Breast Cancer Sourcebook, 2nd Edition

Basic Consumer Health Information about Breast Cancer, Including Facts about Risk Factors, Prevention, Screening and Diagnostic Methods, Treatment Options, Complementary and Alternative Therapies, Post-Treatment Concerns, Clinical Trials, Special Risk Populations, and New Developments in Breast Cancer Research

Along with Breast Cancer Statistics, a Glossary of Related Terms, and a Directory of Resources for Additional Help and Information

Edited by Sandra J. Judd. 595 pages. 2004. 0-7808-0668-9.

"This book will be an excellent addition to public, community college, medical, and academic libraries."
— American Reference Books Annual, 2006

"It would be a useful reference book in a library or on loan to women in a support group."
— Cancer Forum, Mar '03

"Recommended reference source."
— Booklist, American Library Association, Jan '02

"This reference source is highly recommended. It is quite informative, comprehensive and detailed in nature, and yet it offers practical advice in easy-to-read language. It could be thought of as the 'bible' of breast cancer for the consumer." *— E-Streams, Jan '02*

"From the pros and cons of different screening methods and results to treatment options, *Breast Cancer Sourcebook* provides the latest information on the subject."
— Library Bookwatch, Dec '01

"This thoroughgoing, very readable reference covers all aspects of breast health and cancer. . . . Readers will find

much to consider here. Recommended for all public and patient health collections."
— *Library Journal, Sep '01*

SEE ALSO *Cancer Sourcebook for Women, Women's Health Concerns Sourcebook*

■

Breastfeeding Sourcebook

Basic Consumer Health Information about the Benefits of Breastmilk, Preparing to Breastfeed, Breastfeeding as a Baby Grows, Nutrition, and More, Including Information on Special Situations and Concerns Such as Mastitis, Illness, Medications, Allergies, Multiple Births, Prematurity, Special Needs, and Adoption

Along with a Glossary and Resources for Additional Help and Information

Edited by Jenni Lynn Colson. 388 pages. 2002. 0-7808-0332-9.

"Particularly useful is the information about professional lactation services and chapters on breastfeeding when returning to work. . . . *Breastfeeding Sourcebook* will be useful for public libraries, consumer health libraries, and technical schools offering nurse assistant training, especially in areas where Internet access is problematic."
— *American Reference Books Annual, 2003*

SEE ALSO *Pregnancy & Birth Sourcebook*

■

Burns Sourcebook

Basic Consumer Health Information about Various Types of Burns and Scalds, Including Flame, Heat, Cold, Electrical, Chemical, and Sun Burns

Along with Information on Short-Term and Long-Term Treatments, Tissue Reconstruction, Plastic Surgery, Prevention Suggestions, and First Aid

Edited by Allan R. Cook. 604 pages. 1999. 0-7808-0204-7.

"This is an exceptional addition to the series and is highly recommended for all consumer health collections, hospital libraries, and academic medical centers."
— *E-Streams, Mar '00*

"This key reference guide is an invaluable addition to all health care and public libraries in confronting this ongoing health issue."
— *American Reference Books Annual, 2000*

"Recommended reference source."
— *Booklist, American Library Association, Dec '99*

SEE ALSO *Dermatological Disorders Sourcebook*

■

Cancer Sourcebook, 4th Edition

Basic Consumer Health Information about Major Forms and Stages of Cancer, Featuring Facts about Head and Neck Cancers, Lung Cancers, Gastrointestinal Cancers, Genitourinary Cancers, Lymphomas, Blood Cell Cancers, Endocrine Cancers, Skin Cancers, Bone Cancers, Sarcomas, and Others, and Including Information about Cancer Treatments and Therapies,

Identifying and Reducing Cancer Risks, and Strategies for Coping with Cancer and the Side Effects of Treatment

Along with a Cancer Glossary, Statistical and Demographic Data, and a Directory of Sources for Additional Help and Information

Edited by Karen Bellenir. 1,119 pages. 2003. 0-7808-0633-6.

"With cancer being the second leading cause of death for Americans, a prodigious work such as this one, which locates centrally so much cancer-related information, is clearly an asset to this nation's citizens and others."
— *Journal of the National Medical Association, 2004*

"This title is recommended for health sciences and public libraries with consumer health collections."
— *E-Streams, Feb '01*

". . . can be effectively used by cancer patients and their families who are looking for answers in a language they can understand. Public and hospital libraries should have it on their shelves."
— *American Reference Books Annual, 2001*

"Recommended reference source."
— *Booklist, American Library Association, Dec '00*

SEE ALSO *Breast Cancer Sourcebook, Cancer Sourcebook for Women, Pediatric Cancer Sourcebook, Prostate Cancer Sourcebook*

■

Cancer Sourcebook for Women, 3rd Edition

Basic Consumer Health Information about Leading Causes of Cancer in Women, Featuring Facts about Gynecologic Cancers and Related Concerns, Such as Breast Cancer, Cervical Cancer, Endometrial Cancer, Uterine Sarcoma, Vaginal Cancer, Vulvar Cancer, and Common Non-Cancerous Gynecologic Conditions, in Addition to Facts about Lung Cancer, Colorectal Cancer, and Thyroid Cancer in Women

Along with Information about Cancer Risk Factors, Screening and Prevention, Treatment Options, and Tips on Coping with Life after Cancer Treatment, a Glossary of Cancer Terms, and a Directory of Resources for Additional Help and Information

Edited by Amy L. Sutton. 715 pages. 2006. 0-7808-0867-3.

"An excellent addition to collections in public, consumer health, and women's health libraries."
— *American Reference Books Annual, 2003*

"Overall, the information is excellent, and complex topics are clearly explained. As a reference book for the consumer it is a valuable resource to assist them to make informed decisions about cancer and its treatments."
— *Cancer Forum, Nov '02*

"Highly recommended for academic and medical reference collections."
— *Library Bookwatch, Sep '02*

"This is a highly recommended book for any public or consumer library, being reader friendly and containing accurate and helpful information."
— *E-Streams, Aug '02*

"Recommended reference source."
—*Booklist, American Library Association, Jul '02*

SEE ALSO *Breast Cancer Sourcebook, Women's Health Concerns Sourcebook*

■

Cardiovascular Diseases & Disorders Sourcebook, 3rd Edition

Basic Consumer Health Information about Heart and Vascular Diseases and Disorders, Such as Angina, Heart Attacks, Arrhythmias, Cardiomyopathy, Valve Disease, Atherosclerosis, and Aneurysms, with Information about Managing Cardiovascular Risk Factors and Maintaining Heart Health, Medications and Procedures Used to Treat Cardiovascular Disorders, and Concerns of Special Significance to Women

Along with Reports on Current Research Initiatives, a Glossary of Related Medical Terms, and a Directory of Sources for Further Help and Information

Edited by Sandra J. Judd. 713 pages. 2005. 0-7808-0739-1.

"This updated sourcebook is still the best first stop for comprehensive introductory information on cardiovascular diseases."
—*American Reference Books Annual, 2006*

"Recommended for public libraries and libraries supporting health care professionals."
—*E-Streams, Sep '05*

"This should be a standard health library reference."
—*The Bookwatch, Jun '05*

"Recommended reference source."
—*Booklist, American Library Association, Dec '00*

". . . comprehensive format provides an extensive overview on this subject."
—*Choice, Association of College & Research Libraries*

■

Caregiving Sourcebook

Basic Consumer Health Information for Caregivers, Including a Profile of Caregivers, Caregiving Responsibilities and Concerns, Tips for Specific Conditions, Care Environments, and the Effects of Caregiving

Along with Facts about Legal Issues, Financial Information, and Future Planning, a Glossary, and a Listing of Additional Resources

Edited by Joyce Brennfleck Shannon. 600 pages. 2001. 0-7808-0331-0.

"Essential for most collections."
—*Library Journal, Apr 1, 2002*

"An ideal addition to the reference collection of any public library. Health sciences information professionals may also want to acquire the *Caregiving Sourcebook* for their hospital or academic library for use as a ready reference tool by health care workers interested in aging and caregiving." —*E-Streams, Jan '02*

"Recommended reference source."
—*Booklist, American Library Association, Oct '01*

Child Abuse Sourcebook

Basic Consumer Health Information about the Physical, Sexual, and Emotional Abuse of Children, with Additional Facts about Neglect, Munchausen Syndrome by Proxy (MSBP), Shaken Baby Syndrome, and Controversial Issues Related to Child Abuse, Such as Withholding Medical Care, Corporal Punishment, and Child Maltreatment in Youth Sports, and Featuring Facts about Child Protective Services, Foster Care, Adoption, Parenting Challenges, and Other Abuse Prevention Efforts

Along with a Glossary of Related Terms and Resources for Additional Help and Information

Edited by Dawn D. Matthews. 620 pages. 2004. 0-7808-0705-7.

"A valuable and highly recommended resource for school, academic and public libraries whether used on its own or as a starting point for more in-depth research." —*E-Streams, Apr '05*

"Every week the news brings cases of child abuse or neglect, so it is useful to have a source that supplies so much helpful information. . . . Recommended. Public and academic libraries, and child welfare offices."
—*Choice, Association of College & Research Libraries, Mar '05*

"Packed with insights on all kinds of issues, from foster care and adoption to parenting and abuse prevention."
—*The Bookwatch, Nov '04*

SEE ALSO: *Domestic Violence Sourcebook, 2nd Edition*

■

Childhood Diseases & Disorders Sourcebook

Basic Consumer Health Information about Medical Problems Often Encountered in Pre-Adolescent Children, Including Respiratory Tract Ailments, Ear Infections, Sore Throats, Disorders of the Skin and Scalp, Digestive and Genitourinary Diseases, Infectious Diseases, Inflammatory Disorders, Chronic Physical and Developmental Disorders, Allergies, and More

Along with Information about Diagnostic Tests, Common Childhood Surgeries, and Frequently Used Medications, with a Glossary of Important Terms and Resource Directory

Edited by Chad T. Kimball. 662 pages. 2003. 0-7808-0458-9.

"This is an excellent book for new parents and should be included in all health care and public libraries."
—*American Reference Books Annual, 2004*

SEE ALSO: *Healthy Children Sourcebook*

■

Colds, Flu & Other Common Ailments Sourcebook

Basic Consumer Health Information about Common Ailments and Injuries, Including Colds, Coughs, the Flu, Sinus Problems, Headaches, Fever, Nausea and

Vomiting, Menstrual Cramps, Diarrhea, Constipation, Hemorrhoids, Back Pain, Dandruff, Dry and Itchy Skin, Cuts, Scrapes, Sprains, Bruises, and More

Along with Information about Prevention, Self-Care, Choosing a Doctor, Over-the-Counter Medications, Folk Remedies, and Alternative Therapies, and Including a Glossary of Important Terms and a Directory of Resources for Further Help and Information

Edited by Chad T. Kimball. 638 pages. 2001. 0-7808-0435-X.

"A good starting point for research on common illnesses. It will be a useful addition to public and consumer health library collections."
—American Reference Books Annual, 2002

"Will prove valuable to any library seeking to maintain a current, comprehensive reference collection of health resources. . . . Excellent reference."
—The Bookwatch, Aug '01

"Recommended reference source."
—Booklist, American Library Association, Jul '01

Communication Disorders Sourcebook

Basic Information about Deafness and Hearing Loss, Speech and Language Disorders, Voice Disorders, Balance and Vestibular Disorders, and Disorders of Smell, Taste, and Touch

Edited by Linda M. Ross. 533 pages. 1996. 0-7808-0077-X.

"This is skillfully edited and is a welcome resource for the layperson. It should be found in every public and medical library." —Booklist Health Sciences Supplement, American Library Association, Oct '97

Complementary & Alternative Medicine Sourcebook, 3rd Edition

Basic Consumer Health Information about Complementary and Alternative Medical Therapies, Including Acupuncture, Ayurveda, Traditional Chinese Medicine, Herbal Medicine, Homeopathy, Naturopathy, Biofeedback, Hypnotherapy, Yoga, Art Therapy, Aromatherapy, Clinical Nutrition, Vitamin and Mineral Supplements, Chiropractic, Massage, Reflexology, Crystal Therapy, Therapeutic Touch, and More

Along with Facts about Alternative and Complementary Treatments for Specific Conditions Such as Cancer, Diabetes, Osteoarthritis, Chronic Pain, Menopause, Gastrointestinal Disorders, Headaches, and Mental Illness, a Glossary, and a Resource List for Additional Help and Information

Edited by Sandra J. Judd. 657 pages. 2006. 0-7808-0864-9.

"Recommended for public, high school, and academic libraries that have consumer health collections. Hospital libraries that also serve the public will find this to be a useful resource." —E-Streams, Feb '03

"Recommended reference source."
—Booklist, American Library Association, Jan '03

"An important alternate health reference."
—MBR Bookwatch, Oct '02

"A great addition to the reference collection of every type of library." —American Reference Books Annual, 2000

Congenital Disorders Sourcebook

Basic Information about Disorders Acquired during Gestation, Including Spina Bifida, Hydrocephalus, Cerebral Palsy, Heart Defects, Craniofacial Abnormalities, Fetal Alcohol Syndrome, and More

Along with Current Treatment Options and Statistical Data

Edited by Karen Bellenir. 607 pages. 1997. 0-7808-0205-5.

"Recommended reference source."
—Booklist, American Library Association, Oct '97

SEE ALSO Pregnancy & Birth Sourcebook

Consumer Issues in Health Care Sourcebook

Basic Information about Health Care Fundamentals and Related Consumer Issues, Including Exams and Screening Tests, Physician Specialties, Choosing a Doctor, Using Prescription and Over-the-Counter Medications Safely, Avoiding Health Scams, Managing Common Health Risks in the Home, Care Options for Chronically or Terminally Ill Patients, and a List of Resources for Obtaining Help and Further Information

Edited by Karen Bellenir. 618 pages. 1998. 0-7808-0221-7.

"Both public and academic libraries will want to have a copy in their collection for readers who are interested in self-education on health issues."
—American Reference Books Annual, 2000

"The editor has researched the literature from government agencies and others, saving readers the time and effort of having to do the research themselves. Recommended for public libraries."
—Reference and User Services Quarterly, American Library Association, Spring '99

"Recommended reference source."
—Booklist, American Library Association, Dec '98

Contagious Diseases Sourcebook

Basic Consumer Health Information about Infectious Diseases Spread by Person-to-Person Contact through Direct Touch, Airborne Transmission, Sexual Contact, or Contact with Blood or Other Body Fluids, Including Hepatitis, Herpes, Influenza, Lice, Measles, Mumps, Pinworm, Ringworm, Severe Acute Respiratory Syndrome (SARS), Streptococcal Infections, Tuberculosis, and Others

Along with Facts about Disease Transmission, Antimicrobial Resistance, and Vaccines, with a Glossary and Directories of Resources for More Information

Edited by Karen Bellenir. 643 pages. 2004. 0-7808-0736-7.

■

Contagious & Non-Contagious Infectious Diseases Sourcebook

Basic Information about Contagious Diseases like Measles, Polio, Hepatitis B, and Infectious Mononucleosis, and Non-Contagious Infectious Diseases like Tetanus and Toxic Shock Syndrome, and Diseases Occurring as Secondary Infections Such as Shingles and Reye Syndrome

Along with Vaccination, Prevention, and Treatment Information, and a Section Describing Emerging Infectious Disease Threats

Edited by Karen Bellenir and Peter D. Dresser. 566 pages. 1996. 0-7808-0075-3.

SEE ALSO *Infectious Diseases Sourcebook*

■

Death & Dying Sourcebook, 2nd Edition

Basic Consumer Health Information about End-of-Life Care and Related Perspectives and Ethical Issues, Including End-of-Life Symptoms and Treatments, Pain Management, Quality-of-Life Concerns, the Use of Life Support, Patients' Rights and Privacy Issues, Advance Directives, Physician-Assisted Suicide, Caregiving, Organ and Tissue Donation, Autopsies, Funeral Arrangements, and Grief

Along with Statistical Data, Information about the Leading Causes of Death, a Glossary, and Directories of Support Groups and Other Resources

Edited by Joyce Brennfleck Shannon. 653 pages. 2006. 0-7808-0871-1.

"Public libraries, medical libraries, and academic libraries will all find this sourcebook a useful addition to their collections."
　　　　—American Reference Books Annual, 2001

"An extremely useful resource for those concerned with death and dying in the United States."
　　　　—Respiratory Care, Nov '00

"Recommended reference source."
　　　　—Booklist, American Library Association, Aug '00

"This book is a definite must for all those involved in end-of-life care."　　*—Doody's Review Service, 2000*

Dental Care & Oral Health Sourcebook, 2nd Edition

Basic Consumer Health Information about Dental Care, Including Oral Hygiene, Dental Visits, Pain Management, Cavities, Crowns, Bridges, Dental Implants, and Fillings, and Other Oral Health Concerns, Such as Gum Disease, Bad Breath, Dry Mouth, Genetic and Developmental Abnormalities, Oral Cancers, Orthodontics, and Temporomandibular Disorders

Along with Updates on Current Research in Oral Health, a Glossary, a Directory of Dental and Oral Health Organizations, and Resources for People with Dental and Oral Health Disorders

Edited by Amy L. Sutton. 609 pages. 2003. 0-7808-0634-4.

"This book could serve as a turning point in the battle to educate consumers in issues concerning oral health."
　　　　—American Reference Books Annual, 2004

"Unique source which will fill a gap in dental sources for patients and the lay public. A valuable reference tool even in a library with thousands of books on dentistry. Comprehensive, clear, inexpensive, and easy to read and use. It fills an enormous gap in the health care literature."　　*—Reference & User Services Quarterly, American Library Association, Summer '98*

"Recommended reference source."
　　　　—Booklist, American Library Association, Dec '97

■

Depression Sourcebook

Basic Consumer Health Information about Unipolar Depression, Bipolar Disorder, Postpartum Depression, Seasonal Affective Disorder, and Other Types of Depression in Children, Adolescents, Women, Men, the Elderly, and Other Selected Populations

Along with Facts about Causes, Risk Factors, Diagnostic Criteria, Treatment Options, Coping Strategies, Suicide Prevention, a Glossary, and a Directory of Sources for Additional Help and Information

Edited by Karen Belleni. 602 pages. 2002. 0-7808-0611-5.

"*Depression Sourcebook* is of a very high standard. Its purpose, which is to serve as a reference source to the lay reader, is very well served."
　　　　—Journal of the National Medical Association, 2004

"Invaluable reference for public and school library collections alike."　　*—Library Bookwatch, Apr '03*

"Recommended for purchase."
　　　　—American Reference Books Annual, 2003

■

Dermatological Disorders Sourcebook, 2nd Edition

Basic Consumer Health Information about Conditions and Disorders Affecting the Skin, Hair, and Nails, Such as Acne, Rosacea, Rashes, Dermatitis, Pigmentation Disorders, Birthmarks, Skin Cancer, Skin Injuries, Psoriasis, Scleroderma, and Hair Loss, Including Facts about Medications and Treatments for Dermatological

Disorders and Tips for Maintaining Healthy Skin, Hair, and Nails

Along with Information about How Aging Affects the Skin, a Glossary of Related Terms, and a Directory of Resources for Additional Help and Information

Edited by Amy L. Sutton. 645 pages. 2005. 0-7808-0795-2.

"... comprehensive, easily read reference book."
—Doody's Health Sciences Book Reviews, Oct '97

SEE ALSO Burns Sourcebook

Diabetes Sourcebook, 3rd Edition

Basic Consumer Health Information about Type 1 Diabetes (Insulin-Dependent or Juvenile-Onset Diabetes), Type 2 Diabetes (Noninsulin-Dependent or Adult-Onset Diabetes), Gestational Diabetes, Impaired Glucose Tolerance (IGT), and Related Complications, Such as Amputation, Eye Disease, Gum Disease, Nerve Damage, and End-Stage Renal Disease, Including Facts about Insulin, Oral Diabetes Medications, Blood Sugar Testing, and the Role of Exercise and Nutrition in the Control of Diabetes

Along with a Glossary and Resources for Further Help and Information

Edited by Dawn D. Matthews. 622 pages. 2003. 0-7808-0629-8.

"This edition is even more helpful than earlier versions. . . . It is a truly valuable tool for anyone seeking readable and authoritative information on diabetes."
—American Reference Books Annual, 2004

"An invaluable reference." —Library Journal, May '00

Selected as one of the 250 "Best Health Sciences Books of 1999." —Doody's Rating Service, Mar-Apr '00

"Provides useful information for the general public."
—Healthlines, University of Michigan Health Management Research Center, Sep/Oct '99

"... provides reliable mainstream medical information . . . belongs on the shelves of any library with a consumer health collection." —E-Streams, Sep '99

"Recommended reference source."
—Booklist, American Library Association, Feb '99

Diet & Nutrition Sourcebook, 3rd Edition

Basic Consumer Health Information about Dietary Guidelines and the Food Guidance System, Recommended Daily Nutrient Intakes, Serving Proportions, Weight Control, Vitamins and Supplements, Nutrition Issues for Different Life Stages and Lifestyles, and the Needs of People with Specific Medical Concerns, Including Cancer, Celiac Disease, Diabetes, Eating Disorders, Food Allergies, and Cardiovascular Disease

Along with Facts about Federal Nutrition Support Programs, a Glossary of Nutrition and Dietary Terms, and Directories of Additional Resources for More Information about Nutrition

Edited by Joyce Brennfleck Shannon. 633 pages. 2006. 0-7808-0800-2.

"This book is an excellent source of basic diet and nutrition information." —Booklist Health Sciences Supplement, American Library Association, Dec '00

"This reference document should be in any public library, but it would be a very good guide for beginning students in the health sciences. If the other books in this publisher's series are as good as this, they should all be in the health sciences collections."
—American Reference Books Annual, 2000

"This book is an excellent general nutrition reference for consumers who desire to take an active role in their health care for prevention. Consumers of all ages who select this book can feel confident they are receiving current and accurate information." —Journal of Nutrition for the Elderly, Vol. 19, No. 4, 2000

SEE ALSO Digestive Diseases & Disorders Sourcebook, Eating Disorders Sourcebook, Gastrointestinal Diseases & Disorders Sourcebook, Vegetarian Sourcebook

---

Digestive Diseases & Disorders Sourcebook

Basic Consumer Health Information about Diseases and Disorders that Impact the Upper and Lower Digestive System, Including Celiac Disease, Constipation, Crohn's Disease, Cyclic Vomiting Syndrome, Diarrhea, Diverticulosis and Diverticulitis, Gallstones, Heartburn, Hemorrhoids, Hernias, Indigestion (Dyspepsia), Irritable Bowel Syndrome, Lactose Intolerance, Ulcers, and More

Along with Information about Medications and Other Treatments, Tips for Maintaining a Healthy Digestive Tract, a Glossary, and Directory of Digestive Diseases Organizations

Edited by Karen Bellenir. 335 pages. 2000. 0-7808-0327-2.

"This title would be an excellent addition to all public or patient-research libraries."
—American Reference Books Annual, 2001

"This title is recommended for public, hospital, and health sciences libraries with consumer health collections." —E-Streams, Jul-Aug '00

"Recommended reference source."
—Booklist, American Library Association, May '00

SEE ALSO Eating Disorders Sourcebook, Gastrointestinal Diseases & Disorders Sourcebook

---

Disabilities Sourcebook

Basic Consumer Health Information about Physical and Psychiatric Disabilities, Including Descriptions of Major Causes of Disability, Assistive and Adaptive Aids, Workplace Issues, and Accessibility Concerns

Along with Information about the Americans with Disabilities Act, a Glossary, and Resources for Additional Help and Information

Edited by Dawn D. Matthews. 616 pages. 2000. 0-7808-0389-2.

"It is a must for libraries with a consumer health section." — *American Reference Books Annual, 2002*

"A much needed addition to the Omnigraphics Health Reference Series. A current reference work to provide people with disabilities, their families, caregivers or those who work with them, a broad range of information in one volume, has not been available until now. . . . It is recommended for all public and academic library reference collections." — *E-Streams, May '01*

"An excellent source book in easy-to-read format covering many current topics; highly recommended for all libraries." — *Choice, Association of College & Research Libraries, Jan '01*

"Recommended reference source." — *Booklist, American Library Association, Jul '00*

■

Domestic Violence Sourcebook, 2nd Edition

Basic Consumer Health Information about the Causes and Consequences of Abusive Relationships, Including Physical Violence, Sexual Assault, Battery, Stalking, and Emotional Abuse, and Facts about the Effects of Violence on Women, Men, Young Adults, and the Elderly, with Reports about Domestic Violence in Selected Populations, and Featuring Facts about Medical Care, Victim Assistance and Protection, Prevention Strategies, Mental Health Services, and Legal Issues

Along with a Glossary of Related Terms and Resources for Additional Help and Information

Edited by Dawn D. Matthews. 628 pages. 2004. 0-7808-0669-7.

"Educators, clergy, medical professionals, police, and victims and their families will benefit from this realistic and easy-to-understand resource." — *American Reference Books Annual, 2005*

"Recommended for all collections supporting consumer health information. It should also be considered for any collection needing general, readable information on domestic violence." — *E-Streams, Jan '05*

"This sourcebook complements other books in its field, providing a one-stop resource . . . Recommended." — *Choice, Association of College & Research Libraries, Jan '05*

"Interested lay persons should find the book extremely beneficial. . . . A copy of *Domestic Violence and Child Abuse Sourcebook* should be in every public library in the United States." — *Social Science & Medicine, No. 56, 2003*

"This is important information. The Web has many resources but this sourcebook fills an important societal need. I am not aware of any other resources of this type." — *Doody's Review Service, Sep '01*

"Recommended reference source." — *Booklist, American Library Association, Apr '01*

"Important pick for college-level health reference libraries." — *The Bookwatch, Mar '01*

"Because this problem is so widespread and because this book includes a lot of issues within one volume, this work is recommended for all public libraries." — *American Reference Books Annual, 2001*

SEE ALSO Child Abuse Sourcebook

■

Drug Abuse Sourcebook, 2nd Edition

Basic Consumer Health Information about Illicit Substances of Abuse and the Misuse of Prescription and Over-the-Counter Medications, Including Depressants, Hallucinogens, Inhalants, Marijuana, Stimulants, and Anabolic Steroids

Along with Facts about Related Health Risks, Treatment Programs, Prevention Programs, a Glossary of Abuse and Addiction Terms, a Glossary of Drug-Related Street Terms, and a Directory of Resources for More Information

Edited by Catherine Ginther. 607 pages. 2004. 0-7808-0740-5.

"Commendable for organizing useful, normally scattered government and association-produced data into a logical sequence." — *American Reference Books Annual, 2006*

"This easy-to-read volume is recommended for consumer health collections within public or academic libraries." — *E-Streams, Sep '05*

"An excellent library reference." — *The Bookwatch, May '05*

"Containing a wealth of information, this book will be useful to the college student just beginning to explore the topic of substance abuse. This resource belongs in libraries that serve a lower-division undergraduate or community college clientele as well as the general public." — *Choice, Association of College & Research Libraries, Jun '01*

"Recommended reference source." — *Booklist, American Library Association, Feb '01*

SEE ALSO Alcoholism Sourcebook, Substance Abuse Sourcebook

■

Ear, Nose & Throat Disorders Sourcebook, 2nd Edition

Basic Consumer Health Information about Disorders of the Ears, Hearing Loss, Vestibular Disorders, Nasal and Sinus Problems, Throat and Vocal Cord Disorders, and Otolaryngologic Cancers, Including Facts about Ear Infections and Injuries, Genetic and Congenital Deafness, Sensorineural Hearing Disorders, Tinnitus, Vertigo, Ménière Disease, Rhinitis, Sinusitis, Snoring, Sore Throats, Hoarseness, and More

Along with Reports on Current Research Initiatives, a Glossary of Related Medical Terms, and a Directory of Sources for Further Help and Information

Edited by Sandra J. Judd. 659 pages. 2006. 0-7808-0872-X.

"Overall, this sourcebook is helpful for the consumer seeking information on ENT issues. It is recommended for public libraries."
—American Reference Books Annual, 1999

"Recommended reference source."
—Booklist, American Library Association, Dec '98

∎

Eating Disorders Sourcebook

Basic Consumer Health Information about Eating Disorders, Including Information about Anorexia Nervosa, Bulimia Nervosa, Binge Eating, Body Dysmorphic Disorder, Pica, Laxative Abuse, and Night Eating Syndrome

Along with Information about Causes, Adverse Effects, and Treatment and Prevention Issues, and Featuring a Section on Concerns Specific to Children and Adolescents, a Glossary, and Resources for Further Help and Information

Edited by Dawn D. Matthews. 322 pages. 2001. 0-7808-0335-3.

"Recommended for health science libraries that are open to the public, as well as hospital libraries. This book is a good resource for the consumer who is concerned about eating disorders." —E-Streams, Mar '02

"This volume is another convenient collection of excerpted articles. Recommended for school and public library patrons; lower-division undergraduates; and two-year technical program students."
—Choice, Association of College & Research Libraries, Jan '02

"Recommended reference source."
—Booklist, American Library Association, Oct '01

SEE ALSO Diet & Nutrition Sourcebook, Digestive Diseases & Disorders Sourcebook, Gastrointestinal Diseases & Disorders Sourcebook

∎

Emergency Medical Services Sourcebook

Basic Consumer Health Information about Preventing, Preparing for, and Managing Emergency Situations, When and Who to Call for Help, What to Expect in the Emergency Room, the Emergency Medical Team, Patient Issues, and Current Topics in Emergency Medicine

Along with Statistical Data, a Glossary, and Sources of Additional Help and Information

Edited by Jenni Lynn Colson. 494 pages. 2002. 0-7808-0420-1.

"Handy and convenient for home, public, school, and college libraries. Recommended."
— Choice, Association of College & Research Libraries, Apr '03

"This reference can provide the consumer with answers to most questions about emergency care in the United States, or it will direct them to a resource where the answer can be found."
—American Reference Books Annual, 2003

"Recommended reference source."
— Booklist, American Library Association, Feb '03

∎

Endocrine & Metabolic Disorders Sourcebook

Basic Information for the Layperson about Pancreatic and Insulin-Related Disorders Such as Pancreatitis, Diabetes, and Hypoglycemia; Adrenal Gland Disorders Such as Cushing's Syndrome, Addison's Disease, and Congenital Adrenal Hyperplasia; Pituitary Gland Disorders Such as Growth Hormone Deficiency, Acromegaly, and Pituitary Tumors; Thyroid Disorders Such as Hypothyroidism, Graves' Disease, Hashimoto's Disease, and Goiter; Hyperparathyroidism; and Other Diseases and Syndromes of Hormone Imbalance or Metabolic Dysfunction

Along with Reports on Current Research Initiatives

Edited by Linda M. Shin. 574 pages. 1998. 0-7808-0207-1.

"Omnigraphics has produced another needed resource for health information consumers."
—American Reference Books Annual, 2000

"Recommended reference source."
— Booklist, American Library Association, Dec '98

∎

Environmental Health Sourcebook, 2nd Edition

Basic Consumer Health Information about the Environment and Its Effect on Human Health, Including the Effects of Air Pollution, Water Pollution, Hazardous Chemicals, Food Hazards, Radiation Hazards, Biological Agents, Household Hazards, Such as Radon, Asbestos, Carbon Monoxide, and Mold, and Information about Associated Diseases and Disorders, Including Cancer, Allergies, Respiratory Problems, and Skin Disorders

Along with Information about Environmental Concerns for Specific Populations, a Glossary of Related Terms, and Resources for Further Help and Information

Edited by Dawn D. Matthews. 673 pages. 2003. 0-7808-0632-8.

"This recently updated edition continues the level of quality and the reputation of the numerous other volumes in Omnigraphics' Health Reference Series."
—American Reference Books Annual, 2004

"An excellent updated edition."
—The Bookwatch, Oct '03

"Recommended reference source."
— Booklist, American Library Association, Sep '98

"This book will be a useful addition to anyone's library." —Choice Health Sciences Supplement, Association of College & Research Libraries, May '98

"... a good survey of numerous environmentally induced physical disorders ... a useful addition to anyone's library."
— *Doody's Health Sciences Book Reviews, Jan '98*

Environmentally Induced Disorders Sourcebook

SEE *Environmental Health Sourcebook, 2nd Edition*

Ethnic Diseases Sourcebook

Basic Consumer Health Information for Ethnic and Racial Minority Groups in the United States, Including General Health Indicators and Behaviors, Ethnic Diseases, Genetic Testing, the Impact of Chronic Diseases, Women's Health, Mental Health Issues, and Preventive Health Care Services

Along with a Glossary and a Listing of Additional Resources

Edited by Joyce Brennfleck Shannon. 664 pages. 2001. 0-7808-0336-1.

"Recommended for health sciences libraries where public health programs are a priority."
— *E-Streams, Jan '02*

"Not many books have been written on this topic to date, and the *Ethnic Diseases Sourcebook* is a strong addition to the list. It will be an important introductory resource for health consumers, students, health care personnel, and social scientists. It is recommended for public, academic, and large hospital libraries."
— *American Reference Books Annual, 2002*

"Recommended reference source."
— *Booklist, American Library Association, Oct '01*

"Will prove valuable to any library seeking to maintain a current, comprehensive reference collection of health resources.... An excellent source of health information about genetic disorders which affect particular ethnic and racial minorities in the U.S."
— *The Bookwatch, Aug '01*

Eye Care Sourcebook, 2nd Edition

Basic Consumer Health Information about Eye Care and Eye Disorders, Including Facts about the Diagnosis, Prevention, and Treatment of Common Refractive Problems Such as Myopia, Hyperopia, Astigmatism, and Presbyopia, and Eye Diseases, Including Glaucoma, Cataract, Age-Related Macular Degeneration, and Diabetic Retinopathy

Along with a Section on Vision Correction and Refractive Surgeries, Including LASIK and LASEK, a Glossary, and Directories of Resources for Additional Help and Information

Edited by Amy L. Sutton. 543 pages. 2003. 0-7808-0635-2.

"... a solid reference tool for eye care and a valuable addition to a collection."
— *American Reference Books Annual, 2004*

Family Planning Sourcebook

Basic Consumer Health Information about Planning for Pregnancy and Contraception, Including Traditional Methods, Barrier Methods, Hormonal Methods, Permanent Methods, Future Methods, Emergency Contraception, and Birth Control Choices for Women at Each Stage of Life

Along with Statistics, a Glossary, and Sources of Additional Information

Edited by Amy Marcaccio Keyzer. 520 pages. 2001. 0-7808-0379-5.

"Recommended for public, health, and undergraduate libraries as part of the circulating collection."
— *E-Streams, Mar '02*

"Information is presented in an unbiased, readable manner, and the sourcebook will certainly be a necessary addition to those public and high school libraries where Internet access is restricted or otherwise problematic." — *American Reference Books Annual, 2002*

"Recommended reference source."
— *Booklist, American Library Association, Oct '01*

"Will prove valuable to any library seeking to maintain a current, comprehensive reference collection of health resources.... Excellent reference."
— *The Bookwatch, Aug '01*

SEE ALSO *Pregnancy & Birth Sourcebook*

Fitness & Exercise Sourcebook, 2nd Edition

Basic Consumer Health Information about the Fundamentals of Fitness and Exercise, Including How to Begin and Maintain a Fitness Program, Fitness as a Lifestyle, the Link between Fitness and Diet, Advice for Specific Groups of People, Exercise as It Relates to Specific Medical Conditions, and Recent Research in Fitness and Exercise

Along with a Glossary of Important Terms and Resources for Additional Help and Information

Edited by Kristen M. Gledhill. 646 pages. 2001. 0-7808-0334-5.

"This work is recommended for all general reference collections."
— *American Reference Books Annual, 2002*

"Highly recommended for public, consumer, and school grades fourth through college." — *E-Streams, Nov '01*

"Recommended reference source."
— *Booklist, American Library Association, Oct '01*

"The information appears quite comprehensive and is considered reliable. . . . This second edition is a welcomed addition to the series."
— *Doody's Review Service, Sep '01*

Food & Animal Borne Diseases Sourcebook

Basic Information about Diseases That Can Be Spread to Humans through the Ingestion of Contaminated Food or Water or by Contact with Infected Animals and Insects, Such as Botulism, E. Coli, Hepatitis A, Trichinosis, Lyme Disease, and Rabies

Along with Information Regarding Prevention and Treatment Methods, and Including a Special Section for International Travelers Describing Diseases Such as Cholera, Malaria, Travelers' Diarrhea, and Yellow Fever, and Offering Recommendations for Avoiding Illness

Edited by Karen Bellenir and Peter D. Dresser. 535 pages. 1995. 0-7808-0033-8.

"Targeting general readers and providing them with a single, comprehensive source of information on selected topics, this book continues, with the excellent caliber of its predecessors, to catalog topical information on health matters of general interest. Readable and thorough, this valuable resource is highly recommended for all libraries."

— *Academic Library Book Review, Summer '96*

"A comprehensive collection of authoritative information."   — *Emergency Medical Services, Oct '95*

■

Food Safety Sourcebook

Basic Consumer Health Information about the Safe Handling of Meat, Poultry, Seafood, Eggs, Fruit Juices, and Other Food Items, and Facts about Pesticides, Drinking Water, Food Safety Overseas, and the Onset, Duration, and Symptoms of Foodborne Illnesses, Including Types of Pathogenic Bacteria, Parasitic Protozoa, Worms, Viruses, and Natural Toxins

Along with the Role of the Consumer, the Food Handler, and the Government in Food Safety; a Glossary, and Resources for Additional Help and Information

Edited by Dawn D. Matthews. 339 pages. 1999. 0-7808-0326-4.

"This book is recommended for public libraries and universities with home economic and food science programs."   — *E-Streams, Nov '00*

"Recommended reference source."

— *Booklist, American Library Association, May '00*

"This book takes the complex issues of food safety and foodborne pathogens and presents them in an easily understood manner. [It does] an excellent job of covering a large and often confusing topic."

— *American Reference Books Annual, 2000*

■

Forensic Medicine Sourcebook

Basic Consumer Information for the Layperson about Forensic Medicine, Including Crime Scene Investigation, Evidence Collection and Analysis, Expert Testimony, Computer-Aided Criminal Identification, Digital Imaging in the Courtroom, DNA Profiling, Accident Reconstruction, Autopsies, Ballistics, Drugs and

Explosives Detection, Latent Fingerprints, Product Tampering, and Questioned Document Examination

Along with Statistical Data, a Glossary of Forensics Terminology, and Listings of Sources for Further Help and Information

Edited by Annemarie S. Muth. 574 pages. 1999. 0-7808-0232-2.

"Given the expected widespread interest in its content and its easy to read style, this book is recommended for most public and all college and university libraries."

— *E-Streams, Feb '01*

"Recommended for public libraries."

— *Reference & User Services Quarterly, American Library Association, Spring 2000*

"Recommended reference source."

— *Booklist, American Library Association, Feb '00*

"A wealth of information, useful statistics, references are up-to-date and extremely complete. This wonderful collection of data will help students who are interested in a career in any type of forensic field. It is a great resource for attorneys who need information about types of expert witnesses needed in a particular case. It also offers useful information for fiction and nonfiction writers whose work involves a crime. A fascinating compilation. All levels."

— *Choice, Association of College & Research Libraries, Jan '00*

"There are several items that make this book attractive to consumers who are seeking certain forensic data. . . . This is a useful current source for those seeking general forensic medical answers."

— *American Reference Books Annual, 2000*

■

Gastrointestinal Diseases & Disorders Sourcebook, 2nd Edition

Basic Consumer Health Information about the Upper and Lower Gastrointestinal (GI) Tract, Including the Esophagus, Stomach, Intestines, Rectum, Liver, and Pancreas, with Facts about Gastroesophageal Reflux Disease, Gastritis, Hernias, Ulcers, Celiac Disease, Diverticulitis, Irritable Bowel Syndrome, Hemorrhoids, Gastrointestinal Cancers, and Other Diseases and Disorders Related to the Digestive Process

Along with Information about Commonly Used Diagnostic and Surgical Procedures, Statistics, Reports on Current Research Initiatives and Clinical Trials, a Glossary, and Resources for Additional Help and Information

Edited by Sandra J. Judd. 681 pages. 2006. 0-7808-0798-7.

". . . very readable form. The successful editorial work that brought this material together into a useful and understandable reference makes accessible to all readers information that can help them more effectively understand and obtain help for digestive tract problems."

— *Choice, Association of College & Research Libraries, Feb '97*

SEE ALSO *Diet & Nutrition Sourcebook, Digestive Diseases & Disorders, Eating Disorders Sourcebook*

■

Genetic Disorders Sourcebook, 3rd Edition

Basic Consumer Health Information about Hereditary Diseases and Disorders, Including Facts about the Human Genome, Genetic Inheritance Patterns, Disorders Associated with Specific Genes, Such as Sickle Cell Disease, Hemophilia, and Cystic Fibrosis, Chromosome Disorders, Such as Down Syndrome, Fragile X Syndrome, and Turner Syndrome, and Complex Diseases and Disorders Resulting from the Interaction of Environmental and Genetic Factors, Such as Allergies, Cancer, and Obesity

Along with Facts about Genetic Testing, Suggestions for Parents of Children with Special Needs, Reports on Current Research Initiatives, a Glossary of Genetic Terminology, and Resources for Additional Help and Information

Edited by Karen Bellenir. 777 pages. 2004. 0-7808-0742-1.

"This text is recommended for any library with an interest in providing consumer health resources."
— *E-Streams, Aug '05*

"This is a valuable resource for anyone wishing to have an understandable description of any of the topics or disorders included. The editor succeeds in making complex genetic issues understandable."
— *Doody's Book Review Service, May '05*

"A good acquisition for public libraries."
— *American Reference Books Annual, 2005*

"Excellent reference." — *The Bookwatch, Jan '05*

"Recommended reference source."
— *Booklist, American Library Association, Apr '01*

"Important pick for college-level health reference libraries." — *The Bookwatch, Mar '01*

■

Head Trauma Sourcebook

Basic Information for the Layperson about Open-Head and Closed-Head Injuries, Treatment Advances, Recovery, and Rehabilitation

Along with Reports on Current Research Initiatives

Edited by Karen Bellenir. 414 pages. 1997. 0-7808-0208-X.

■

Headache Sourcebook

Basic Consumer Health Information about Migraine, Tension, Cluster, Rebound and Other Types of Headaches, with Facts about the Cause and Prevention of Headaches, the Effects of Stress and the Environment, Headaches during Pregnancy and Menopause, and Childhood Headaches

Along with a Glossary and Other Resources for Additional Help and Information

Edited by Dawn D. Matthews. 362 pages. 2002. 0-7808-0337-X.

"Highly recommended for academic and medical reference collections." — *Library Bookwatch, Sep '02*

■

Health Insurance Sourcebook

Basic Information about Managed Care Organizations, Traditional Fee-for-Service Insurance, Insurance Portability and Pre-Existing Conditions Clauses, Medicare, Medicaid, Social Security, and Military Health Care

Along with Information about Insurance Fraud

Edited by Wendy Wilcox. 530 pages. 1997. 0-7808-0222-5.

"Particularly useful because it brings much of this information together in one volume. This book will be a handy reference source in the health sciences library, hospital library, college and university library, and medium to large public library."
— *Medical Reference Services Quarterly, Fall '98*

Awarded "Books of the Year Award"
— *American Journal of Nursing, 1997*

"The layout of the book is particularly helpful as it provides easy access to reference material. A most useful addition to the vast amount of information about health insurance. The use of data from U.S. government agencies is most commendable. Useful in a library or learning center for healthcare professional students."
— *Doody's Health Sciences Book Reviews, Nov '97*

■

Healthy Aging Sourcebook

Basic Consumer Health Information about Maintaining Health through the Aging Process, Including Advice on Nutrition, Exercise, and Sleep, Help in Making Decisions about Midlife Issues and Retirement, and Guidance Concerning Practical and Informed Choices in Health Consumerism

Along with Data Concerning the Theories of Aging, Different Experiences in Aging by Minority Groups, and Facts about Aging Now and Aging in the Future; and Featuring a Glossary, a Guide to Consumer Help, Additional Suggested Reading, and Practical Resource Directory

Edited by Jenifer Swanson. 536 pages. 1999. 0-7808-0390-6.

"Recommended reference source."
— *Booklist, American Library Association, Feb '00*

SEE ALSO Physical & Mental Issues in Aging Sourcebook

■

Healthy Children Sourcebook

Basic Consumer Health Information about the Physical and Mental Development of Children between the Ages of 3 and 12, Including Routine Health Care, Preventative Health Services, Safety and First Aid, Healthy Sleep, Dental Care, Nutrition, and Fitness, and Featuring Parenting Tips on Such Topics as Bed-

wetting, Choosing Day Care, Monitoring TV and Other Media, and Establishing a Foundation for Substance Abuse Prevention

Along with a Glossary of Commonly Used Pediatric Terms and Resources for Additional Help and Information.

Edited by Chad T. Kimball. 647 pages. 2003. 0-7808-0247-0.

"It is hard to imagine that any other single resource exists that would provide such a comprehensive guide of timely information on health promotion and disease prevention for children aged 3 to 12."
—*American Reference Books Annual, 2004*

"The strengths of this book are many. It is clearly written, presented and structured."
—*Journal of the National Medical Association, 2004*

SEE ALSO Childhood Diseases & Disorders Sourcebook

■

Healthy Heart Sourcebook for Women

Basic Consumer Health Information about Cardiac Issues Specific to Women, Including Facts about Major Risk Factors and Prevention, Treatment and Control Strategies, and Important Dietary Issues

Along with a Special Section Regarding the Pros and Cons of Hormone Replacement Therapy and Its Impact on Heart Health, and Additional Help, Including Recipes, a Glossary, and a Directory of Resources

Edited by Dawn D. Matthews. 336 pages. 2000. 0-7808-0329-9.

"A good reference source and recommended for all public, academic, medical, and hospital libraries."
—*Medical Reference Services Quarterly, Summer '01*

"Because of the lack of information specific to women on this topic, this book is recommended for public libraries and consumer libraries."
—*American Reference Books Annual, 2001*

"Contains very important information about coronary artery disease that all women should know. The information is current and presented in an easy-to-read format. The book will make a good addition to any library."
—*American Medical Writers Association Journal, Summer '00*

"Important, basic reference."
—*Reviewer's Bookwatch, Jul '00*

SEE ALSO Cardiovascular Diseases & Disorders Sourcebook, Women's Health Concerns Sourcebook

■

Heart Diseases & Disorders Sourcebook

SEE Cardiovascular Diseases & Disorders Sourcebook, 3rd Edition

Hepatitis Sourcebook

Basic Consumer Health Information about Hepatitis A, Hepatitis B, Hepatitis C, and Other Forms of Hepatitis, Including Autoimmune Hepatitis, Alcoholic Hepatitis, Nonalcoholic Steatohepatitis, and Toxic Hepatitis, with Facts about Risk Factors, Screening Methods, Diagnostic Tests, and Treatment Options

Along with Information on Liver Health, Tips for People Living with Chronic Hepatitis, Reports on Current Research Initiatives, a Glossary of Terms Related to Hepatitis, and a Directory of Sources for Further Help and Information

Edited by Sandra J. Judd. 597 pages. 2005. 0-7808-0749-9.

"Highly recommended."
—*American Reference Books Annual, 2006*

■

Household Safety Sourcebook

Basic Consumer Health Information about Household Safety, Including Information about Poisons, Chemicals, Fire, and Water Hazards in the Home

Along with Advice about the Safe Use of Home Maintenance Equipment, Choosing Toys and Nursery Furniture, Holiday and Recreation Safety, a Glossary, and Resources for Further Help and Information

Edited by Dawn D. Matthews. 606 pages. 2002. 0-7808-0338-8.

"This work will be useful in public libraries with large consumer health and wellness departments."
—*American Reference Books Annual, 2003*

"As a sourcebook on household safety this book meets its mark. It is encyclopedic in scope and covers a wide range of safety issues that are commonly seen in the home."
—*E-Streams, Jul '02*

■

Hypertension Sourcebook

Basic Consumer Health Information about the Causes, Diagnosis, and Treatment of High Blood Pressure, with Facts about Consequences, Complications, and Co-Occurring Disorders, Such as Coronary Heart Disease, Diabetes, Stroke, Kidney Disease, and Hypertensive Retinopathy, and Issues in Blood Pressure Control, Including Dietary Choices, Stress Management, and Medications

Along with Reports on Current Research Initiatives and Clinical Trials, a Glossary, and Resources for Additional Help and Information

Edited by Dawn D. Matthews and Karen Bellenir. 613 pages. 2004. 0-7808-0674-3.

"Academic, public, and medical libraries will want to add the *Hypertension Sourcebook* to their collections."
—*E-Streams, Aug '05*

"The strength of this source is the wide range of information given about hypertension."
—*American Reference Books Annual, 2005*

Immune System Disorders Sourcebook, 2nd Edition

Basic Consumer Health Information about Disorders of the Immune System, Including Immune System Function and Response, Diagnosis of Immune Disorders, Information about Inherited Immune Disease, Acquired Immune Disease, and Autoimmune Diseases, Including Primary Immune Deficiency, Acquired Immunodeficiency Syndrome (AIDS), Lupus, Multiple Sclerosis, Type 1 Diabetes, Rheumatoid Arthritis, and Graves' Disease

Along with Treatments, Tips for Coping with Immune Disorders, a Glossary, and a Directory of Additional Resources.

Edited by Joyce Brennfleck Shannon. 671 pages. 2005. 0-7808-0748-0

"Highly recommended for academic and public libraries." — *American Reference Books Annual, 2006*

"The updated second edition is a 'must' for any consumer health library seeking a solid resource covering the treatments, symptoms, and options for immune disorder sufferers. . . . An excellent guide."
— *MBR Bookwatch, Jan '06*

■

Infant & Toddler Health Sourcebook

Basic Consumer Health Information about the Physical and Mental Development of Newborns, Infants, and Toddlers, Including Neonatal Concerns, Nutrition Recommendations, Immunization Schedules, Common Pediatric Disorders, Assessments and Milestones, Safety Tips, and Advice for Parents and Other Caregivers

Along with a Glossary of Terms and Resource Listings for Additional Help

Edited by Jenifer Swanson. 585 pages. 2000. 0-7808-0246-2.

"As a reference for the general public, this would be useful in any library." — *E-Streams, May '01*

"Recommended reference source."
— *Booklist, American Library Association, Feb '01*

"This is a good source for general use."
— *American Reference Books Annual, 2001*

■

Infectious Diseases Sourcebook

Basic Consumer Health Information about Non-Contagious Bacterial, Viral, Prion, Fungal, and Parasitic Diseases Spread by Food and Water, Insects and Animals, or Environmental Contact, Including Botulism, E. Coli, Encephalitis, Legionnaires' Disease, Lyme Disease, Malaria, Plague, Rabies, Salmonella, Tetanus, and Others, and Facts about Newly Emerging Diseases, Such as Hantavirus, Mad Cow Disease, Monkeypox, and West Nile Virus

Along with Information about Preventing Disease Transmission, the Threat of Bioterrorism, and Current

Research Initiatives, with a Glossary and Directory of Resources for More Information

Edited by Karen Bellenir. 634 pages. 2004. 0-7808-0675-1.

"This reference continues the excellent tradition of the *Health Reference Series* in consolidating a wealth of information on a selected topic into a format that is easy to use and accessible to the general public."
— *American Reference Books Annual, 2005*

"Recommended for public and academic libraries."
— *E-Streams, Jan '05*

■

Injury & Trauma Sourcebook

Basic Consumer Health Information about the Impact of Injury, the Diagnosis and Treatment of Common and Traumatic Injuries, Emergency Care, and Specific Injuries Related to Home, Community, Workplace, Transportation, and Recreation

Along with Guidelines for Injury Prevention, a Glossary, and a Directory of Additional Resources

Edited by Joyce Brennfleck Shannon. 696 pages. 2002. 0-7808-0421-X.

"This publication is the most comprehensive work of its kind about injury and trauma."
— *American Reference Books Annual, 2003*

"This sourcebook provides concise, easily readable, basic health information about injuries. . . . This book is well organized and an easy to use reference resource suitable for hospital, health sciences and public libraries with consumer health collections."
— *E-Streams, Nov '02*

"Practitioners should be aware of guides such as this in order to facilitate their use by patients and their families." — *Doody's Health Sciences Book Review Journal, Sep-Oct '02*

"Recommended reference source."
— *Booklist, American Library Association, Sep '02*

"Highly recommended for academic and medical reference collections." — *Library Bookwatch, Sep '02*

■

Kidney & Urinary Tract Diseases & Disorders Sourcebook

SEE Urinary Tract & Kidney Diseases & Disorders Sourcebook, 2nd Edition

■

Learning Disabilities Sourcebook, 2nd Edition

Basic Consumer Health Information about Learning Disabilities, Including Dyslexia, Developmental Speech and Language Disabilities, Non-Verbal Learning Disorders, Developmental Arithmetic Disorder, Developmental Writing Disorder, and Other Conditions That Impede Learning Such as Attention Deficit/ Hyperac-

tivity Disorder, Brain Injury, Hearing Impairment, Kline-felter Syndrome, Dyspraxia, and Tourette's Syndrome

Along with Facts about Educational Issues and Assistive Technology, Coping Strategies, a Glossary of Related Terms, and Resources for Further Help and Information

Edited by Dawn D. Matthews. 621 pages. 2003. 0-7808-0626-3.

"The second edition of Learning Disabilities Sourcebook far surpasses the earlier edition in that it is more focused on information that will be useful as a consumer health resource."
— American Reference Books Annual, 2004

"Teachers as well as consumers will find this an essential guide to understanding various syndromes and their latest treatments. [An] invaluable reference for public and school library collections alike."
— Library Bookwatch, Apr '03

Named "Outstanding Reference Book of 1999."
— New York Public Library, Feb 2000

"An excellent candidate for inclusion in a public library reference section. It's a great source of information. Teachers will also find the book useful. Definitely worth reading."
— Journal of Adolescent & Adult Literacy, Feb 2000

"Readable . . . provides a solid base of information regarding successful techniques used with individuals who have learning disabilities, as well as practical suggestions for educators and family members. Clear language, concise descriptions, and pertinent information for contacting multiple resources add to the strength of this book as a useful tool."
— Choice, Association of College & Research Libraries, Feb '99

"Recommended reference source."
— Booklist, American Library Association, Sep '98

"A useful resource for libraries and for those who don't have the time to identify and locate the individual publications."
— Disability Resources Monthly, Sep '98

Leukemia Sourcebook

Basic Consumer Health Information about Adult and Childhood Leukemias, Including Acute Lymphocytic Leukemia (ALL), Chronic Lymphocytic Leukemia (CLL), Acute Myelogenous Leukemia (AML), Chronic Myelogenous Leukemia (CML), and Hairy Cell Leukemia, and Treatments Such as Chemotherapy, Radiation Therapy, Peripheral Blood Stem Cell and Marrow Transplantation, and Immunotherapy

Along with Tips for Life During and After Treatment, a Glossary, and Directories of Additional Resources

Edited by Joyce Brennfleck Shannon. 587 pages. 2003. 0-7808-0627-1.

"Unlike other medical books for the layperson, . . . the language does not talk down to the reader. . . . This volume is highly recommended for all libraries."
— American Reference Books Annual, 2004

"... a fine title which ranges from diagnosis to alternative treatments, staging, and tips for life during and after diagnosis."
— The Bookwatch, Dec '03

Liver Disorders Sourcebook

Basic Consumer Health Information about the Liver and How It Works; Liver Diseases, Including Cancer, Cirrhosis, Hepatitis, and Toxic and Drug Related Diseases; Tips for Maintaining a Healthy Liver; Laboratory Tests, Radiology Tests, and Facts about Liver Transplantation

Along with a Section on Support Groups, a Glossary, and Resource Listings

Edited by Joyce Brennfleck Shannon. 591 pages. 2000. 0-7808-0383-3.

"A valuable resource."
— American Reference Books Annual, 2001

"This title is recommended for health sciences and public libraries with consumer health collections."
— E-Streams, Oct '00

"Recommended reference source."
— Booklist, American Library Association, Jun '00

Lung Disorders Sourcebook

Basic Consumer Health Information about Emphysema, Pneumonia, Tuberculosis, Asthma, Cystic Fibrosis, and Other Lung Disorders, Including Facts about Diagnostic Procedures, Treatment Strategies, Disease Prevention Efforts, and Such Risk Factors as Smoking, Air Pollution, and Exposure to Asbestos, Radon, and Other Agents

Along with a Glossary and Resources for Additional Help and Information

Edited by Dawn D. Matthews. 678 pages. 2002. 0-7808-0339-6.

"This title is a great addition for public and school libraries because it provides concise health information on the lungs."
— American Reference Books Annual, 2003

"Highly recommended for academic and medical reference collections."
— Library Bookwatch, Sep '02

SEE ALSO Respiratory Diseases & Disorders Sourcebook

Medical Tests Sourcebook, 2nd Edition

Basic Consumer Health Information about Medical Tests, Including Age-Specific Health Tests, Important Health Screenings and Exams, Home-Use Tests, Blood and Specimen Tests, Electrical Tests, Scope Tests, Genetic Testing, and Imaging Tests, Such as X-Rays, Ultrasound, Computed Tomography, Magnetic Resonance Imaging, Angiography, and Nuclear Medicine

Along with a Glossary and Directory of Additional Resources

Edited by Joyce Brennfleck Shannon. 654 pages. 2004. 0-7808-0670-0.

"Recommended for hospital and health sciences libraries with consumer health collections."
— *E-Streams, Mar '00*

"This is an overall excellent reference with a wealth of general knowledge that may aid those who are reluctant to get vital tests performed."
— *Today's Librarian, Jan '00*

"A valuable reference guide."
— *American Reference Books Annual, 2000*

■

Men's Health Concerns Sourcebook, 2nd Edition

Basic Consumer Health Information about the Medical and Mental Concerns of Men, Including Theories about the Shorter Male Lifespan, the Leading Causes of Death and Disability, Physical Concerns of Special Significance to Men, Reproductive and Sexual Concerns, Sexually Transmitted Diseases, Men's Mental and Emotional Health, and Lifestyle Choices That Affect Wellness, Such as Nutrition, Fitness, and Substance Use

Along with a Glossary of Related Terms and a Directory of Organizational Resources in Men's Health

Edited by Robert Aquinas McNally. 644 pages. 2004. 0-7808-0671-9.

"A very accessible reference for non-specialist general readers and consumers." — *The Bookwatch, Jun '04*

"This comprehensive resource and the series are highly recommended."
— *American Reference Books Annual, 2000*

"Recommended reference source."
— *Booklist, American Library Association, Dec '98*

■

Mental Health Disorders Sourcebook, 3rd Edition

Basic Consumer Health Information about Mental and Emotional Health and Mental Illness, Including Facts about Depression, Bipolar Disorder, and Other Mood Disorders, Phobias, Post-Traumatic Stress Disorder (PTSD), Obsessive-Compulsive Disorder, and Other Anxiety Disorders, Impulse Control Disorders, Eating Disorders, Personality Disorders, and Psychotic Disorders, Including Schizophrenia and Dissociative Disorders

Along with Statistical Information, a Special Section Concerning Mental Health Issues in Children and Adolescents, a Glossary, and Directories of Resources for Additional Help and Information

Edited by Karen Bellenir. 661 pages. 2005. 0-7808-0747-2.

"Recommended for public libraries and academic libraries with an undergraduate program in psychology."
— *American Reference Books Annual, 2006*

"Recommended reference source."
— *Booklist, American Library Association, Jun '00*

■

Mental Retardation Sourcebook

Basic Consumer Health Information about Mental Retardation and Its Causes, Including Down Syndrome, Fetal Alcohol Syndrome, Fragile X Syndrome, Genetic Conditions, Injury, and Environmental Sources

Along with Preventive Strategies, Parenting Issues, Educational Implications, Health Care Needs, Employment and Economic Matters, Legal Issues, a Glossary, and a Resource Listing for Additional Help and Information

Edited by Joyce Brennfleck Shannon. 642 pages. 2000. 0-7808-0377-9.

"Public libraries will find the book useful for reference and as a beginning research point for students, parents, and caregivers."
— *American Reference Books Annual, 2001*

"The strength of this work is that it compiles many basic fact sheets and addresses for further information in one volume. It is intended and suitable for the general public. This sourcebook is relevant to any collection providing health information to the general public."
— *E-Streams, Nov '00*

"From preventing retardation to parenting and family challenges, this covers health, social and legal issues and will prove an invaluable overview."
— *Reviewer's Bookwatch, Jul '00*

■

Movement Disorders Sourcebook

Basic Consumer Health Information about Neurological Movement Disorders, Including Essential Tremor, Parkinson's Disease, Dystonia, Cerebral Palsy, Huntington's Disease, Myasthenia Gravis, Multiple Sclerosis, and Other Early-Onset and Adult-Onset Movement Disorders, Their Symptoms and Causes, Diagnostic Tests, and Treatments

Along with Mobility and Assistive Technology Information, a Glossary, and a Directory of Additional Resources

Edited by Joyce Brennfleck Shannon. 655 pages. 2003. 0-7808-0628-X.

". . . a good resource for consumers and recommended for public, community college and undergraduate libraries." — *American Reference Books Annual, 2004*

■

Muscular Dystrophy Sourcebook

Basic Consumer Health Information about Congenital, Childhood-Onset, and Adult-Onset Forms of Muscular Dystrophy, Such as Duchenne, Becker, Emery-Dreifuss, Distal, Limb-Girdle, Facioscapulohumeral (FSHD), Myotonic, and Ophthalmoplegic Muscular Dystro-

phies, Including Facts about Diagnostic Tests, Medical and Physical Therapies, Management of Co-Occurring Conditions, and Parenting Guidelines

Along with Practical Tips for Home Care, a Glossary, and Directories of Additional Resources

Edited by Joyce Brennfleck Shannon. 577 pages. 2004. 0-7808-0676-X.

"This book is highly recommended for public and academic libraries as well as health care offices that support the information needs of patients and their families."
— E-Streams, Apr '05

"Excellent reference." — The Bookwatch, Jan '05

■

Obesity Sourcebook

Basic Consumer Health Information about Diseases and Other Problems Associated with Obesity, and Including Facts about Risk Factors, Prevention Issues, and Management Approaches

Along with Statistical and Demographic Data, Information about Special Populations, Research Updates, a Glossary, and Source Listings for Further Help and Information

Edited by Wilma Caldwell and Chad T. Kimball. 376 pages. 2001. 0-7808-0333-7.

"The book synthesizes the reliable medical literature on obesity into one easy-to-read and useful resource for the general public."
— American Reference Books Annual, 2002

"This is a very useful resource book for the lay public."
— Doody's Review Service, Nov '01

"Well suited for the health reference collection of a public library or an academic health science library that serves the general population." — E-Streams, Sep '01

"Recommended reference source."
— Booklist, American Library Association, Apr '01

"Recommended pick both for specialty health library collections and any general consumer health reference collection." — The Bookwatch, Apr '01

■

Ophthalmic Disorders Sourcebook

SEE Eye Care Sourcebook, 2nd Edition

■

Oral Health Sourcebook

SEE Dental Care & Oral Health Sourcebook, 2nd Edition

■

Osteoporosis Sourcebook

Basic Consumer Health Information about Primary and Secondary Osteoporosis and Juvenile Osteoporosis and Related Conditions, Including Fibrous Dysplasia,

Gaucher Disease, Hyperthyroidism, Hypophosphatasia, Myeloma, Osteopetrosis, Osteogenesis Imperfecta, and Paget's Disease

Along with Information about Risk Factors, Treatments, Traditional and Non-Traditional Pain Management, a Glossary of Related Terms, and a Directory of Resources

Edited by Allan R. Cook. 584 pages. 2001. 0-7808-0239-X.

"This would be a book to be kept in a staff or patient library. The targeted audience is the layperson, but the therapist who needs a quick bit of information on a particular topic will also find the book useful."
— Physical Therapy, Jan '02

"This resource is recommended as a great reference source for public, health, and academic libraries, and is another triumph for the editors of Omnigraphics."
— American Reference Books Annual, 2002

"Recommended for all public libraries and general health collections, especially those supporting patient education or consumer health programs."
— E-Streams, Nov '01

"Will prove valuable to any library seeking to maintain a current, comprehensive reference collection of health resources. . . . From prevention to treatment and associated conditions, this provides an excellent survey."
— The Bookwatch, Aug '01

"Recommended reference source."
— Booklist, American Library Association, Jul '01

SEE ALSO Healthy Aging Sourcebook, Physical & Mental Issues in Aging Sourcebook, Women's Health Concerns Sourcebook

■

Pain Sourcebook, 2nd Edition

Basic Consumer Health Information about Specific Forms of Acute and Chronic Pain, Including Muscle and Skeletal Pain, Nerve Pain, Cancer Pain, and Disorders Characterized by Pain, Such as Fibromyalgia, Shingles, Angina, Arthritis, and Headaches

Along with Information about Pain Medications and Management Techniques, Complementary and Alternative Pain Relief Options, Tips for People Living with Chronic Pain, a Glossary, and a Directory of Sources for Further Information

Edited by Karen Bellenir. 670 pages. 2002. 0-7808-0612-3.

"A source of valuable information. . . . This book offers help to nonmedical people who need information about pain and pain management. It is also an excellent reference for those who participate in patient education."
— Doody's Review Service, Sep '02

"Highly recommended for academic and medical reference collections." — Library Bookwatch, Sep '02

"The text is readable, easily understood, and well indexed. This excellent volume belongs in all patient education libraries, consumer health sections of public libraries, and many personal collections."
— American Reference Books Annual, 1999

"The information is basic in terms of scholarship and is appropriate for general readers. Written in journalistic style . . . intended for non-professionals. Quite thorough in its coverage of different pain conditions and summarizes the latest clinical information regarding pain treatment." — *Choice, Association of College and Research Libraries, Jun '98*

"Recommended reference source."
— *Booklist, American Library Association, Mar '98*

■

Pediatric Cancer Sourcebook

Basic Consumer Health Information about Leukemias, Brain Tumors, Sarcomas, Lymphomas, and Other Cancers in Infants, Children, and Adolescents, Including Descriptions of Cancers, Treatments, and Coping Strategies

Along with Suggestions for Parents, Caregivers, and Concerned Relatives, a Glossary of Cancer Terms, and Resource Listings

Edited by Edward J. Prucha. 587 pages. 1999. 0-7808-0245-4.

"An excellent source of information. Recommended for public, hospital, and health science libraries with consumer health collections." — *E-Streams, Jun '00*

"Recommended reference source."
— *Booklist, American Library Association, Feb '00*

"A valuable addition to all libraries specializing in health services and many public libraries."
— *American Reference Books Annual, 2000*

SEE ALSO *Childhood Diseases & Disorders Sourcebook, Healthy Children Sourcebook*

■

Physical & Mental Issues in Aging Sourcebook

Basic Consumer Health Information on Physical and Mental Disorders Associated with the Aging Process, Including Concerns about Cardiovascular Disease, Pulmonary Disease, Oral Health, Digestive Disorders, Musculoskeletal and Skin Disorders, Metabolic Changes, Sexual and Reproductive Issues, and Changes in Vision, Hearing, and Other Senses

Along with Data about Longevity and Causes of Death, Information on Acute and Chronic Pain, Descriptions of Mental Concerns, a Glossary of Terms, and Resource Listings for Additional Help

Edited by Jenifer Swanson. 660 pages. 1999. 0-7808-0233-0.

"This is a treasure of health information for the layperson." — *Choice Health Sciences Supplement, Association of College & Research Libraries, May '00*

"Recommended for public libraries."
— *American Reference Books Annual, 2000*

"Recommended reference source."
— *Booklist, American Library Association, Oct '99*

SEE ALSO *Healthy Aging Sourcebook*

Podiatry Sourcebook

Basic Consumer Health Information about Foot Conditions, Diseases, and Injuries, Including Bunions, Corns, Calluses, Athlete's Foot, Plantar Warts, Hammertoes and Clawtoes, Clubfoot, Heel Pain, Gout, and More

Along with Facts about Foot Care, Disease Prevention, Foot Safety, Choosing a Foot Care Specialist, a Glossary of Terms, and Resource Listings for Additional Information

Edited by M. Lisa Weatherford. 380 pages. 2001. 0-7808-0215-2.

"Recommended reference source."
— *Booklist, American Library Association, Feb '02*

"There is a lot of information presented here on a topic that is usually only covered sparingly in most larger comprehensive medical encyclopedias."
— *American Reference Books Annual, 2002*

■

Pregnancy & Birth Sourcebook, 2nd Edition

Basic Consumer Health Information about Conception and Pregnancy, Including Facts about Fertility, Infertility, Pregnancy Symptoms and Complications, Fetal Growth and Development, Labor, Delivery, and the Postpartum Period, as Well as Information about Maintaining Health and Wellness during Pregnancy and Caring for a Newborn

Along with Information about Public Health Assistance for Low-Income Pregnant Women, a Glossary, and Directories of Agencies and Organizations Providing Help and Support

Edited by Amy L. Sutton. 626 pages. 2004. 0-7808-0672-7.

"Will appeal to public and school reference collections strong in medicine and women's health. . . . Deserves a spot on any medical reference shelf."
— *The Bookwatch, Jul '04*

"A well-organized handbook. Recommended."
— *Choice, Association of College & Research Libraries, Apr '98*

"Recommended reference source."
— *Booklist, American Library Association, Mar '98*

"Recommended for public libraries."
— *American Reference Books Annual, 1998*

SEE ALSO *Breastfeeding Sourcebook, Congenital Disorders Sourcebook, Family Planning Sourcebook*

■

Prostate Cancer Sourcebook

Basic Consumer Health Information about Prostate Cancer, Including Information about the Associated Risk Factors, Detection, Diagnosis, and Treatment of Prostate Cancer

Along with Information on Non-Malignant Prostate Conditions, and Featuring a Section Listing Support and Treatment Centers and a Glossary of Related Terms

Edited by Dawn D. Matthews. 358 pages. 2001. 0-7808-0324-8.

"A valuable resource for health care consumers seeking information on the subject. . . . All text is written in a clear, easy-to-understand language that avoids technical jargon. Any library that collects consumer health resources would strengthen their collection with the addition of the Prostate Cancer Sourcebook."
— *American Reference Books Annual, 2002*

SEE ALSO *Men's Health Concerns Sourcebook*

Prostate & Urological Disorders Sourcebook

Basic Consumer Health Information about Urogenital and Sexual Disorders in Men, Including Prostate and Other Andrological Cancers, Prostatitis, Benign Prostatic Hyperplasia, Testicular and Penile Trauma, Cryptorchidism, Peyronie Disease, Erectile Dysfunction, and Male Factor Infertility, and Facts about Commonly Used Tests and Procedures, Such as Prostatectomy, Vasectomy, Vasectomy Reversal, Penile Implants, and Semen Analysis

Along with a Glossary of Andrological Terms and a Directory of Resources for Additional Information

Edited by Karen Bellenir. 631 pages. 2005. 0-7808-0797-9.

Public Health Sourcebook

Basic Information about Government Health Agencies, Including National Health Statistics and Trends, Healthy People 2000 Program Goals and Objectives, the Centers for Disease Control and Prevention, the Food and Drug Administration, and the National Institutes of Health

Along with Full Contact Information for Each Agency

Edited by Wendy Wilcox. 698 pages. 1998. 0-7808-0220-9.

"This consumer guide provides welcome assistance in navigating the maze of federal health agencies and their data on public health concerns."
— *SciTech Book News, Sep '98*

Reconstructive & Cosmetic Surgery Sourcebook

Basic Consumer Health Information on Cosmetic and Reconstructive Plastic Surgery, Including Statistical Information about Different Surgical Procedures, Things to Consider Prior to Surgery, Plastic Surgery Techniques and Tools, Emotional and Psychological Considerations, and Procedure-Specific Information

Along with a Glossary of Terms and a Listing of Resources for Additional Help and Information

Edited by M. Lisa Weatherford. 374 pages. 2001. 0-7808-0214-4.

"An excellent reference that addresses cosmetic and medically necessary reconstructive surgeries. . . . The style of the prose is calm and reassuring, discussing the many positive outcomes now available due to advances in surgical techniques."
— *American Reference Books Annual, 2002*

"Recommended for health science libraries that are open to the public, as well as hospital libraries that are open to the patients. This book is a good resource for the consumer interested in plastic surgery."
— *E-Streams, Dec '01*

Rehabilitation Sourcebook

Basic Consumer Health Information about Rehabilitation for People Recovering from Heart Surgery, Spinal Cord Injury, Stroke, Orthopedic Impairments, Amputation, Pulmonary Impairments, Traumatic Injury, and More, Including Physical Therapy, Occupational Therapy, Speech/Language Therapy, Massage Therapy, Dance Therapy, Art Therapy, and Recreational Therapy

Along with Information on Assistive and Adaptive Devices, a Glossary, and Resources for Additional Help and Information

Edited by Dawn D. Matthews. 531 pages. 1999. 0-7808-0236-5.

"This is an excellent resource for public library reference and health collections."
— *American Reference Books Annual, 2001*

Respiratory Diseases & Disorders Sourcebook

Basic Information about Respiratory Diseases and Disorders, Including Asthma, Cystic Fibrosis, Pneumonia, the Common Cold, Influenza, and Others, Featuring Facts about the Respiratory System, Statistical and Demographic Data, Treatments, Self-Help Management Suggestions, and Current Research Initiatives

Edited by Allan R. Cook and Peter D. Dresser. 771 pages. 1995. 0-7808-0037-0.

"Designed for the layperson and for patients and their families coping with respiratory illness. . . . an extensive array of information on diagnosis, treatment, management, and prevention of respiratory illnesses for the general reader." — *Choice, Association of College & Research Libraries, Jun '96*

"A highly recommended text for all collections. It is a comforting reminder of the power of knowledge that good books carry between their covers."
— *Academic Library Book Review, Spring '96*

676

"A comprehensive collection of authoritative information presented in a nontechnical, humanitarian style for patients, families, and caregivers."
—*Association of Operating Room Nurses, Sep/Oct '95*

SEE ALSO *Lung Disorders Sourcebook*

Sexually Transmitted Diseases Sourcebook, 3rd Edition

Basic Consumer Health Information about Chlamydial Infections, Gonorrhea, Hepatitis, Herpes, HIV/AIDS, Human Papillomavirus, Pubic Lice, Scabies, Syphilis, Trichomoniasis, Vaginal Infections, and Other Sexually Transmitted Diseases, Including Facts about Risk Factors, Symptoms, Diagnosis, Treatment, and the Prevention of Sexually Transmitted Infections

Along with Updates on Current Research Initiatives, a Glossary of Related Terms, and Resources for Additional Help and Information

Edited by Amy L. Sutton. 629 pages. 2006. 0-7808-0824-X.

"Recommended for consumer health collections in public libraries, and secondary school and community college libraries."
—*American Reference Books Annual, 2002*

"Every school and public library should have a copy of this comprehensive and user-friendly reference book."
—*Choice, Association of College & Research Libraries, Sep '01*

"This is a highly recommended book. This is an especially important book for all school and public libraries."
—*AIDS Book Review Journal, Jul-Aug '01*

"Recommended reference source."
—*Booklist, American Library Association, Apr '01*

Skin Disorders Sourcebook

SEE *Dermatological Disorders Sourcebook, 2nd Edition*

Sleep Disorders Sourcebook, 2nd Edition

Basic Consumer Health Information about Sleep and Sleep Disorders, Including Insomnia, Sleep Apnea, Restless Legs Syndrome, Narcolepsy, Parasomnias, and Other Health Problems That Affect Sleep, Plus Facts about Diagnostic Procedures, Treatment Strategies, Sleep Medications, and Tips for Improving Sleep Quality

Along with a Glossary of Related Terms and Resources for Additional Help and Information

Edited by Amy L. Sutton. 567 pages. 2005. 0-7808-0743-X.

"This book will be useful for just about everybody, especially the 40 million Americans with sleep disorders."
—*American Reference Books Annual, 2006*

"Recommended for public libraries and libraries supporting health care professionals." —*E-Streams, Sep '05*

"... key medical library acquisition."
—*The Bookwatch, Jun '05*

Smoking Concerns Sourcebook

Basic Consumer Health Information about Nicotine Addiction and Smoking Cessation, Featuring Facts about the Health Effects of Tobacco Use, Including Lung and Other Cancers, Heart Disease, Stroke, and Respiratory Disorders, Such as Emphysema and Chronic Bronchitis

Along with Information about Smoking Prevention Programs, Suggestions for Achieving and Maintaining a Smoke-Free Lifestyle, Statistics about Tobacco Use, Reports on Current Research Initiatives, a Glossary of Related Terms, and Directories of Resources for Additional Help and Information

Edited by Karen Bellenir. 621 pages. 2004. 0-7808-0323-X.

"Provides everything needed for the student or general reader seeking practical details on the effects of tobacco use." —*The Bookwatch, Mar '05*

"Public libraries and consumer health care libraries will find this work useful."
—*American Reference Books Annual, 2005*

Sports Injuries Sourcebook, 2nd Edition

Basic Consumer Health Information about the Diagnosis, Treatment, and Rehabilitation of Common Sports-Related Injuries in Children and Adults

Along with Suggestions for Conditioning and Training, Information and Prevention Tips for Injuries Frequently Associated with Specific Sports and Special Populations, a Glossary, and a Directory of Additional Resources

Edited by Joyce Brennfleck Shannon. 614 pages. 2002. 0-7808-0604-2.

"This is an excellent reference for consumers and it is recommended for public, community college, and undergraduate libraries."
—*American Reference Books Annual, 2003*

"Recommended reference source."
—*Booklist, American Library Association, Feb '03*

Stress-Related Disorders Sourcebook

Basic Consumer Health Information about Stress and Stress-Related Disorders, Including Stress Origins and Signals, Environmental Stress at Work and Home, Mental and Emotional Stress Associated with Depression, Post-Traumatic Stress Disorder, Panic Disorder, Suicide, and the Physical Effects of Stress on the Cardiovascular, Immune, and Nervous Systems

Along with Stress Management Techniques, a Glossary, and a Listing of Additional Resources

Edited by Joyce Brennfleck Shannon. 610 pages. 2002. 0-7808-0560-7.

"Well written for a general readership, the *Stress-Related Disorders Sourcebook* is a useful addition to the health reference literature."
— *American Reference Books Annual, 2003*

"I am impressed by the amount of information. It offers a thorough overview of the causes and consequences of stress for the layperson. . . . A well-done and thorough reference guide for professionals and nonprofessionals alike." — *Doody's Review Service, Dec '02*

Stroke Sourcebook

Basic Consumer Health Information about Stroke, Including Ischemic, Hemorrhagic, Transient Ischemic Attack (TIA), and Pediatric Stroke, Stroke Triggers and Risks, Diagnostic Tests, Treatments, and Rehabilitation Information

Along with Stroke Prevention Guidelines, Legal and Financial Information, a Glossary, and a Directory of Additional Resources

Edited by Joyce Brennfleck Shannon. 606 pages. 2003. 0-7808-0630-1.

"This volume is highly recommended and should be in every medical, hospital, and public library."
— *American Reference Books Annual, 2004*

"Highly recommended for the amount and variety of topics and information covered." — *Choice, Nov '03*

Substance Abuse Sourcebook

Basic Health-Related Information about the Abuse of Legal and Illegal Substances Such as Alcohol, Tobacco, Prescription Drugs, Marijuana, Cocaine, and Heroin; and Including Facts about Substance Abuse Prevention Strategies, Intervention Methods, Treatment and Recovery Programs, and a Section Addressing the Special Problems Related to Substance Abuse during Pregnancy

Edited by Karen Bellenir. 573 pages. 1996. 0-7808-0038-9.

"A valuable addition to any health reference section. Highly recommended."
— *The Book Report, Mar/Apr '97*

". . . a comprehensive collection of substance abuse information that's both highly readable and compact. Families and caregivers of substance abusers will find the information enlightening and helpful, while teachers, social workers and journalists should benefit from the concise format. Recommended."
— *Drug Abuse Update, Winter '96/'97*

SEE ALSO *Alcoholism Sourcebook, Drug Abuse Sourcebook*

Surgery Sourcebook

Basic Consumer Health Information about Inpatient and Outpatient Surgeries, Including Cardiac, Vascular, Orthopedic, Ocular, Reconstructive, Cosmetic, Gynecologic, and Ear, Nose, and Throat Procedures and More

Along with Information about Operating Room Policies and Instruments, Laser Surgery Techniques, Hospital Errors, Statistical Data, a Glossary, and Listings of Sources for Further Help and Information

Edited by Annemarie S. Muth and Karen Bellenir. 596 pages. 2002. 0-7808-0380-9.

"Large public libraries and medical libraries would benefit from this material in their reference collections."
— *American Reference Books Annual, 2004*

"Invaluable reference for public and school library collections alike." — *Library Bookwatch, Apr '03*

Thyroid Disorders Sourcebook

Basic Consumer Health Information about Disorders of the Thyroid and Parathyroid Glands, Including Hypothyroidism, Hyperthyroidism, Graves Disease, Hashimoto Thyroiditis, Thyroid Cancer, and Parathyroid Disorders, Featuring Facts about Symptoms, Risk Factors, Tests, and Treatments

Along with Information about the Effects of Thyroid Imbalance on Other Body Systems, Environmental Factors That Affect the Thyroid Gland, a Glossary, and a Directory of Additional Resources

Edited by Joyce Brennfleck Shannon. 599 pages. 2005. 0-7808-0745-6.

"Recommended for consumer health collections."
— *American Reference Books Annual, 2006*

"Highly recommended pick for basic consumer health reference holdings at all levels."
— *The Bookwatch, Aug '05*

Transplantation Sourcebook

Basic Consumer Health Information about Organ and Tissue Transplantation, Including Physical and Financial Preparations, Procedures and Issues Relating to Specific Solid Organ and Tissue Transplants, Rehabilitation, Pediatric Transplant Information, the Future of Transplantation, and Organ and Tissue Donation

Along with a Glossary and Listings of Additional Resources

Edited by Joyce Brennfleck Shannon. 628 pages. 2002. 0-7808-0322-1.

"Along with these advances [in transplantation technology] have come a number of daunting questions for potential transplant patients, their families, and their health care providers. This reference text is the best single tool to address many of these questions. . . . It will be a much-needed addition to the reference collections in health care, academic, and large public libraries."
— *American Reference Books Annual, 2003*

678

"Recommended for libraries with an interest in offering consumer health information." — *E-Streams, Jul '02*

"This is a unique and valuable resource for patients facing transplantation and their families."
— *Doody's Review Service, Jun '02*

■

Traveler's Health Sourcebook

Basic Consumer Health Information for Travelers, Including Physical and Medical Preparations, Transportation Health and Safety, Essential Information about Food and Water, Sun Exposure, Insect and Snake Bites, Camping and Wilderness Medicine, and Travel with Physical or Medical Disabilities

Along with International Travel Tips, Vaccination Recommendations, Geographical Health Issues, Disease Risks, a Glossary, and a Listing of Additional Resources

Edited by Joyce Brennfleck Shannon. 613 pages. 2000. 0-7808-0384-1.

"Recommended reference source."
— *Booklist, American Library Association, Feb '01*

"This book is recommended for any public library, any travel collection, and especially any collection for the physically disabled."
— *American Reference Books Annual, 2001*

SEE ALSO *Worldwide Health Sourcebook*

■

Urinary Tract & Kidney Diseases & Disorders Sourcebook, 2nd Edition

Basic Consumer Health Information about the Urinary System, Including the Bladder, Urethra, Ureters, and Kidneys, with Facts about Urinary Tract Infections, Incontinence, Congenital Disorders, Kidney Stones, Cancers of the Urinary Tract and Kidneys, Kidney Failure, Dialysis, and Kidney Transplantation

Along with Statistical and Demographic Information, Reports on Current Research in Kidney and Urologic Health, a Summary of Commonly Used Diagnostic Tests, a Glossary of Related Terms, and a Directory of Resources for Additional Help and Information

Edited by Ivy L. Alexander. 649 pages. 2005. 0-7808-0750-2.

"A good choice for a consumer health information library or for a medical library needing information to refer to their patients."
— *American Reference Books Annual, 2006*

■

Vegetarian Sourcebook

Basic Consumer Health Information about Vegetarian Diets, Lifestyle, and Philosophy, Including Definitions of Vegetarianism and Veganism, Tips about Adopting Vegetarianism, Creating a Vegetarian Pantry, and Meeting Nutritional Needs of Vegetarians, with Facts Regarding Vegetarianism's Effect on Pregnant and Lactating Women, Children, Athletes, and Senior Citizens

Along with a Glossary of Commonly Used Vegetarian Terms and Resources for Additional Help and Information

Edited by Chad T. Kimball. 360 pages. 2002. 0-7808-0439-2.

"Organizes into one concise volume the answers to the most common questions concerning vegetarian diets and lifestyles. This title is recommended for public and secondary school libraries." — *E-Streams, Apr '03*

"Invaluable reference for public and school library collections alike." — *Library Bookwatch, Apr '03*

"The articles in this volume are easy to read and come from authoritative sources. The book does not necessarily support the vegetarian diet but instead provides the pros and cons of this important decision. The Vegetarian Sourcebook is recommended for public libraries and consumer health libraries."
— *American Reference Books Annual, 2003*

SEE ALSO *Diet & Nutrition Sourcebook*

■

Women's Health Concerns Sourcebook, 2nd Edition

Basic Consumer Health Information about the Medical and Mental Concerns of Women, Including Maintaining Health and Wellness, Gynecological Concerns, Breast Health, Sexuality and Reproductive Issues, Menopause, Cancer in Women, Leading Causes of Death and Disability among Women, Physical Concerns of Special Significance to Women, and Women's Mental and Emotional Health

Along with a Glossary of Related Terms and Directories of Resources for Additional Help and Information

Edited by Amy L. Sutton. 746 pages. 2004. 0-7808-0673-5.

"This is a useful reference book, which makes the reader knowledgeable about several issues that concern women's health. It is recommended for public libraries and home library collections." — *E-Streams, May '05*

"A useful addition to public and consumer health library collections."
— *American Reference Books Annual, 2005*

"A highly recommended title."
— *The Bookwatch, May '04*

"Handy compilation. There is an impressive range of diseases, devices, disorders, procedures, and other physical and emotional issues covered . . . well organized, illustrated, and indexed." — *Choice, Association of College & Research Libraries, Jan '98*

SEE ALSO *Breast Cancer Sourcebook, Cancer Sourcebook for Women, Healthy Heart Sourcebook for Women, Osteoporosis Sourcebook*

Workplace Health & Safety Sourcebook

Basic Consumer Health Information about Workplace Health and Safety, Including the Effect of Workplace Hazards on the Lungs, Skin, Heart, Ears, Eyes, Brain, Reproductive Organs, Musculoskeletal System, and Other Organs and Body Parts

Along with Information about Occupational Cancer, Personal Protective Equipment, Toxic and Hazardous Chemicals, Child Labor, Stress, and Workplace Violence

Edited by Chad T. Kimball. 626 pages. 2000. 0-7808-0231-4.

"As a reference for the general public, this would be useful in any library." *—E-Streams, Jun '01*

"Provides helpful information for primary care physicians and other caregivers interested in occupational medicine. . . . General readers; professionals."
— Choice, Association of College & Research Libraries, May '01

"Recommended reference source."
—Booklist, American Library Association, Feb '01

"Highly recommended." *— The Bookwatch, Jan '01*

Worldwide Health Sourcebook

Basic Information about Global Health Issues, Including Malnutrition, Reproductive Health, Disease Dispersion and Prevention, Emerging Diseases, Risky Health Behaviors, and the Leading Causes of Death

Along with Global Health Concerns for Children, Women, and the Elderly, Mental Health Issues, Research and Technology Advancements, and Economic, Environmental, and Political Health Implications, a Glossary, and a Resource Listing for Additional Help and Information

Edited by Joyce Brennfleck Shannon. 614 pages. 2001. 0-7808-0330-2.

"Named an Outstanding Academic Title."
— Choice, Association of College & Research Libraries, Jan '02

"Yet another handy but also unique compilation in the extensive Health Reference Series, this is a useful work because many of the international publications reprinted or excerpted are not readily available. Highly recommended." *— Choice, Association of College & Research Libraries, Nov '01*

"Recommended reference source."
—Booklist, American Library Association, Oct '01

SEE ALSO *Traveler's Health Sourcebook*

Teen Health Series
Helping Young Adults Understand, Manage, and Avoid Serious Illness

List price $65 per volume. **School and library price $58 per volume.**

Alcohol Information for Teens
Health Tips about Alcohol and Alcoholism
Including Facts about Underage Drinking, Preventing Teen Alcohol Use, Alcohol's Effects on the Brain and the Body, Alcohol Abuse Treatment, Help for Children of Alcoholics, and More

Edited by Joyce Brennfleck Shannon. 370 pages. 2005. 0-7808-0741-3.

"Boxed facts and tips add visual interest to the well-researched and clearly written text."
— *Curriculum Connection, Apr '06*

■

Allergy Information for Teens
Health Tips about Allergic Reactions Such as Anaphylaxis, Respiratory Problems, and Rashes
Including Facts about Identifying and Managing Allergies to Food, Pollen, Mold, Animals, Chemicals, Drugs, and Other Substances

Edited by Karen Bellenir. 410 pages. 2006. 0-7808-0799-5.

■

Asthma Information for Teens
Health Tips about Managing Asthma and Related Concerns
Including Facts about Asthma Causes, Triggers, Symptoms, Diagnosis, and Treatment

Edited by Karen Bellenir. 386 pages. 2005. 0-7808-0770-7.

"Highly recommended for medical libraries, public school libraries, and public libraries."
— *American Reference Books Annual, 2006*

"It is so clearly written and well organized that even hesitant readers will be able to find the facts they need, whether for reports or personal information. . . . A succinct but complete resource."
— *School Library Journal, Sep '05*

■

Cancer Information for Teens
Health Tips about Cancer Awareness, Prevention, Diagnosis, and Treatment
Including Facts about Frequently Occurring Cancers, Cancer Risk Factors, and Coping Strategies for Teens Fighting Cancer or Dealing with Cancer in Friends or Family Members

Edited by Wilma R. Caldwell. 428 pages. 2004. 0-7808-0678-6.

"Recommended for school libraries, or consumer libraries that see a lot of use by teens."
— *E-Streams, May 2005*

"A valuable educational tool."
— *American Reference Books Annual, 2005*

"Young adults and their parents alike will find this new addition to the *Teen Health Series* an important reference to cancer in teens."
— *Children's Bookwatch, Feb '05*

■

Diabetes Information for Teens
Health Tips about Managing Diabetes and Preventing Related Complications
Including Information about Insulin, Glucose Control, Healthy Eating, Physical Activity, and Learning to Live with Diabetes

Edited by Sandra Augustyn Lawton. 410 pages. 2006. 0-7808-0811-8.

■

Diet Information for Teens, 2nd Edition
Health Tips about Diet and Nutrition
Including Facts about Dietary Guidelines, Food Groups, Nutrients, Healthy Meals, Snacks, Weight Control, Medical Concerns Related to Diet, and More

Edited by Karen Bellenir. 432 pages. 2006. 0-7808-0820-7.

"Full of helpful insights and facts throughout the book. . . . An excellent resource to be placed in public libraries or even in personal collections."
— *American Reference Books Annual, 2002*

"Recommended for middle and high school libraries and media centers as well as academic libraries that educate future teachers of teenagers. It is also a suitable addition to health science libraries that serve patrons who are interested in teen health promotion and education." — *E-Streams, Oct '01*

"This comprehensive book would be beneficial to collections that need information about nutrition, dietary guidelines, meal planning, and weight control. . . . This reference is so easy to use that its purchase is recommended." — *The Book Report, Sep-Oct '01*

"This book is written in an easy to understand format describing issues that many teens face every day, and then provides thoughtful explanations so that teens can make informed decisions. This is an interesting book that provides important facts and information for today's teens." — *Doody's Health Sciences Book Review Journal, Jul-Aug '01*

"A comprehensive compendium of diet and nutrition. The information is presented in a straightforward, plain-spoken manner. This title will be useful to those working on reports on a variety of topics, as well as to general readers concerned about their dietary health." — *School Library Journal, Jun '01*

■

Drug Information for Teens, 2nd Edition

Health Tips about the Physical and Mental Effects of Substance Abuse

Including Information about Marijuana, Inhalants, Club Drugs, Stimulants, Hallucinogens, Opiates, Prescription and Over-the-Counter Drugs, Herbal Products, Tobacco, Alcohol, and More

Edited by Sandra Augustyn Lawton. 468 pages. 2006. 0-7808-0862-2.

"A clearly written resource for general readers and researchers alike." — *School Library Journal*

"This book is well-balanced. . . . a must for public and school libraries." — *VOYA: Voice of Youth Advocates, Dec '03*

"The chapters are quick to make a connection to their teenage reading audience. The prose is straightforward and the book lends itself to spot reading. It should be useful both for practical information and for research, and it is suitable for public and school libraries." — *American Reference Books Annual, 2003*

"Recommended reference source." — *Booklist, American Library Association, Feb '03*

"This is an excellent resource for teens and their parents. Education about drugs and substances is key to discouraging teen drug abuse and this book provides this much needed information in a way that is interesting and factual." — *Doody's Review Service, Dec '02*

■

Eating Disorders Information for Teens

Health Tips about Anorexia, Bulimia, Binge Eating, and Other Eating Disorders

Including Information on the Causes, Prevention, and Treatment of Eating Disorders, and Such Other Issues as Maintaining Healthy Eating and Exercise Habits

Edited by Sandra Augustyn Lawton. 337 pages. 2005. 0-7808-0783-9.

"An excellent resource for teens and those who work with them." — *VOYA: Voice of Youth Advocates, Apr '06*

"A welcome addition to high school and undergraduate libraries." — *American Reference Books Annual, 2006*

"This book covers the topic in a lucid manner but delves deeper into every aspect of an eating disorder. A solid addition for any nonfiction or reference collection." — *School Library Journal, Dec '05*

■

Fitness Information for Teens

Health Tips about Exercise, Physical Well-Being, and Health Maintenance

Including Facts about Aerobic and Anaerobic Conditioning, Stretching, Body Shape and Body Image, Sports Training, Nutrition, and Activities for Non-Athletes

Edited by Karen Bellenir. 425 pages. 2004. 0-7808-0679-4.

"Another excellent offering from Omnigraphics in their *Teen Health Series*. . . . This book will be a great addition to any public, junior high, senior high, or secondary school library." — *American Reference Books Annual, 2005*

■

Learning Disabilities Information for Teens

Health Tips about Academic Skills Disorders and Other Disabilities That Affect Learning

Including Information about Common Signs of Learning Disabilities, School Issues, Learning to Live with a Learning Disability, and Other Related Issues

Edited by Sandra Augustyn Lawton. 337 pages. 2005. 0-7808-0796-0.

"This book provides a wealth of information for any reader interested in the signs, causes, and consequences of learning disabilities, as well as related legal rights and educational interventions. . . . Public and academic libraries should want this title for both students and general readers." — *American Reference Books Annual, 2006*

■

Mental Health Information for Teens, 2nd Edition

Health Tips about Mental Wellness and Mental Illness

Including Facts about Mental and Emotional Health, Depression and Other Mood Disorders, Anxiety Disorders, Behavior Disorders, Self-Injury, Psychosis, Schizophrenia, and More

Edited by Karen Bellenir. 400 pages. 2006. 0-7808-0863-0.

"In both language and approach, this user-friendly entry in the *Teen Health Series* is on target for teens needing information on mental health concerns." — *Booklist, American Library Association, Jan '02*

"Readers will find the material accessible and informative, with the shaded notes, facts, and embedded glos-

sary insets adding appropriately to the already interesting and succinct presentation."
— *School Library Journal, Jan '02*

"This title is highly recommended for any library that serves adolescents and parents/caregivers of adolescents."
— *E-Streams, Jan '02*

"Recommended for high school libraries and young adult collections in public libraries. Both health professionals and teenagers will find this book useful."
— *American Reference Books Annual, 2002*

"This is a nice book written to enlighten the society, primarily teenagers, about common teen mental health issues. It is highly recommended to teachers and parents as well as adolescents."
— *Doody's Review Service, Dec '01*

■

Sexual Health Information for Teens

Health Tips about Sexual Development, Human Reproduction, and Sexually Transmitted Diseases

Including Facts about Puberty, Reproductive Health, Chlamydia, Human Papillomavirus, Pelvic Inflammatory Disease, Herpes, AIDS, Contraception, Pregnancy, and More

Edited by Deborah A. Stanley. 391 pages. 2003. 0-7808-0445-7.

"This work should be included in all high school libraries and many larger public libraries. . . . highly recommended."
— *American Reference Books Annual, 2004*

"Sexual Health approaches its subject with appropriate seriousness and offers easily accessible advice and information."
— *School Library Journal, Feb '04*

■

Skin Health Information for Teens

Health Tips about Dermatological Concerns and Skin Cancer Risks

Including Facts about Acne, Warts, Hives, and Other Conditions and Lifestyle Choices, Such as Tanning, Tattooing, and Piercing, That Affect the Skin, Nails, Scalp, and Hair

Edited by Robert Aquinas McNally. 429 pages. 2003. 0-7808-0446-5.

"This volume, as with others in the series, will be a useful addition to school and public library collections."
— *American Reference Books Annual, 2004*

"There is no doubt that this reference tool is valuable."
— *VOYA: Voice of Youth Advocates, Feb '04*

"This volume serves as a one-stop source and should be a necessity for any health collection."
— *Library Media Connection*

Sports Injuries Information for Teens

Health Tips about Sports Injuries and Injury Protection

Including Facts about Specific Injuries, Emergency Treatment, Rehabilitation, Sports Safety, Competition Stress, Fitness, Sports Nutrition, Steroid Risks, and More

Edited by Joyce Brennfleck Shannon. 405 pages. 2003. 0-7808-0447-3.

"This work will be useful in the young adult collections of public libraries as well as high school libraries."
— *American Reference Books Annual, 2004*

■

Suicide Information for Teens

Health Tips about Suicide Causes and Prevention

Including Facts about Depression, Risk Factors, Getting Help, Survivor Support, and More

Edited by Joyce Brennfleck Shannon. 368 pages. 2005. 0-7808-0737-5.

Health Reference Series